Residential Ventilation Handbook - V3

Home Ventilation Management

Paul H. Raymer

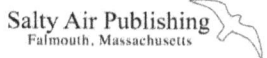

Contents

1. INTRODUCTION ... 1
   - Why a home needs a mechanical ventilation system ... 2
   - A few quick ventilation thoughts: ... 4
   - How to use this book ... 5

2. CHOOSING RESIDENTIAL VENTILATION SYSTEMS ... 9
   - Choosing ventilation systems for a new home ... 11
   - Ventilation system design for an existing home ... 17
   - Totaling up the ventilation in the house ... 18
   - How to read a fan box ... 20

3. BASIC APPLICATIONS, AIRFLOW, AND SIZING GUIDELINES ... 23
   - House as a system—rooms as ducts ... 24
   - Fan System Choices ... 26
   - Airflow Considerations for the Whole Dwelling Ventilation System ... 28
   - Whole Dwelling System Sizing ... 29
   - Distributed Ventilation Sizing ... 34
   - Spot/Local Exhaust Ventilation ... 34
   - *Bath Fan sizing* ... 36
   - Kitchen Exhaust Fans ... 38
   - *Kitchen Fan Sizing* ... 40
   - A Word About Clothes Dryers ... 42
   - Other Ventilation System Sizing ... 43

4. SYSTEM DESIGN CHOICES ... 44
   - Exhaust-Centered (Exhaust-only) Whole Dwelling Ventilation System ... 45
   - Supply-Centered Whole Dwelling Ventilation System ... 48
   - Balanced and Distributed Whole Dwelling Ventilation System ... 50
   - Balanced with Heat or Energy Recovery Whole Dwelling Ventilation System - HRVs and ERVs ... 51
   - Circulation and Distribution Basics ... 56
   - System Documentation ... 66

5. SOUND	67
General Sound Considerations	68
Sound Considerations for the Whole Dwelling Ventilation System	73
Sound Considerations for bath fans	75
Sound considerations for kitchen fans	77
Sound Considerations for Radon/Soil Gas Exhaust Fans	79
6. INSTALLATION DETAILS	81
System Design Overview	81
Ducting	84
Duct Joints and Mastics and Duct Tapes	88
Calculating the Effect on Performance	95
Termination Fittings	101
Dampers	103
System Commissioning and Documentation	107
Replacing an existing bathroom fan	108
Replacing an existing range hood	109
Installing a Radon/Soil Gas Mitigation System	110
7. HOUSE PRESSURES	112
Building Pressures	112
Leaky Ducts and Air Handling Equipment	116
Effects of Pressure on Backdrafting	117
Attached Garages	119
House Tightness or Building Tightness Limits (BTL)	120
8. PASSIVE INLETS, OUTLETS, TRANSFER GRILLES AND MAKEUP AIR	123
Over, Under and Through-wall Circulation	124
Inlets and Outlets	128
Design and Tempering the Make-up Air	131
9. COMMISSIONING AND TESTING	135
Flow Testing Processes and Equipment	135
Installed System Testing and Balancing	142
Flow testing supply-centered systems	148
Flow testing balanced systems	153
Using an Averaging Flow Station (AFS) to measure airflow	153
Commissioning and owner education	155
Product Testing and Laboratories	157

10. SYSTEM TROUBLESHOOTING, SERVICE, AND
    MAINTENANCE   163
    My system isn't moving any air   163
    My system is too noisy/too quiet   166
    My system is too drafty   169
    My system doesn't clear the moisture off the mirror   170
    Ventilation system maintenance   171
    Bath fan system maintenance   172
    HRV/ERV system maintenance   173

11. COSTS OF VENTILATION   174
    First Cost   175
    Electrical costs   179
    Conditioned Air Cost   181
    Motor Life/Replacement Cost   184
    Ventilation Cost Summary   186
    "Selling" the Ventilation System   187

12. VENTILATION CODES   190
    2024 *International Energy Conservation Code*   213
    2024 International Building Code   218
    2024 International Residential Code   223
    2024 International Property Maintenance Code   237
    State Ventilation Codes   238
    California   238
    Florida   246
    Massachusetts   247
    Minnesota   250
    Vermont   257
    Washington State   258
    Safety Testing and Performance Certification   258

13. PROGRAM REQUIREMENTS AND OPPORTUNITIES   262
    Contractor Training and Certification Programs   264
    In Person Training   266
    On-line Training   269
    Green Building Programs   272
    University Programs   273
    ASHRAE Standards   273
    Ventilation & Health: Healthy Housing Programs   275

14. FAN TYPES AND APPLICATIONS — 278
    Fan Laws — 278
    Axial Fans — 280
    Centrifugal Fans — 282
    Motorized impellers — 285
    Tangential Blowers — 286

15. SPECIAL APPLICATION VENTILATION — 287
    Fireplaces and wood stoves — 287
    Radon ventilation systems — 289
    Crawl Space Ventilation — 293
    Passive Ventilation — 294
    Garage Ventilation — 298
    Displacement Ventilation — 303

16. VENTILATION FOR COOLING — 304
    Ridge and Soffit Vents — 305
    Attic Fans (Powered Attic Ventilators) — 308
    Whole House Comfort Ventilators (Whole House Fans) — 311
    Pedestal and Box Fans — 317
    Ceiling Fans — 319
    Cooling Tubes — 321
    Evaporative Coolers — 322

17. HUMIDIFIERS, DEHUMIDIFIERS, FILTERS, AND VENTILATION ACCESSORIES — 324
    Relative Humidity (RH) and Dew Point — 324
    Humidifiers and dehumidifiers — 325
    Room Air Filters — 328
    Room Air Cleaners/Purifiers — 329
    Ventilation and furnace filters — 330

18. INDOOR AIR/ENVIRONMENTAL QUALITY CONCERNS — 337
    Moisture — 341
    Carbon Monoxide — 343
    PM 2.5 Particles — 347
    Other Pollutants — 348
    Comfortable Air — 350
    DALY - Disability Adjusted Life Year — 352

19. THE FUTURE OF THE RESIDENTIAL VENTILATION ARTS — 354
    Airflow Rates — 356
    Fresh Air Sources — 357
    Equipment & Installation — 358

Other Ventilation Related Equipment	358
Controls	360
Airflow Measurement	361
Occupant Knowledge	362
AI version—Crystal Ball	363
Appendix A - Acronyms and Abbreviations	367
Appendix B - Useful Formulas, Values, and Multipliers	373
Appendix C - Glossary	375
Appendix D - References	393
Appendix E - Organizations & Resources	399
Appendix F - Equipment Sources	411
Appendix G - Digital Tools & Applications	423
Appendix H - Manual BV	427
Acknowledgments	471
Paul H. Raymer	473
Salty Air Publishing Newsletter & Website	475

Copyright © 2025 by Paul H. Raymer.

Salty Air Publishing values and supports copyright. Copyright fuels creativity, encourages diverse voices, promotes free speech, and creates a vibrant culture. Thank you for buying an authorized edition of this book and for complying with copyright laws by not reproducing, scanning, or distributing any part of it in any form without permission. You are supporting writers and allowing us to continue publishing for any reader. All rights reserved. No part of this publication may be reproduced, distributed or transmitted in any form or by any means, including photocopying, recording, or other electronic or mechanical methods, without the prior written permission of the Salty Air Publishing, except in the case of brief quotations embodied in critical reviews and certain other noncommercial uses permitted by copyright law. For permission requests, write to Salty Air Publishing, addressed "Attention: Permissions Coordinator," at the address below.

Paul H. Raymer/Salty Air Publishing

157 Palmer Ave.

Falmouth, MA 02540

www.paulhraymer.com

Ordering Information:

Quantity sales. Special discounts are available on quantity purchases by corporations, associations, and others. For details, contact the "Special Sales Department" at the address above.

Residential Ventilation Handbook V3/ Paul H. Raymer. —1st ed.c

ISBN: Print 979-8-9904850-2-0

ISBN: eBook: 979-8-9904850-3-7

❦ Created with Vellum

This book is dedicated to John Tooley who kicked the residential ventilation challenge into my head.

Chapter 1

Introduction

Residential ventilation is the movement of air. It is just that simple. It is the process of moving the polluted air out of the home and replacing it with fresh, breathable air in order to keep the occupants healthy. Since we've known that for a very long time, why is it necessary to have an entire book about it? Why is it necessary to have conferences, meetings, arguments, and societies to discuss and debate it? Don't we know it all already?

The reason for this book are the changes brought about by a confluence of issues – tighter construction, more time indoors, money, Covid-19, indoor air quality research, and the impacts on health. Breathing 'bad' air is intuitively a bad thing, but what is 'bad' air? How bad is it? How much air do we have to move to make it better? How quickly do we need to move it? What device should we use to initiate that movement?

Intuition is good, but it isn't good enough to know the answers to these questions. Believe it or not, there is a scientific community that thinks about the answers every single day. As we learn more, we develop better tools to go even farther and learn even more. This book contains a lot of the answers to those residential ventilation questions, and it contains links that reach out to connect to even more answers.

Why a home needs a mechanical ventilation system

The air in homes is not perfect. Usually acceptable, but not always. It is a varying soup of gases, chemicals, and particulates that ebb and flow with the convective breezes driven by pressure changes, mechanical equipment, and door and window openings. A house is a system that interacts with the occupants and the exterior conditions. To save energy, homes are built increasingly tightly to the point where combustion gases don't always go up the chimney. Turning on a powerful kitchen exhaust fan to solve the problem of burning onions may cause the carbon monoxide generated by a car in the attached garage to be pulled into the house.

Homes are not air tight – but they're getting close to it. If a home were just a single story, air tight, empty box of air constructed of benign, non-volatile materials and there were no people in it, there wouldn't be an issue with ventilation. But houses are places to shelter people, and as soon as you move people into the box along with all their "stuff" you add air pollution. An adult human breathes approximately 66 pounds of air per day, approximately 880 cubic feet.[1] We breathe out carbon dioxide (along with a bunch of other stuff), and we breathe in whatever is in the air. If we don't change the air in the space, we end up inhaling the stuff we just exhaled.

***

A NEW YORK STATE study of a small random selection of homes built before 1940 averaged about 1.1 air changes per hour (ach).[2] In a larger study of new houses in New York State the average was only 0.23 ach.[3] The Northwest Infiltration Study[4] revealed that for a random group of houses built after 1982 some of which were designed to be "energy efficient" the average natural leakage rate was 0.4 ach, just above the current minimum ventilation standard of 0.35. To achieve the average, half of these homes had to be above the average and half below.

---

1. Indoor Air – The Silent Killer, Yberg, Ingvar; Svensk Ventilation, 2004; page 11
2. An Investigation of Infiltration and Indoor Air Quality, Rizzuto, J.; NYSERDA 90-11;1989
3. Indoor Air Quality, Infiltration and Ventilation in Residential Buildings, Rizzuto, J., Nitchke, Traynor, Wadach, Clarkin, and Clark; NYSERDA 85-10;1985
4. The Northwest Infiltration Survey, Palmiter and Brown; ECOTOPE; Aug. 5, 1989, Prepared for the Washington State Energy Office

Introduction 3

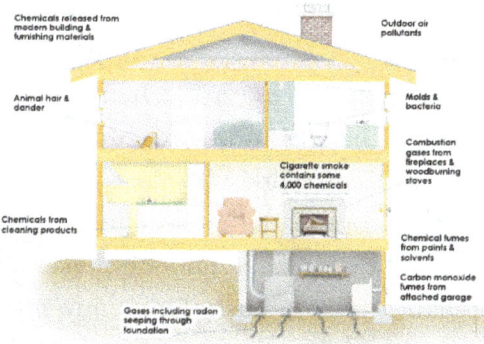

Figure 1.1 Indoor pollutants (Panasonic/Morrissey)

Most homes have more than people in them. They have all the things that people bring with them like furniture and wall and floor coverings and cleaning products. These objects impact the indoor air evidenced by the new carpet or fresh paint smells. There are also the devices that we add for activities like cooking. The stoves and the food and the cooking process all add to the interior, chemical soup that we are brewing. And we get fancy adding vented and unvented fireplaces and lighting candles for romantic interludes. Then there are the devices that keep us warm in the winter and cool in the summer and heat the water for the showers and the laundry. We try to vent the combustion appliances to the outdoors, but the air doesn't always flow in the right direction through the pipes. So sometimes those combustion products get added to the air in the living space. We park cars in the garage, and garages are commonly attached to houses and that air may get sucked into the house.

Then there is humidity, humidity from people and plants and cooking and combustion appliances and laundry and showers. An average family of four generates two to three gallons of water per day from these activities.[5] In a house with one air change per hour, air moving through the house will carry away about ten gallons of water. With that great an air change, the energy costs would be high and the house might feel too dry, dropping the winter relative humidity (RH) uncomfortably to less than 30%. If the air change rate drops to 0.25 ach, however, only two gallons of water will be carried out of the house. The house may feel damp, moisture will condense on cool surfaces (like windows) and mold is likely to flourish.

---

5. Understanding Ventilation; Bower, John, The Healthy House Institute, 1995, page 55

It is clear that there are pollutants in the air in our houses and those pollutants are not good for us.

The only other reason not to use a mechanical ventilation system in a house would be if the air changes frequently enough naturally. Natural or passive ventilation strategies can work with the right designs in the right locations in the right conditions, but all of that is complex. For the air to move into and out of the house there needs to be enough holes in the right places and there needs to be a reliable force to push the air into and out of those holes – infiltration and exfiltration. The general physics of this is covered in Chapter 7 in this book, but suffice it to say that these conditions don't happen reliably and the majority of people don't want a chilling breeze moving through their homes in winter.

One more thing; there is attic ventilation and there is living space ventilation. They're not the same. Although there is some interaction between the two, they need to be thought about independently. Just because there are soffit, gable, or ridge vents, doesn't mean that the air in the living space will be acceptable.

So there are pollutants, we all need to breathe good air to stay healthy, and adequate air changes don't happen reliably or comfortably naturally. That means our homes need mechanical ventilation systems and that is what this book is about.

A few quick ventilation thoughts:

- Don't point infrared motion detectors at heating outlets. It will confuse the detector.
- Don't locate a thermostat over heating vents.
- Humidistats/dehumidistats need to sense humidity. Don't hide them and don't let them sense the humidity in the wall cavity behind them.
- Do put in some sort of control with a high quality, quiet fan. You can't rely on passive ventilation.
- No control will compensate for a poor fan installation.
- A tight seal on a bathroom door will cut the flow through the fan by as much as 35%. For best performance, let some air into the room.

- Venting several rooms with the same fan cuts down on the number of outlets from the house. It also cuts down on the occupants' ability to control the system.
- Remember: controls are there to improve performance, durability, health, and COMFORT.
- Houses and people need ventilation and ventilation means fans.
- Fans won't work if they aren't run.
- Fans need to run longer than the time people spend in the bathroom.
- People don't like running the fan all the time.
- Ventilation controls are necessary because conditions in a house change constantly.
- Humidity and air quality (IAQ) controls are confusing for most people.

* * *

How to use this book

People need to breathe. There have been thousands of conferences, studies and educated articles, papers, and books on ventilation in commercial buildings. Providing good air for people and productivity is an accepted and well-documented concern.

Residential ventilation, however, is a much less certain subject. Although dozens of ventilation issues have been studied, conferences held, and papers written, it remains an area of remarkable contention. There are very few books on residential ventilation, and there are those who believe that purposefully moving fresh air through homes is not a concern. They believe that the volume of the house is too large and there is enough air moving in and out naturally through leaks and holes to satisfy any ventilation requirement. That isolationist sentiment has shifted recently with the Covid-19 pandemic and people working from home, but there is still an attitude of "if you can't see it, it won't hurt you."

Since a home is essentially a box of conditioned air that we trap with the walls, floors, and ceilings, we can keep the air in a range of conditions that are comfortable for the occupants. The better we build the box, the less energy it will take to maintain the right air temperature conditions. As we tighten the box, things we put into the box have an ever-greater effect on the quality of the air in the box. An architect who specialized in underground houses said that having eight people in his home was enough to heat it. He went on to say that if he got two of those people in a fight, he could send four people home. People generate about a hundred watts of heat and expel humidity and a lot of other things. There are chemicals and glues and gases that are emitted by the objects we bring into our homes that add together to create a chemical "mélange" in the air. Radon seeps out of the ground and out of our granite counter tops. Mold grows in places we can't always see. We park cars in our garages and store our paints in the utility closet with the air handler. There are combustion by-products from gas stoves, fireplaces, furnaces and water heaters. And we continue to tighten up our "boxes", our homes, to save energy, aiming to live more comfortably physically and economically.

Admittedly the levels of most of these pollutants are generally small and appear to be tolerated by the majority of the population. The most obvious health effects are seen in the very young and the very old and people with heightened chemical sensitivities. But as we learn more about the effects of low-level exposure to many of these pollutants, we realize the value of a well-designed, installed and operated mechanical ventilation system in a home. We wouldn't want to keep reusing the same water in the shower over and over, and we definitely wouldn't want to keep re-breathing the air in our homes.

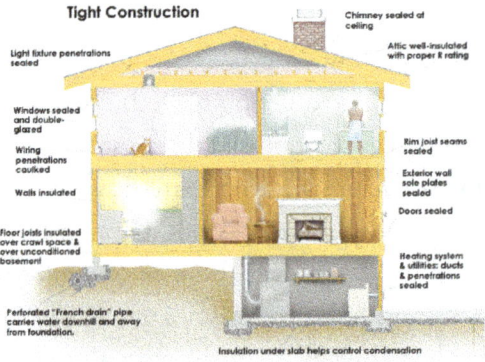

Figure 1.2: *Tight construction details. (Panasonic/Morrissey)*

One fact is clear: as houses become tighter, reaching for better energy efficiency and comfort, the adage that "a house is a system" becomes ever more critical. Contractors and practitioners must understand the interaction between elements. If you burn the bacon, it's a natural reaction to turn on the range hood or open the windows to get rid of the smoke. Strong odors in the bathroom beg for the activation of an effective bathroom fan. The object of both of these ventilating activities is to dilute the polluted air in the home with fresher, outdoor air. Occupants generally only think about the exhausting side of the equation, accepting that the outdoor air will sneak back in from somewhere. But as all those cracks and holes and leaks are sealed up to improve energy efficiency, the various exhaust systems in the house compete for the make-up air. It doesn't always enter by the best route, sometimes coming down through the water heater vent or down the fireplace chimney.

This guide is meant to be useful. It would be nice to think that an Oscar winning movie could be made from this book, but that seems less likely than a snake with elbows. It's just not the sort of popular subject that would cause many people to read it straight through from cover to cover. I have tried to provide a practical approach. If you are interested in installing or replacing a bathroom fan, for example, you should be able to get the information you need to select the proper fan, install it so that it operates correctly, and test that operation if you are so inclined and know if it is doing anything. If you are interested in just getting the job done, there are enough details to accomplish it. If you are interested in going into greater depth about indoor environmental quality (IEQ) or engineering, you will be able to find that information (or at least some of it) as well. (In the Appendices there are a lot of great resources for going further.) There are lots of references and footnotes to websites, but those are almost out of date before they appear on paper so you might have to do a bit of searching. But the web makes that pretty easy to do.

The early chapters of the book discuss fundamental design and sizing issues and describe system choices. The chapters flow on to installation issues and design and from there to installed system testing, and from there to code requirements, technical fan types, fan laws, and special ventilation applications like garages and radon ventilation and ventilation for cooling.

One would think that since houses have been around for so long residential ventilation techniques should have been resolved long ago. The Romans were pretty good at it. The ancient Egyptians noticed that stone carvers working indoors had more respiratory problems than the ones working outdoors. They attributed it to dust.[6] The fact is that we are still learning (or

---

6. Janssen, John E., "The History of Ventilation and Temperature Control", ASHRAE Journal, September, 1999

remembering what we have forgotten) about the subject. We are beginning to appreciate the relationships between all building components and systems and that leads to new information, new codes and new standards. Although I have sought to use the most up-to-date information in putting this book together, things are changing even as I write it. Yet there are a couple of books in Appendix E that were written in 1889 and 1891 that deal with surprisingly similar topics that face us today. And they didn't have electric motors! The fundamentals are still fundamental (as the Romans and Egyptians understood), but how they are applied, the rules for the their use, and the equipment for testing their performance are constantly changing. Luckily we now have the Internet where you can find the latest information. Hopefully this book will give you a road map of what to look for.

There is an expression that is commonly thrown about: "Build it tight. Ventilate it right." It's simple to say, but not simple to accomplish. Ventilating a house correctly is dependent on many variables not the least of which is the climate. Products and technologies are changing. New answers and new questions are arising every day.

There is a great deal of information about residential ventilation from conferences and technical papers, articles and books. Much of that information and wisdom is referenced in this book. There is no single solution to the ventilation for a home that will fit every home in every climate condition with every occupant. If you bring a group of people into a room and ask them for their opinion on the condition of the air, you would certainly not get the same answer from every one of them. The American Society of Heating Refrigerating and Air Conditioning Engineers (ASHRAE) in their residential ventilation standard defines acceptable indoor air quality as, "air toward which a substantial majority of occupants express no dissatisfaction with respect to odor and sensory irritation and in which there are not likely to be contaminants at concentrations that are known to pose a health risk."[7] Such a condition is difficult to measure.

---

7. ASHRAE Standard 62.2-2025 "Ventilation and Acceptable Indoor Air Quality in Low-Rise Residential Buildings"; page 3

Chapter 2

Choosing Residential Ventilation Systems

Working with a large production builder, I noticed that the location of the toilet paper holder was carefully detailed on the plans, but there was no notation regarding the location or ducting design or control for the bathroom fan. "Everyone knows where the fan goes," he said. For a new house, designing the ventilation system should be as much a part of the design process as selecting the windows or the location of the rooms. It is much easier to visualize and design the whole ventilation plan as the house is being designed than it is to do it as an after-thought.

Changing the ventilation in an existing house is more difficult in the sense that the "system" wasn't planned in the first place. On the other hand, it can be relatively simple to make modest improvements, such as using a better bathroom fan, improving the ducting layout, or upgrading the control.

There are several ventilation requirements in a home:

- Ventilation for people—this is the air the people need to breathe and live healthy lives;
- Ventilation for combustion appliances—this is the air that is needed to have combustion appliances operate safely and effectively;
- Ventilation for specialty purposes such as radon mitigation or garage exhaust;

- Ventilation for cooling—this includes elements such as ceiling/paddle fans, whole house fans, and attic exhaust fans;
- Ventilation for the attic to prevent ice dams and meet code - (although this should more properly be termed 'venting' when it is not mechanical.)

These systems work together because everything in the house works together one way or another. Other systems such as clothes dryers and central vacuums also draw on the air in the house and vent it to the outside. They should be included in adding up the total air moving through the house.

Some combustion appliances can be isolated from the home. There are combustion based space and water heaters (called sealed combustion) that draw in their own combustion air and vent their exhaust fumes to the outside. The air they use is completely isolated from the air in the house. Homes with sealed combustion appliances such as these don't have to include combustion air in their ventilation calculations, as long as they are installed correctly and are working properly.

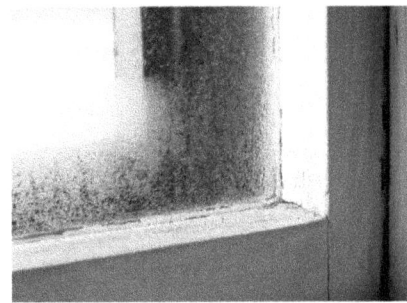

Figure 2.1: Window Condensation

Some homes, like all-electric homes, don't have combustion appliances—no gas range or clothes dryer or water heater or fireplace. Obviously, if they aren't there, they don't have to be figured into the system calculation either!

If there is no attached garage, that would eliminate it from the ventilation system designs—as long as the air barrier between the house and garage is carefully sealed (including the access door).

Perhaps surprisingly, homes with ducted heating and cooling systems need to consider those devices as part of the ventilation system. Duct systems are commonly covered under the term HVAC or Heating, Ventilating and Air Conditioning system. Most of the time they have been installed with little or no intentional connection to "Ventilating", but it is very common for the ducting to be run through unconditioned spaces such as attics or crawl spaces and to have joints that are not completely sealed. Those holes and gaps suck in or blow out air, pressurizing or depressurizing the home and inadvertently "ventilating" it. In the Pacific Northwest, it was found that when the ducts running under the "bellies" of manufactured homes were carefully sealed, ventilation rates in the homes dropped to practically nothing, requiring the addition of mechanical ventilation systems.

Paddle or ceiling fans that are used to cool the occupants of the house by creating gentle, convective breezes commonly only move the air in a room and have no connection to moving the air into or out of the home. Whole house fans (or whole house comfort ventilators) that are used for cooling will purposely depressurize or suck the overheated air out of the house through open windows and vent it out through the attic to the outside. If these powerful fans are used at the wrong time or when the windows are closed, they will seek to draw the air from any other source, including chimneys, and will interfere with other components in the overall ventilation system.

The ventilation for people component can be divided into primary or whole dwelling ventilation and "spot" ventilation. Whole dwelling ventilation must run long enough to keep all the air in the home at an acceptable indoor air quality or IAQ level. "Spot" ventilation can be at a "polluting" source such as a kitchen or bathroom and will draw out the worst of the contaminated air quickly, before the pollutants can be circulated throughout the house.

Smells from garbage that has been left to molder in a trashcan undisturbed may not be immediately noticed. The smells are the symptom. Some or all the items in the trashcan are the cause as bacteria eats away at the contents. The longer the can sits there, the more the smells blend with the household air. This is a "spot" source. The cause of the problem can easily be removed from the house by emptying the trashcan. The offensive odors in the air can be diluted with general household ventilation. Or if the can has its own exhaust fan, the immediate spot could be exhausted, removing most of the contaminant smells at the source before they blended in with the rest of the air in the house.

* * *

Choosing ventilation systems for a new home

The first step in deciding on the ventilation system for a new home is to consider all the components that will move the air in or out of the house— where they will be located and how much air they will move. Such a list must include the bath and kitchen fans, clothes dryers, central vacuums, and combustion appliances such as fireplaces, water heaters, and furnaces. (A gas clothes dryer is also a combustion appliance.) The system should also consider attic fans, whole house fans, radon fans, and garage exhaust fans. The fundamental object of this exercise is to provide a safe and comfortable condition in any room in the home in any weather condition. This summary must be assembled by thinking about the SYSTEM, including the house and all of its components and making a ventilation plan.

Chapter 3 discusses how much air the ventilation system for people should move. Chapter 4 discusses the types of systems that are most applicable. Bathroom and kitchen fans are considered "spot ventilation" fans since they are located close to spots or sources of pollutants—odors, smoke, and moisture.

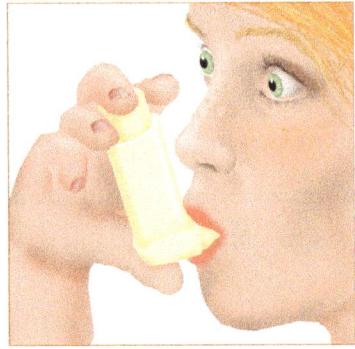

Figure 2.2 Bad IAQ and Asthma Are Not a Good Mix

When working with a new home design, all the options for ventilation are available. The ventilation component is as important or more important than the heating system or the type of windows or style of flooring. Good ventilation will keep the people healthy. It is difficult to quantify the effects of low-grade pollutants such as carbon monoxide (CO) or formaldehyde (H_2CO) on people's health, but it is clear from the studies that have been done,[1] that keeping the air fresh in the house is an important component to people's physical and mental well-being. The system can be as simple as dedicated exhaust fans with fresh air intakes into rooms or into the return side of the HVAC system or as complex as a fully ducted supply or exhaust system, heat or

---

1. Occupant Health Benefits of Residential Energy Efficiency, November 2016, E4TheFuture, https://e4thefuture.org/resources/publications/

energy recovery ventilator (HRV or ERV). New houses are much tighter and energy efficient than houses built in the past. We can no longer take for granted that breezes and drafts will blow through and rattling the window frames or in through the basement or crawl space. Tighter houses are designed to trap the air inside. That air must be conditioned—heated, cooled, filtered, exchanged, humidified, or dehumidified to keep the building and the occupants safe, comfortable, and healthy.

The Whole Dwelling Ventilation System should be selected to gently and continuously change all the air in the house at a rate reasonably ensuring the health of the occupants and the building. It should be designed in a way that will provide air circulation and distribution through all the rooms in the house, including the bedrooms. In still air, pollutants can accumulate around the occupants. If the air motion is excessive, the occupants will be bothered by drafts and discomfort. Tight houses are remarkably quiet, so the system has to be virtually silent. The quality of the motors in the whole dwelling ventilation system needs to be high because the system should run continuously.

Since it is important to circulate the ventilation air around the people in the house, the rooms, and hallways will probably serve as ducting. Air may enter or leave through the mechanical system with grilles and vents in strategic places, but the primary air passages will be the living spaces. There must be provisions for circulating air from room to room no matter how the building is being used, whether interior doors are open or closed. The house should be thought of as a large ducting system with the doors operating as dampers.

Outside air entering the system will be at a different temperature than the inside air. How will it be conditioned? Where will it enter so that it will not cause discomfort? One cubic foot of air moving into the house must be balanced by one cubic foot of air leaving the house.

> **Rule 1 of air motion:** One cubic foot of air (cfm) moves into a house only if one cubic foot of air moves out of the house. 1 cfm out = 1 cfm in (This is easy to say and hard to believe.)

A high-quality bathroom fan can serve as the whole dwelling ventilation system if it is centrally located in a place where it can draw air from the house continuously most of the time. It shouldn't be in a primary bathroom inside a primary bedroom where the air will need to circumvent several closed doors.

Remember that an exhaust fan works by lowering the pressure in the house and that may affect other appliances and systems.

Particular thought should be given to how the air is going to get from the outside into the bedrooms and out of the bedrooms to the whole dwelling ventilation system. Houses last a long time and usually have numerous owners. Not all of them are going to open the windows at night in January when the temperature outside is 0°F!

A fully ducted, balanced ventilation approach such as a heat or energy recovery ventilator (HRV or ERV)[2], will supply air to bedrooms and extract exhaust air from bathrooms via the ducting. Air will move effectively through the rooms, from the inlets to the outlets. Conditioning will occur in the exchanger element. This is the ideal, no compromise approach.

Spot ventilation systems complement the whole dwelling ventilation system, taking the air out of the spaces that are the primary polluting sources —moisture in bathrooms and cooking by-products in kitchens. By locating the fans close to the pollutant source, the fans can be less powerful and the pollutants are removed before they mix with the general air in the house and get circulated. These fans should be quiet enough so that they are used, but since the fans are likely to be operated intermittently, motor quality doesn't need to be as high as the primary ventilation system. In fact, in some bathrooms, a little fan noise is accepted as a good thing.

Any mechanical system will need to be serviced at some point, and the ventilation system design should allow for access to the mechanical components so that filters can be changed and motors can be replaced. The systems should not be buried in walls or attics. The systems should be "commissioned" after installation to make sure that they work as they were designed. Airflows should be measured. It is surprising how many of these systems are not commissioned by the installers or designers to make sure that the ducting is all connected, as it should be, that filters are installed correctly, that switches and controls are programmed.

---

2. See Chapter 4 and Appendix H

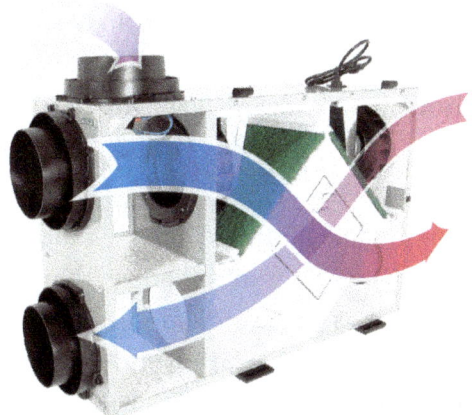

Figure 2.3 Typical Cross-Flow Heat Recovery Ventilator (HRV)
(Greentek)

The homeowner should not be expected to be a ventilation expert. They should be informed as to why the system was designed the way it was, how it is supposed to work, and how it should be maintained. Without that information, homeowners are likely to be concerned that the system is running too much and may try to defeat it and stuff the fresh air inlets full of socks to prevent air from leaking in or out!

After the whole dwelling ventilation system and the spot ventilation systems, other ventilation systems should be considered. It is much easier to install a radon mitigation system (and some jurisdictions require it) during construction. These systems will ensure that not only radon but also other soil gases are removed before they can enter the home. The pipe will run all the way from the slab at the base of the house all the way up through the roof. There should be a monitoring system that will alert the homeowner if the fan stops running.

Detailed research has been performed to determine the optimum approach for removing the pollutants from an attached residential garage.[3] For many years, building codes required a 100 cfm exhaust fan in a garage, and it turns out, after extensive research, that was the right approach. This should be done if there are no atmospherically vented combustion appliances in the garage that might be back-drafted by an exhaust fan. If the air pressure

---

3. https://technologyportal.ashrae.org/Report/Detail/682

in the garage is lower than the air pressure in the house, any pollutants in the garage will "flow" toward the outside and not into the house.

Rule 2 of air motion: Air always flows from higher pressure to lower pressure.

A whole-house fan (whole house comfort ventilator) can be used for cooling the house when it is warmer in the house than it is outside. The traditional design is a large fan that sits in the middle of the top floor, drawing the air in through open windows and venting the house air into the attic and forcing it out through the attic vents. Some of these systems have motorized and insulated doors that block undesirable heat loss when the system is not in use. Others are ducted, removing air from multiple rooms and venting it directly to the outside, avoiding pressurizing the attic.

An attic exhaust fan, or PAV (Powered Attic Ventilator), vents the air from the attic directly outside. These fans will remove excess heat and humidity from the attic. The connection between the house and the attic must be carefully sealed for these systems to work effectively and not draw more moisture from the house into the attic. Like the whole house comfort ventilator, PAVs can have unintended consequences on the pressures in the house and should be thoughtfully designed. They can impact the combustion appliances in the house. They can draw moisture up into the attic. They can make it difficult to perform whole building leakage testing, among other effects. (See Chapter 16 for more information on attic ventilation.)

So FOR A NEW HOME, the ventilation systems, in order of importance that should be integrated into the design, are:
1. Whole Dwelling Ventilation System
2. Spot ventilation systems (bathroom and kitchen fans)
3. Radon/Soil gas ventilation system
4. Garage ventilation system
5. Attic ventilation

* * *

Ventilation system design for an existing home

The same system priorities apply to an existing house, particularly if it has been air sealed, reducing the natural infiltration rate. When a house reaches predetermined levels of tightness known as building tightness limits or BTL, weatherization programs require mechanical ventilation to be certain that acceptable levels of air quality will be maintained.[4] (Note that this is just a system check. More information on this process can be found in Chapter 7.)

Often in an existing home, one is replacing an existing component like a broken bath fan or addressing a specific issue such as radon. You need to keep in mind the system nature of the house. A radon mitigation system, for example, is likely to include a fan drawing the air out of the space under the slab. As long as the path from the ground to the space under the slab through the fan to the outside is a completely sealed system, there should not be any interference with other elements in the house. But if there is a sump pump in the basement's floor or a crack in the floor that connects the basement air to the space underneath it, it is possible that air will be drawn from the house into the radon mitigation system. If air is drawn from the basement that is needed for the draft of the water heater, air could be drawn back down the chimney, and so on and so on. It is important to think through all the possibilities.

Replacing a component such as a broken or annoying bath fan should begin by evaluating the initial installation. The design of the existing ductwork should be checked for a straight and smooth path to the outdoors. The external hood should be checked for the function of its backdraft damper and whether any birds or other creatures have lived in the ducting. A bathroom fan exhaust duct that runs through an uninsulated space in a cold climate should be replaced with insulated ducting and possibly rerouted. It is common for significant moisture to collect in uninsulated ducting.

Before removing the offending device, try to determine its performance. This will give you an idea of the effectiveness of the existing installation and serve as a reference to recheck after the product has been replaced. Get what information you can from the label in the fan. Scrape it off and find the cfm (cubic feet per minute) rating and maybe the sound rating in sones. If it was

---

4. Karg, Rick, "Survey of Tightness Limits for Residential Buildings, July, 2001", For the Chicago Regional Diagnostics Working Group, https://www.redcalc.com/wp-content/uploads/2022/02/Survey-of-BTL.pdf

originally rated as quiet (2 sones or less), why was it noisy? That could indicate an installation problem. Check to determine if any air is moving through the product. Hold a tissue up to the grille and see if there is enough airflow to pull it in. If it's a bath fan, try it with the bathroom door open and the bathroom door closed. (Testing methods are described in Chapter 9.) Check the outside of the house at the grille or termination fitting, with the fan running to see if the damper is being pushed open by the airflow.

Airflow is remarkably lazy. It is not eager to work. It will always seek the path of least resistance. It has to be pushed to get anything done.

Rule 3 of air motion: Moving air will always seek the path of least resistance.

Having made the initial observations regarding the installation of the existing product, refer to Chapter 6 to select, install, and test the replacement.

* * *

Totaling up the ventilation in the house

Fundamental rule of ventilation number two: one cubic foot of air coming into the house MUST be balanced by one cubic foot of air leaving the house. Don't be fooled into thinking that just because a fan is running and making a noise that it is moving air. If you covered up one side of a "box" fan (one of those fans that people put in their windows in the summer), the fan blade wouldn't stop spinning, but the air would stop moving except a small amount in the neighborhood of the fan, stirred up by the spinning blades.

Ventilation is not just the exhaust fans, particularly the kitchen and bath fans, but as previously stated, there are other systems that affect the flow of air through a house. The infiltration and exfiltration of the air is driven by pressures inside and outside of the house, naturally moving the air. Then there are the chimneys designed to be exhaust systems to guide the exhaust air from combustion appliances (water heater, furnace, fireplace, etc.) out of the house. The clothes dryer is also an exhaust system, sometimes quite a powerful one.

Central vacuums should take air out of the house as well. The mechanical systems, for example[5]:

Two small bath fans @ 50 cfm	100 cfm
Range hood @ 400 cfm	400cfm
Clothes dryer @ 200 cfm	200cfm
Central vacuum @ 150 cfm	150cfm
Total mechanical exhaust	850 cfm

Table 2.1 Total Ventilation in the House

This means that if all these systems were running simultaneously, 850 cfm would have to be "leaking" into the house somewhere just for them to work. If the air doesn't come in at these rates, it won't be leaving at these rates no matter what the label on the fan says. All of these mechanical devices will compete for incoming air, and remember, air is lazy. It takes the path of least resistance. If the closest, biggest hole is a window, that's where the air is going to come from. If the closest, biggest hole is the fireplace chimney, that's where the air is going to come from. If you close the bathroom door, the fan will seek to pull the air into the room from any opening—the crack under the door, the ceiling light fixture, the wall outlets, or the plumbing chases. If there is a control that responds to air quality issues such as humidity, the sensor in the control may respond to the humidity in the wall cavity and not to the humidity in the room.

Besides the mechanical ventilation devices, there are the passive or natural ventilation devices like gas fired water heaters that rely on the "stack effect" or the natural effect of rising warm air to draw the combustion fumes up the flue. It doesn't take much for the mechanical systems to overcome the natural systems and have the air flow the wrong way down the combustion exhaust pipe and into the house.

The goal is to know where the air is coming from and where it is going. It is much simpler and more effective to build a tight house with controlled and intentional airflows than it is to rely on natural air motion into and out of the house at the right times.

---

5. cfm means cubic feet per minute

* * *

How to read a fan box

There is some basic information printed on fan boxes you find in the electrical products aisle that says more about the product than its manufacturer's name and the price. Understanding the basic specifications is critical to selecting the right product. The following is the information for an exhaust fan product, but the fundamental information will apply to all residential ventilation products.

Besides the brand and the bar code and the color of the grille, is information like:

AIR FLOW: 70 cfm

This means that the fan can move 70 cubic feet of air per minute (cfm) under certain standard, prescribed conditions. If the fan is capable of multiple speed setting, that would be listed as 50/70/110. If the company has its products tested and certified under those prescribed conditions, the test laboratory's symbol should also be on the box like HVI (Home Ventilating Institute) or AMCA (Air Movement and Control Association). That airflow marking on the box will only provide an approximation of how the fan will perform once it has been installed. Remember: air is lazy. It doesn't like to push its way around corners or bump over the segments of flexible ducting or squeeze through small diameter ducting or push open the damper in the hood. All of those things resist the flow of air. Since every installation is different, the manufacturers had to agree on a common resistance or a test point so that all tested and certified products could be compared to each other. That test point (0.1 iwg) was set low enough so that any product that is appropriate for a task (like ventilating a bathroom) could meet it. Since the test point indicates low resistance to the airflow, the installed performance will be lower (sometimes significantly lower) than what is marked on the box. Some manufacturers supply a second rating point (0.25 iwg), reflecting performance at a higher resistance. Some programs (such as ENERGY STAR) require the fans to be tested and rated at a higher resistance. (Certified fan product manufacturers generate graphs of the fan performance at different resistances called "fan curves". These are sometimes included in the product literature and sometimes you have to request them.)

Not every fan box will include all this information, but here is some other information that you might find:

Noise Rating: 4 Sones

A sone is a linear indicator of sound level. One sone is approximately the sound a quiet refrigerator makes in a quiet kitchen. Two sones are twice as loud as one sone. The quietest fans are rated at < 0.3 sones. If it's a multi-speed fan, the noise level at each speed might be listed as <0.3/0.3/0.8. (More on Sound in Chapter 5.)

For baths up to 65 sq. ft, other rooms to 85 sq. ft.

This is another way of reflecting the airflow capability of the fan. The Home Ventilating Institute recommends 8 air changes per hour for a bathroom to remove all the moisture that is generated from showers and other pollutants. If the bathroom has a floor area of 65 square feet and the ceiling is 8 feet high, the volume of the bath is 65 square feet times 8 feet or 520 cubic feet. Changing all that air 8 times means multiplying the cubic feet by 8 or 4,160 cubic feet of air. Dividing that by 60 minutes comes out to 69.33 cubic feet per minute (pretty close to 70 cfm). Other rooms need fewer air changes (HVI recommends 6 air changes per hour in rooms other than bathrooms) because they have fewer polluting sources. Remember that the performance numbers on the box are based on the fan performing at a low resistance point. Also, remember that to achieve 6 or 8 air changes in an hour, the fan has to actually run for an hour.

Ceiling or wall installation

This is an indicator of how the backdraft damper in the fan is installed and product safety. If the damper is counter weighted for ceiling applications, it won't close properly if it is installed in a wall. (This may also indicate how the bearings in the fan motor are lubricated. Installing a ceiling-only fan in a wall may reduce the fan's life.) Fans that have been safety rated for installation in a wall have been tested to be sure that fingers cannot be inserted through the grille and impact moving parts.

UL Listed

This is indicates that the fan has been tested by a safety testing laboratory, in this case Underwriter Laboratories. (Other safety laboratories that do similar tests are ETL, CSA, and MET Lab.) These are privately operated companies that charge manufacturers to test their products according to established, standardized, safety test criteria.

HVI Certified

This is the Home Ventilating Institute. This is a trade association for residential fan product manufacturers. They establish the test criteria for fans and related products so that the information on product performance can be easily and accurately compared. At this point, there is no obligation by the manufacturers to join HVI or test their products to these standards, although some programs (such as ENERGY STAR) require certified performance results.

* * *

ARMED WITH THIS INFORMATION, it should be possible to select the right ventilation products, install them correctly, and test them to be sure they are operating properly. A good ventilation system will operate effectively for a long time, maintaining a livable level of indoor air quality and protecting the house that shelters the people.

Chapter 3

Basic Applications, Airflow, and Sizing Guidelines

"Gentlemen know that fresh air should be kept in its proper place—out of doors—and that, God having given us indoors and out-of-doors, we should not attempt to do away with this distinction." Rose Macaulay (1881 – 1958) (British poet, novelist, and essayist)

The point of this whole process, of course, is moving the air around. If that's not happening, then not much ventilation is happening! It is important to understand how air moves in a house. Everyone seems to have a grasp on the concept that "warm air rises". Why is that? Is all the air in the house the same and just at different temperatures? If you don't use fans or open windows or turn on the HVAC, would the air just sit there? People talk about air changes. There is continuous debate amongst building science experts about what the rate of change should be. Does that mean all the air changes in the house? (That would be a rather spectacular process with all the air suddenly leaving the house to be replaced by a completely new batch!)

The advent of the "Blower Door" has given us a tool for determining a close approximation of what the natural air change rate of a home is. A blower door is a large fan that is temporarily installed in an outside door of the house exhausting air. The flow rate is increased to a point that overcomes any natural air transfer, and the resulting number can be adjusted to reflect a natural air change rate showing where the house can be tightened up and how much mechanical ventilation might be needed.

* * *

House as a system—rooms as ducts

Air is very interesting stuff. The air in our houses comprises a variety of gases. "Standard Air" consists of nitrogen, oxygen, argon, carbon dioxide, neon, helium, and other gases.[1] (It also contains a bunch of pollutants at varying levels.) Originally, it all came from the outside. When the house was built, the air that was there was encapsulated. When the windows are opened or the fans turned on, some of the old air is moved out and new air is drawn in somewhere else. The volume of airflow is measured in the U.S. in cubic feet per minute or cfm. (In other parts of the world, it is measured in cubic meters per second or cubic liters per hour.)

Imagine an invisible box—a box of air, one foot by one foot by one foot, floating there in front of you. Because it's in the same room, it's about the same temperature and full of about the same particles and gases that you are breathing. There are a finite number of air molecules in the box. If the temperature increased, the air molecules would expand and fewer of them could fit into the box, the box would get lighter, and it would move upward. If the temperature in the box went down, more air molecules could fit in the box, the box would get heavier, and it would sink. Or think of a hot-air balloon filled with warm air, light enough to lift the balloon, basket, and occupants up into the sky and float on the winds.

Molecules of air carry moisture. If the number of molecules of air in the invisible, one cubic foot box rises (because the temperature went down), the amount of moisture relative to the amount of air would also rise. That's why the outside air in the winter can be quite cold and yet have a high, relative humidity or RH. In the summer, there may not be many air molecules in the cubic foot box, but with a high RH, it can be saturated because the amount of moisture relative to the number of air molecules may be high. The hotter the air is, the more moisture it can contain. One hundred percent relative humidity means that the air is totally saturated. It can't hold any more water,

---

1. http://www.engineeringtoolbox.com/air-composition-d_212.html

creating the probability of rain, snow, or fog... or condensation. At high levels of RH, the air can't carry away the moisture generated by our bodies, and we feel uncomfortable. At a point where warm, moist air touches a cooler surface, a surface that is cooler than the dew point temperature, the moisture in the air will condense on that surface, changing from a gas to a liquid. The dew point can occur on the surface of grass in the morning or somewhere inside a wall or on the surface of a glass of ice water.

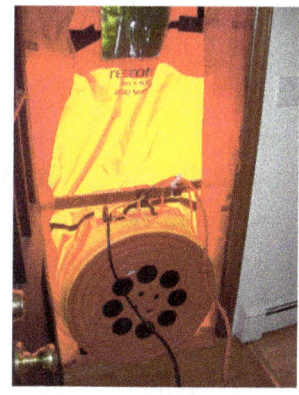

Figure 3.1 Blower Door

There are a lot of other things in a cubic foot of "air" that can upset the make-up of "standard air"—other gases like carbon dioxide (which we breathe out), carbon monoxide (from burning things or cars in the garage), ozone, formaldehyde, and other chemicals of daily life. And there are lots of particulates, both small and large, floating around in the air. (See Chapter 18 for information about Indoor Air Quality (IAQ))

Residential ventilation strategies are based on the assumption that the outside air is cleaner than the inside air. Mothers say, "Go outside and get a breath of fresh air." Sometimes that isn't true, when we are advised to stay indoors, but residential ventilation strategies assume that the polluted air is in the house and needs to be changed with outside air and most of the time in most places, this is true.

> The U.S. EPA has a website that provides an indication of the outdoor air daily at www.AirNow.gov. For Canada, there is the Air Quality Health Index that provides a daily outdoor environmental conditions for various communities across Canada. There are times and locations when the outdoor air should be treated with caution, particularly for people who are susceptible to compromised conditions.

A thermostat only "knows" that when it gets cold, the heating system can be turned on and heat will be produced. We don't know what the outdoor air contains at any moment. We assume the outdoor air is better than indoor air when we operate the ventilation system.

When the air in the house is changed by the ventilation system, not all the air gets changed at once. Each "complete" air change will reduce the pollutant level by one half (1/2). Pour a cup of black coffee into a container. If a cup of clean water is added, the liquid in the container is now half as "polluted". Empty one cup of liquid out of the container and add another cup of clear water. The liquid is now one quarter as polluted as it was at the beginning, and so on and so on. As long as no new "pollutant" or coffee is added to the container, the liquid will become increasingly diluted or less polluted. Because the amount of fresh liquid is equal to the amount of "polluted" liquid, this is equivalent to a 50% change rate. "The solution to pollution is dilution."

In terms of air, if the air changes in the house are continuous, the air will stay acceptable. If the natural air changes (what is called air changes per hour or ACH) are too great, the air may be fresher, but the energy cost will be high. If the ACH is too low, the air in the house will be stale and possibly unhealthy. The trick is to find the balance between the two. There are standards and suggested rates (see Chapters 12 and 13), but a great deal depends on the house, the location, and the occupants. Some people like to open their windows all year 'round. Some people never open their windows. Some people live in climates where natural breezes are welcomed. Some homes are in places where everything possible must be done to keep the outside... outside.

***

Fan System Choices

The most efficient location for exhausting the air from a home is to remove it from the places where the most pollutants are generated, like the bathrooms, kitchen, garage, and from the ground under the slab. Fresh air should be introduced into places where people spend the most time, like the bedrooms, living room, family room, or TV room. The most common fans are fans that mount in the ceiling like a typical bath fan and fans that are mounted in the range hood. Paddle fans hanging from the ceiling help to stir up the air in both summer for cooling and in winter for pushing the warm air back down. Window or box fans, pedestal fans, oscillating fans, and hassock fans are used for cooling people by generating a breeze or pushing warm air out of a hot house. Down-drafting range fans are an alternative to the traditional capture hood. Ventilation air doesn't always have to rise!

There are other, less familiar choices of fans. There are "in-line" fans that are used to pull and push air through a duct. They can be mounted remotely from the space they are venting with the advantage of removing the fan noise from the space. As "work-horse" fans, they can be used for hauling radon or soil gas, polluted air from under a slab or increasing the length of the duct run from a dryer.

There are large, propeller fans that are used as cooling systems in homes (see Chapter 16). These are called "whole house comfort ventilators", although they are more commonly referred to as "whole house fans". Propeller fans are also used as attic fans (known as powered attic ventilators or PAVs), mounted in the roof or gable end of the attic and pushing the hot air out.

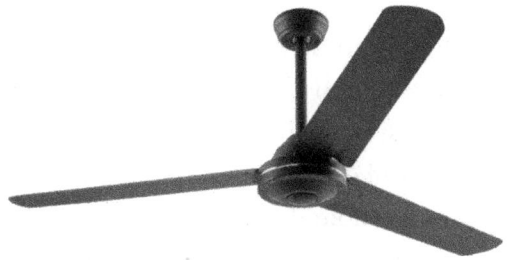

Figure 3.2 Ceiling Fan (Broan)

There is the blower in the air handler that pushes the heated or cooled air around through the ducts to condition the space. These are the most powerful and energy consuming fans in the house as they move the most air, but they circulate air throughout the house and, coupled with a fresh air intake, can be used as the whole dwelling ventilation system.

Window air conditioners, aside from providing cooling, often have an operable vent to the outside that will bring in outside air. Ductless or mini-split heat pump systems have internal blowers that push air around the room they are mounted in. These don't have fresh air intake connections, so they don't exchange the inside and outside air.[2]

Different ventilation components have different jobs to do and should be sized and selected in response to their purpose. Although some ventilating tasks can be combined, in most homes, multiple systems will be required. Always keep in mind, however, that *the house and the occupants are a system.*

---

2. Packaged Terminal Air Handlers (PTAC) units are commonly located in hotel rooms under windows. These usually do have outside air connections.

Airflow Considerations for the Whole Dwelling Ventilation System

The ventilation system that continuously changes all the air in the house is called the 'Whole Dwelling' ventilation system[3]. Its purpose is to make sure that adequate air is effectively moving continuously throughout the house. The secondary systems are the "spot" or "local" exhaust systems that quickly remove pollutants at the source from bathrooms and kitchens. The two functions can be combined, but they both need to be there.

The bathrooms and the kitchen are known sources of moisture and other pollutants. Those pollutants can be exhausted immediately from the "source" by exhausting those points when the bathrooms or kitchen are being used, which is why this is called "spot" or "local" ventilation. But the people and the materials in the house produce other, more widely dispersed pollutants that also need to be exhausted. Whole dwelling, or whole house, air quality ventilation systems are dedicated to improving the air quality of the whole house. These systems must be run continuously or intermittently at a rate that is functionally equivalent to running continuously.

Permanent materials in the house, such as cabinets and flooring, continue to "out-gas" long after they have been installed. Carpeting and furniture have chemicals that are added to the air. Cleaning materials, paints, deodorants, pets, and people all continuously add to the gases and particles in the air. Some of these sources occur intermittently. People might not be in the house all the time. Some pollutants increase and decrease throughout the day. The whole dwelling ventilation system needs to deal with all of that in order to keep the air acceptable to the occupants of the house.

The ASHRAE 62.2 ventilation standard defines acceptable indoor air quality as "air toward which a substantial majority of occupants express no dissatisfaction with respect to odor and sensory irritation and in which there are not likely to be contaminants at concentrations that are known to pose a health risk."[4] These are subjective measurements, but there are certainly

---

3. In some programs, these are known as "ASHRAE fans" and some vendors actually advertise selling "ASHRAE 62.2 fans".
4. ASHRAE Standard 62.2 https://www.energy.gov/eere/buildings/articles/ashrae-standard-622-ventilation-and-acceptable-indoor-air-quality-low-rise

objective measurements in indoor air that need to be controlled as well. By running a whole dwelling, whole house, air quality ventilation system regularly or continuously, the level of the pollutants in the house may not build up and become uncontrollable. (See Chapter 18 regarding Disability Adjusted Life Years (DALY)).

* * *

Whole Dwelling System Sizing

A great deal of work has been done to determine what that optimum, continuous, whole dwelling ventilation rate should be. Calculating the requisite airflow of this system is not as simple as figuring out what size fan to install in the bathroom or kitchen. This is one of those occasions where "one size does not fit all". One airflow number or fan size will not satisfy all the local conditions—house size, occupancy, climate, etc. There are a number of approaches that can arrive at a number "in the ballpark". The flow rates vary from 30 cfm for a small, one-bedroom house to 165 cfm for a large, seven-bedroom house. If the flow rate is too small, its ventilating effects will be inconsequential. If the flow rate is too large, it will put an unnecessary cost burden on conditioning the air. Occupants have different sensitivities to air quality conditions. They bring different materials into their homes. They participate in different activities for different lengths of time. And they live in different places, with different weather in homes that have been constructed differently, with different levels of tightness. On top of all that, the installed performance of systems will vary.

Ideally, the ventilation rate would be determined by detrimental health effects that have been <u>avoided</u> or the number of diseases that <u>didn't</u> happen because of adequate ventilation! Although there have been several studies on the relationship between health, indoor air quality, and ventilation, it is only the most extreme cases that can be quantified. The effects of the myriad of every-day, low-level pollutants on the health of the home's occupants are virtually unknown. We spend about 90% of our lives indoors and know that levels of chemicals such as formaldehyde, chloroform, and styrene are two to 50 times higher indoors than outdoors.[5]

---

5. https://www.latimes.com/archives/la-xpm-2006-jun-22-me-teenair22-story.html

Odors are the one thing that will get people to operate ventilation systems and windows. If the ventilation rate drops below 5 cfm per person for more than a couple of hours, occupants will be bothered by odors.

As ventilation rates increase, so does the cost of conditioning the air. The impact of energy costs fluctuates with the interest in tightening up homes and the increasing cost and declining availability of heating fuels. This cost is relatively low, however.

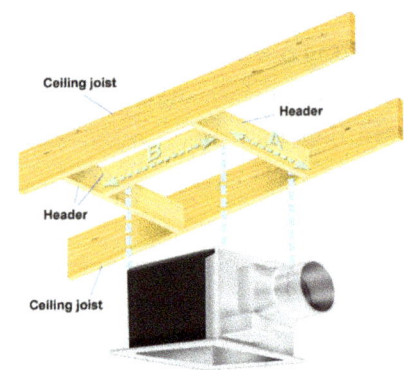

Figure 3.3 Ceiling exhaust fan (Panasonic)

A quick approximation of adequate mechanical airflow is to design the ventilation system to provide 0.3 or one third of a natural air change per hour. A 1,500 square foot house with 8-foot ceilings would require approximately 60 cfm of continuous flow. (See Chapter 7 for a discussion of why you can't rely on natural leakage to provide continuous ventilation.)

A more accurate calculation of flow rate sizing is to use the number of bedrooms as the guiding factor, estimating that the number of bedrooms is a reasonable guide to the number of people that will live in the house, estimating two people in the primary bedroom and one in each other bedroom. ASHRAE proposes that each person be allowed 7.5 cfm along with 0.03 cfm per hundred square feet of floor area. So a two-bedroom 1,500 square foot house would require roughly 70 cubic feet of air moving through it continuously.

Since houses are different and they are in different places and they are built differently, this rate can be further refined. If the house has been leak tested with a blower door, that leakage number could compensate for the height and location of the building and its tightness. If you don't have access to a blower door result, you could reduce the total flow rate by approximately two cfm per one hundred square feet of floor area. That would reduce the total required cfm for our 1,500 square foot house to approximately forty cfm running continuously.

If the house is built tightly, does not have a conditioned air HVAC system, or it is a time of the year when that system isn't running, it is not likely to be that leaky. To be sure of adequate ventilation, it is preferable to size, design and install the mechanical ventilation system to handle the whole load.

Note that these numbers are rates of airflow only. They do not refer to DIRECTION or TYPE of airflow. The direction of flow will affect whether the house will be positively or negatively pressurized and that will have a major effect on moisture and building durability. (See Chapter 7 on House Pressures.)

As a general rule of thumb, if the home is in a hot and humid climate and relies on air conditioning to keep the living space comfortable, a positive ventilation approach is preferable, pushing outside air into the house.

Not that long ago sizing the ventilation system to the ASHRAE standards required referring to tables and doing a bunch of math (which I have included here). But it you don't want to do all the math, you can refer to the web tool from Residential Energy Dynamics or RED at https://www.redcalc.com/redcalc-free/ and just plug in the required values.[6]

ASHRAE offers both a formula based on the floor area of the house and the number of bedrooms,[7] as well as tables that can be used without doing any math. For square foot measurements:

$$Q_{fan} = 0.03 A_{floor} + 7.5(N_{br} + 1)$$

where:
Q_{fan} = fan flow rate in cfm (cubic feet per minute)
A_{floor} = floor area in square feet
N_{br} = number of bedrooms (not less than one)

---

6. RedCalc has a lot of other very useful tools there as well. RedCalc is available for free the Building America Solution Center: https://basc.pnnl.gov/redcalc
7. ASHRAE Standard 62.2 https://www.energy.gov/eere/buildings/articles/ashrae-standard-622-ventilation-and-acceptable-indoor-air-quality-low-rise

Floor Area (ft²)	1 Bedrooms	2	3	4	5
<500	30	38	45	53	60
501-1000	45	53	60	68	75
1001-1500	60	68	75	83	90
1501-2000	75	83	90	98	105
2001-2500	90	98	105	113	120
2501-3000	105	113	120	128	135
3001-3500	120	128	135	143	150
3501-4000	135	143	150	158	165
4001-4500	150	158	165	173	180
4501-5000	165	173	180	188	195

Table 3.1a From ASHRAE 62.2 Table 4.1a (I-P) Ventilation Air Requirements in CFM

For metric measurements:

$$Q_{fan} = 0.15 A_{floor} + 3.5(N_{br} + 1)$$

where:

Q_{fan} = fan flow rate in L/s (liters per second)
A_{floor} = floor area in square meters
N_{br} = number of bedrooms (not less than one)

Floor Area (m²)	1 Bedrooms	2	3	4	5
<47	14	18	21	25	28
47-93	21	24	28	31	35
94-139	28	31	35	38	42
140-186	35	38	42	45	49
187-232	42	45	49	52	56
233-279	49	572	56	59	63
280-325	56	59	63	66	70
326-372	63	66	70	73	77
373-418	70	73	77	80	84
419-465	77	80	84	87	91

Table 3.1b From ASHRAE 62.2 Table 4.1b (SI) Ventilation Air Requirements in L/s

Using the table is pretty straightforward: select the floor area and the number of bedrooms and the intersection is the amount of airflow required for the whole dwelling ventilation system. A 2,000 square foot house with 2 bedrooms, for example, would require 60 cfm of airflow. (ASHRAE 62.2 will be discussed in more detail in Chapter 13.)

The credit for the leakage and height and location of the building can be calculated by using the blower door measurement with the following formula:

$$Q_i = \text{blower door result} \times 0.052 \times s \times wsf$$

where
Q_i = infiltration credit
s = a factor for the height of the building

# of stories	S factor
1	1
1.5	1.16
2	1.31
2.5	1.43
3	1.54

Table 3.2 Height factor (s)

wsf = weather shielding factor based on the location. (There are approximately 1,100 of these in the ASHRAE Standard.)

City	Wsf
Boston	0.66
New York	0.61
Washington, D.C.	0.51
Chicago	0.56
Dallas	0.53
Denver	0.59
Seattle	0.56
San Francisco	0.60

Table 3.3 Weather Shield Factors (wsf) for Major Cities

Distributed Ventilation Sizing

An alternative approach to whole dwelling system sizing is to size the system based on the room use, similar to approach in the Canadian F326 Standard. This approach applies different flow rates to different rooms based on their use. Rooms like kitchens, bathrooms, and utility rooms are designated as exhaust rooms, or Category B rooms. Rooms like bedrooms, living rooms, and family rooms are designated as supply rooms or Category A rooms. The primary bedroom would require 20 cfm and a family room would require 10 cfm of supply air. The kitchen would require 100 cfm of intermittent exhaust and a bathroom, 50 cfm.

This process requires totaling up the cfm supply requirements of the Category A rooms and the exhaust requirements of the Category B rooms to arrive at the total amount of air that needs to be moved through the house. This approach recognizes the air flow requirements by the room use rather than just picking one number for the whole house. There is considerably more information about this approach in the balanced ventilation design in Appendix H.

Spot/Local Exhaust Ventilation

Bath Fans

Besides the furnace blower, the most common fan in the house is the bath fan. It is surprising to find bathrooms that don't have fans. There has been a long battle about whether every bathroom should have a fan mandated by code. Some of that conflict was generated by a definition of the purpose of the bath fan. For many people, the purpose is to provide "masking noise" not to move the air. There are still those who think that if there is a window in the bathroom, a fan isn't necessary. There are many reasons not to open a window in a bathroom—from climate to neighbors. And even if the window is open, it doesn't mean that the air will move effectively through it (particularly if the bathroom door is closed) and in the desired flow direction! Because of the window option, for many years, bathroom fan manufacturers weren't particularly concerned about how noisy the fans were. In fact, it was almost considered, "The noisier the better".

Fans are sometimes run on their own wall switch, but more commonly, the same switch that controls the lights operates the fan. To make that even easier, fan manufacturers added the lights to the fan, so the customer bought everything in a single package. By having the fan come on when the light turned on, there would be at least some mechanical ventilation in the bathroom (and it made the installation simple). The occupant could avoid using the noisy fan only by functioning in the dark. The light switch was a crude "occupancy sensor".

The fan is mounted in the ceiling to get the light up there and to facilitate the duct running from the fan to the outside.

These ceiling mounted fans are commonly a complete package with the fan, the light, the grille, the mounting system, and the duct connection with a backdraft damper to keep the cold drafts from coming back into the room from the outside. These dampers rely on air motion to open and gravity to close, which is why fans designed for ceiling mounting should be installed in ceilings. If the bathroom design calls for the fan to be wall mounted, the fan's description should state that the fan is designed for "wall mounting".

As houses became tighter during the energy disruptions in the early 1970s, building scientists recognized that ventilation played an important role in occupant health and comfort and building durability, and it seemed obvious that the bath fan could be used for more than masking the noises in the bathroom. The fan could improve the air quality in the bathroom and the house, but it would need to be run longer and to do that, fans would need to be quieter.

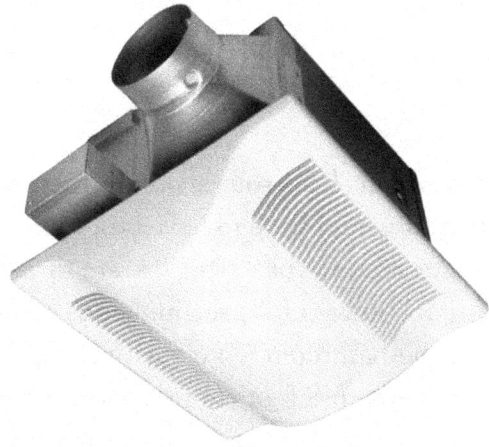

Figure 3.4 Bath fan with a light (Panasonic)

The bath fan doesn't have to actually be in the bathroom. All that's needed is to get the bad air out of there and to the outside. So the fan can be remotely mounted with just a grille in the bathroom. "In-line" fans are ideal for this sort of installation. They can be installed virtually anywhere in the duct line, removing their operating noises from the bathroom and allowing for an array of grille choices. The grilles can be mounted in the ceiling or wall, high up or low down. They can be mounted in a shower area or behind a toilet. They can be mounted in the frame of the mirror to keep the fogging to a minimum. The important thing is that the opening in the bathroom should match the capability of the fan to draw air through it.

Fans can be mounted at the end of the ducting, on the outside surface of the home. It is important that in such installations a backdraft damper be added to the ducting, preferably near the fan, to prevent unconditioned outside air from flowing back into the house when the fan isn't running. The fan itself may not include the damper, although there may be one in the external hood.

There are also fans that can be mounted in an exterior wall of the bathroom, venting through the wall directly to the outside. Some can be mounted in the glass of a window. These are less common in the U.S. with the difficulty of cutting a round hole in a piece of insulated glass. The advantage of these direct exhaust applications is that there is no ducting to be concerned about and the installed performance should equal the rated performance. A disadvantage is that the through-wall opening is bigger than the opening for a ceiling mounted fan and the closure system has to be more positive to prevent air flowing back into the house.

Bath Fan sizing

The proximity of the bath fan to the source of moisture means that it can have a lower airflow rate than it would have to have otherwise. There are a number of considerations in determining the "size" or rate of airflow for a bath fan. The Home Ventilating Institute (HVI) recommends a bath fan be capable of changing all the air in the bathroom (8) eight times an hour. So if the bathroom is 8 feet by 5 feet with an 8-foot ceiling: 8 x 5 x 8 = 320 cubic feet. To change that air eight times in an hour multiplies the volume by eight or 2,560 cubic feet of air to move each hour. Since there are 60 minutes in an hour, dividing 2,560 by 60 results in a 42 cfm rated fan. (Another way to calculate this is to allow for 1 cfm per square foot. So this 40 square foot bathroom would need a 40 cfm fan. Just about the same.)

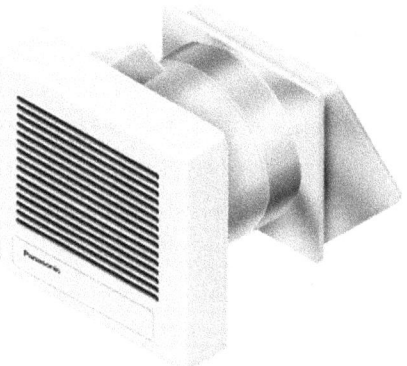

Figure 3.5 Through-wall exhaust fan (Panasonic/Morrissey)

For a larger bathroom (over 100 square feet), HVI recommends sizing the ventilation by the appliances:[8]

Toilet	50 cfm
Shower	50 cfm
Bath Tub	50 cfm
Jetted Tub	100 cfm

Table 3.4 Recommended Airflow per Bath Appliance

For example, if the bathroom had a toilet, a separate shower, and a bathtub, it would require 50 plus 50 plus 50 or 150 cfm. These areas could be vented separately with separate fans or with a single, remote fan with multiple inlets or with a single, 150 cfm ceiling fan.

ASHRAE in Standard 62.2-2025 offers two numbers for bathroom fans— 20 cfm (10L/s) if the fan is to be operated continuously and 50 cfm (25L/s) if it is to be operated intermittently or on demand.

It is important that the fan runs long enough to accomplish a reasonable air change. That is one reason HVI suggests higher airflows. If the 42 cfm fan

---

8. https://www.hvi.org/resources/publications/bathroom-exhaust-fans/

is on for only 20 minutes in the 320 cubic foot bathroom, it will only accomplish about two and a half air changes. A more powerful fan will change the air in the bathroom more quickly and will not need to run as long as a fan with a lower cfm capability. Of course, exhausting more air from the house has an energy penalty to it, but that is small. (For a fan that moves 150 cfm running for 20 minutes when it's 30 degrees outside and 70 degrees inside, the energy required to heat the air is about 2,160 BTUs or $0.004 (at $0.21/kWh). Remember though, that the bath fan is just one part of the total ventilation inventory in the house, and as its exhaust airflow increases the amount of make-up air needed also increases (remember Rule 1 in Chapter 2: 1 cfm out = 1 cfm in).

Just running a more powerful fan for a shorter time is not necessarily the equivalent of running a smaller fan for a longer period. It takes a long time for the moisture on the walls of the shower or the moisture absorbed by the towels to evaporate. It is likely to require hours depending on how much moisture there already is in the air - its relative humidity or RH.

It is also important that the installation of the fan complies with the manufacturer's specifications. The manuals that come with these fans are good at offering installation details, but who reads installation manuals? Long, twisting runs of flexible ducting will greatly reduce the actual installed performance of the fan. Air is lazy.

Kitchen Exhaust Fans

Range hoods are designed to trap or "entrain" the fumes and smoke and moisture from cooking and sweep them out of the room before they pollute the rest of the house. Their ability to accomplish this is called "capture efficiency". The higher the capture efficiency, the lower the volume of airflow has to be. Kitchen exhaust fans are commonly located or associated with a range hood that is mounted over the stove. Some hoods have the fan installed in the hood and some have the fan installed remotely. In an attempt to ease installation, recirculating hoods are designed simply to draw the air in, pass it through a "filter", and then vent it back out into the kitchen. The filter in the hood is designed to trap the grease and odors using an odor "absorbing" material, such as charcoal or carbon. Grease will coat the carbon, making it ineffective, so these "traps" need to be replaced regularly. Because these recirculating fans do not vent to the outside, they have little impact on the quality of the air in the house.

As an alternative to the range hood mounted fans, there are "down-drafting" vents that pull the air down and out. There are also fans that are used as "general" kitchen fans, exhausting through a wall or window or from the ceiling of the kitchen.

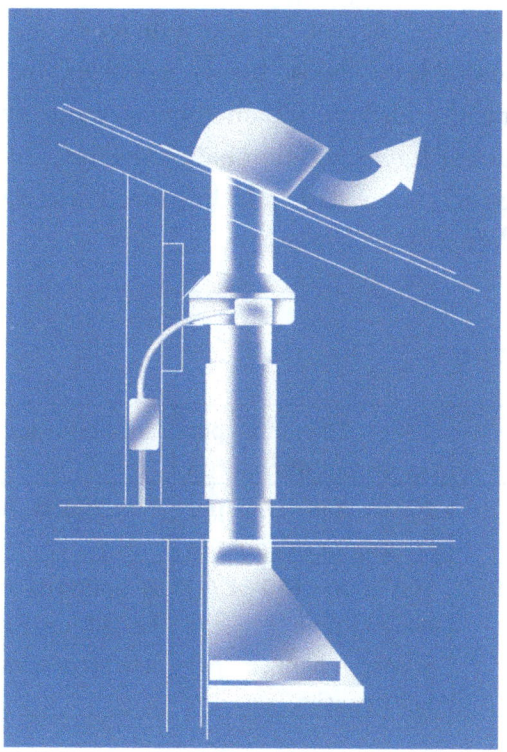

Figure 3.6 Remote range hood (Fantech)

There has been a trend toward installing commercial appliances in the kitchen under the "bigger-and-more-powerful-is-better" philosophy. With commercial stoves installed, the inclination is to employ commercial range hoods as well, making a significant statement about size and prestige and power. In commercial applications, there are strict code requirements regarding airflow and make-up air. Commercial hoods need an adequate amount of airflow power to draw the air through the filter system at a high enough velocity to entrain the grease and other particulates and limit their settling on other parts of the kitchen and serving as a source for grease fires. A higher airflow velocity will keep the particles suspended and allow them to be vented out of the kitchen. The Uniform Mechanical Code (UMC) requires makeup air for commercial kitchens, but with few exceptions,[9] residential code requirements are less restrictive. But if a commercial hood is used in a residential application, the commercial codes should be applied in order for the product to work properly.

With a kitchen range hood, what is truly important is the ability of the hood to capture the effluents produced by the cooking. The most desirable range hood will have the highest capture efficiency and the lowest power consumption and noise level. Most hoods, however, increase their capture ability by increasing the airflow, which increases the noise and the power consumption. Studies at Lawrence-Berkeley Labs in California are underway to develop a capture efficiency scale and improved criteria for selecting range hoods for optimum efficiency.

Kitchen Fan Sizing

HVI	40 to 100 cfm per linear foot of cooktop	For hoods located against a wall
	50 to 150 cfm per linear foot of cooktop	For "island" hoods
ASHRAE 62.2-2025	100 cfm (50 L/s) intermittent 5 Air changes per hour continuous	If operated continuously, it can be all or part of the primary ventilation system

Table 3.4 Minimum recommended sizes for range hoods

By HVI's criteria, a typical four burner, 30-inch wide range would require a 100 to 250 cfm exhaust fan. Commercial criteria commonly call for 300 cfm per linear foot! This would indicate the need for a 750 cfm exhaust fan. Although there are limited code requirements regarding makeup air, remember that 1 cfm out equals 1 cfm in. For the larger, commercial sized range hood fans to work properly, they will require some means of supplying

---

9. IMC 505.2 "Exhaust hood systems capable of exhausting in excess of 400 cfm (0.19 m3/s) shall be provided with make-up air at a rate approximately equal to the exhaust air rate."

makeup air whether or not makeup is a local code requirement. (See Section 8.3)

Backdrafting is an important consideration in sizing any fan, but particularly a kitchen range hood, because of the potential power. A casual over-sizing of the fan in order to satisfy the "bigger-is-better" need can lead to potentially disastrous consequences. Imagine a winter party with a cozy fire in the fireplace. The host flips on the range hood fan when he burns some hors d'oeuvres and the house fills with smoke from the back drafting fireplace. At the same time, the gas water heater in the basement backdrafts, drawing in carbon monoxide and other combustion by-products. As houses become tighter, it takes less and less negative pressure to cause problems with combustion appliances seeking to use the same air. It is best to use a less powerful fan and test the performance to make sure.

ASHRAE 62.2-2025 requires 100 cfm of venting from the range hood if there isn't a kitchen exhaust fan running continuously that is capable of 5 air changes per hour. For example, a 300 square foot, enclosed kitchen would require a 200 cfm fan exhausting continuously. Kitchens that are not enclosed (open to the rest of the house) cannot meet the Standard with a continuously running fan, primarily because of the difficulty of defining the boundaries of the kitchen.

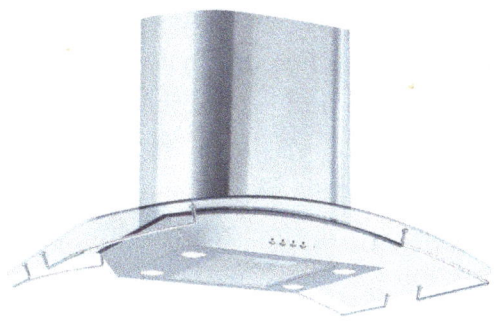

Figure 3.7 Island range hood (Air King)

There is another sizing suggestion of 1 cfm per 100 BTU rating of the cooktop. This would put the commercial cooktops in a completely different sizing category, since they are rated in excess of 10,000 BTUs, some as high as

280,000 BTUs. The thing to remember is that, hopefully, all those burners won't be operating at the same time. Using the linear approach for sizing the fan (meaning a fan of only 600 cfm) will be adequate in the vast majority of applications.

The hood should be at least as wide as the cooktop, preferably an inch or two wider on each side and mounted between 20" and 30" above the cooking surface. When the hood is closer to the cooking surface, the capture efficiency is improved. It should be simple to maintain. Some hoods have fan blades that can be removed and washed in the dishwasher. The grease filters should also be cleaned regularly.

Extra information on kitchen range hoods was created by the Building Performance Workshop and the HomeChem project.[10]

A Word About Clothes Dryers

The fundamental purpose of a clothes dryer is to dry the clothes! It is designed to accomplish that using heat and airflow. The air is usually drawn in at the bottom of the device and pushed through a filter to a duct designed to transport the air to the outside of the building. The air is heated to allow it to carry the moisture in the air stream. (Warm air can hold more moisture than cold air.) If the air is heated with a gas-fired flame, then the exhaust air also carries the combustion gases and the duct functions as the flue.

If clothes are piled around the base of the dryer, it will restrict the easy flow of air into the dryer and extend the drying time.

If the duct is bent around numerous ninety-degree turns and full of lint, it will restrict the easy flow of air and extend the trying time and may trap and pool condensed moisture.

And if the dryer is in a congested space and tries to move over 200 cfm, by code,[11] it needs an easy flow path from the building or at least from the main body of the house.

The fact is that if the air flow path into, through, and out of the dryer is smooth and easy, the clothes will dry more quickly, are less likely to "cook" in the dryer, will last longer, and the whole process will use less energy.

Note that heat pump clothes dryers don't vent to the outdoors so they

---

10. https://buildingperformanceworkshop.com/blog/kitchen-exhaust
11. IMC § 504.6 Makeup air

don't impact the pressures in the house. The waste water in them, however, must be connected to a drain.

Other Ventilation System Sizing

Other ventilation systems will be discussed in more detail in Chapter 15, but they should be considered as a part of the total ventilation "inventory" in determining the total airflow.

Radon or soil gas mitigation systems suck the air from under the basement slab or crawl space floor and from around the foundation walls and blow it to the outside. These systems should run continuously, but they draw very little air from the inside of the house except through cracks or gaps in the floor.

Attached garages can also add pollutants to the house. If the pressure in the house is lower than the pressure in the garage, air will flow from the garage to the house carrying with it all the pollutants that are in the garage air. A garage exhaust fan can mitigate this problem, but care must be taken to be sure that a fan blowing out of and depressurizing the garage will not affect any combustion appliance in the garage or the house. The right airflow for a garage exhaust fan will vary by the tightness of the garage and by the runtime. If the garage is tightly constructed and the fan is run continuously, a small airflow will depressurize it—flows as small as 20 cfm. A typical garage with intermittent operation needs 100 cfm per bay or 0.75 cfm per square foot.

Chapter 4

System Design Choices

The best point to select a ventilation system design is when the house is being designed, when the ducting, wiring, and plumbing are being laid out. At that time, all the options are open and there is an opportunity to think through how the systems (and their installers) will work together. It is the time to think about how the systems will first be used and how they might be used after the first occupants leave and another family moves in. It is a time to think about what might happen in the future, both in terms of modifications to the house, but also in terms of maintenance of the systems. Houses have lasted for hundreds of years. It is the best use of the materials. Parts of the house that will last for two hundred years should not have to be ripped out to repair or replace parts that will only last ten or twenty years. If the ventilation system is not designed properly in the first place, it is likely to shorten the life of the building. If poor equipment is used, it may need to be serviced regularly or replaced sooner. If good equipment is purchased and a good system is designed but it is installed poorly, the system won't be effective, and it will need to be serviced. The unfortunate fact is that any mechanical system, no matter how beautifully designed and manufactured, will need to be repaired or replaced at some point. Burying fan systems in wall or ceiling cavities with no access guarantees that someone in the future is going to have to rip that wall or ceiling apart for even a simple adjustment or repair.

This certainly doesn't mean that an existing ventilation system cannot be repaired or replaced or improved in an existing house. It's just more of a challenge. Running ducting through existing walls and ceilings is not as simple as snaking a wire (and even that can be a challenge).

The options are essentially based on where and how the mechanical components of the system are placed. Pollutant source control requires limiting the sources as a first step, keeping the materials that contain significant, harmful chemical components out of the building—like formaldehyde and carbon monoxide. Radon and soil gas mitigation fans and bath and kitchen fans are near the source of pollutants and provide the activity related ventilation control. They do not have to be powerful because they are near the polluting source. The distance the air needs to move is relatively small, and, like a local whirlpool, they will suck in what is around them. These devices are part of the ventilation system, but, as discussed in the previous chapter, they need to be accompanied by a whole house, air quality, whole dwelling ventilation system.

Exhaust-Centered (Exhaust-only) Whole Dwelling Ventilation System

An exhaust-centered[1] system locates the mechanical component on the exhaust side, like a bathroom fan, blowing air out of the house. The exhaust-centered approach depressurizes the house, sucking the air out of it, relying on leaks and cracks and gaps in the building shell to let the air back in. The exhaust fan may do double duty and be located where pollutants are generated, like in a bathroom, or it may be centrally located in a hallway. Inlet air "leaks", however, will be spread about the house and may (or may not) effectively draw fresh air into all the rooms, particularly bedrooms where people spend the most time.

---

1. I'm calling this exhaust-centered whole dwelling ventilation rather than *exhaust-only* whole dwelling ventilation because *exhaust-only* implies that the air is only moving one way.

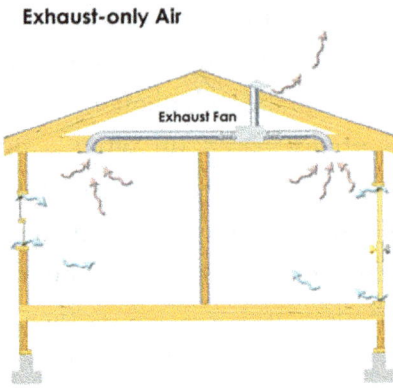

Figure 4.1 Exhaust-centered Whole Dwelling Ventilation (Panasonic/Morrissey)

This is the most basic, standard ventilation system. It grew out of the concept of putting a fan in the bathroom to remove odors and a fan in the kitchen to remove cooking smoke and smell. When houses were fairly "leaky", this worked well, although they could still feel stuffy, particularly in the winter. There is certainly an advantage to using the same fan that exhausts bathroom pollutants to serve as the whole dwelling ventilation system. The fan does double duty.

For this strategy to work, the fan has to run constantly, or at least part of every hour. That requires a quiet, energy efficient fan, otherwise it will be defeated, shut off, and stuffed full of socks. And, equally important, the occupant needs to understand and appreciate why it is running all the time or it will be defeated, shut off, and stuffed full of socks.

> How long can a fan run before it breaks down? The number of hours that a fan can run depends primarily on the lubricants in the bearings of the motor. If a fan motor is rated to run 60,000 hours, it is equivalent to 6.8 years of continuous operation. Although there are many green building programs and residential ventilation codes that require the use of fans "rated for continuous operation", there is no standardized test, group, or agency that provides such a rating. It is up to the manufacturer to provide that information.

Since the fan is running continuously and it is quiet, the home occupants will not know that it is on and, conversely, won't know if it is off or stops running. Why do you need a fan running all the time anyway? Many of the forces of nature are very, very slow. Imagine a stoppered bathroom sink with a leaky faucet, a single drip every 15 seconds. It's just a drop; a tiny amount of water, but after 8 hours there will be more than a pint of water in the sink. After a day, it will be approaching a gallon and perhaps the edge of the sink. A small amount of condensation occurring somewhere in a wall will gradually grow mold, encouraged as it will be by that slow, inexorable drip.

Pollutant materials can out-gas over a long period of time. The average ventilation rate is different from the effective ventilation rate. The effective ventilation rate 'ε' is defined as the inverse of the steady-state concentration of the pollutant, i.e. the removal of the pollutant from the air in the home.

Consider two identical homes. One is mechanically ventilated continuously at 0.35 air changes per hour (0.35 ACH). The other assumes a low, natural ventilation or infiltration rate of 0.22 ACH for 23 hours a day and one hour of high, mechanical ventilation at 3.4 ACH.

System description	**System 1** Continuous venting at 0.35 ACH, 24 hours/day	**System 2** Natural 0.22 ACH for 23 hours, and one hour of mechanical ventilation at 3.4 ACH
Average ACH	$\frac{0.35 \text{ ACH} \times 24 \text{hrs}}{24 \text{ hrs}} = 0.35$ ACH	$\frac{(0.22 \text{ ACH} \times 23 \text{ hrs}) + (3.4 \text{ACH} \times 1 \text{ hr})}{24 \text{ hrs}} = 0.35$ ACH

Table 4.1 Air Change Rate Comparison

The average ventilation rate, or ACH, describes the average amount of air moving through the house. System 1 is a continuously operating, mechanical system with a total ACH of 0.35, including both natural and mechanical ventilation. System 2 relies on a natural, continuous 0.22 ACH for 23 hours, along with one high exhaust hour at 3.4 ACH. The resulting average ventilation rate is the same over 24 hours.

The effective ventilation rate, for the two homes in this example, can be defined by considering a pollutant source like rotting shrimp out-gassing continuously over a long period. For this example, the source strength is divided into equal parts of Shrimp per hour.

	System 1	**System 2**
Pollutant Source Strength	1 Shrimp (Sp)/hour (Continuous ventilation)	1 Shrimp (Sp)/hour (Ventilation at 0.22 ACH for 23 hours, then 3.4 ACH for 1 hour)
Average Concentration	$\dfrac{1 Sp/hr}{0.35 ACH} = \dfrac{2.86 Sp}{Volume}$	$\dfrac{1 Sp/hr}{0.22 ACH} \times \dfrac{23}{24} + \dfrac{1 Sp/hr}{3.4 ACH} \times \dfrac{1}{24} = \dfrac{4.37 Sp}{Volume}$
Effective (D) ACH	$\dfrac{1 Sp/hr}{2.86 Sp/vol} = 0.35 ACH$	$\dfrac{1 Sp/hr}{4.37 Sp/vol} = 0.23 ACH$

Table 4.2 Effective ACH (Sp = Shrimp)

The average daily pollution concentration in the home with the continuous ventilation (System 1) is about half as much as the home with intermittent ventilation (2.86 Shrimp/air volume as opposed to 4.37 Shrimp/air volume). If the pollutant source is continuous throughout the day, continuous ventilation has a greater impact on the effective ventilation performance, even though the heat loss from the two buildings because of the average ventilation rate will be the same.

If the house is ventilated continuously, the occupants would come home to a much lower level of odor than if they came home and turned a big exhaust fan on for an hour to get rid of the stink that had built up. The stink would still have been there because the shrimp were still there. Removing the source of the pollution is the first step in any indoor air quality control approach. Exhausting air from near the polluting source provides the shortest path from the pollutant to the outside and the least amount of mixing with the room air. Exhaust-centered ventilation "sucks" the air out of the house, slightly deflating it. Outside, unconditioned air slips back in through gaps and cracks. If it is hot and humid outside and air-conditioned inside, the moisture in the incoming unconditioned but humid air may condense on some surface in the wall or ceiling structure. Although bath and kitchen fans are necessary to extract the immediate pollutants in any climate, exhaust-centered ventilation is not the best primary ventilation strategy for hot and humid climates.

Supply-Centered Whole Dwelling Ventilation System

Supply-centered ventilation is another whole dwelling ventilation strategy. It is not for spot or source ventilation. It wouldn't work well to have a range hood blowing in, blowing the smoke in the cook's face! Supply-centered ventilation works best if it is distributed to the rooms that are occupied for most of the time, like bedrooms where people spend about eight hours per day sleeping. A steady, low flow of fresh air to the bedrooms and perhaps other living areas is balanced by leakage from the house and by mechanical airflow through spot exhaust fans.

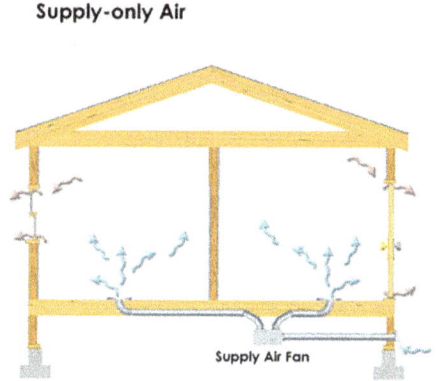

Figure 4.2 Supply-centered Whole Dwelling Ventilation
(Panasonic/Morrissey)

Because the air is not coming in randomly through cracks and holes in the house, it can be controlled. It can be filtered and tempered, and the rate of flow can be adjusted.

A number of systems are available that supply air directly into the return side of the HVAC air handler. Some of these systems have controllers that monitor the runtime of the air handler for heating or cooling and subtract that from the run time required for ventilation. Some of them have motorized dampers that close when outside air is not required. Others have flow restrictors in the inlet pipe that limit the amount of air that is drawn into the system depending on building and system pressures. These are all essentially supply-centered systems because they are mechanically adding ventilation air to the building.

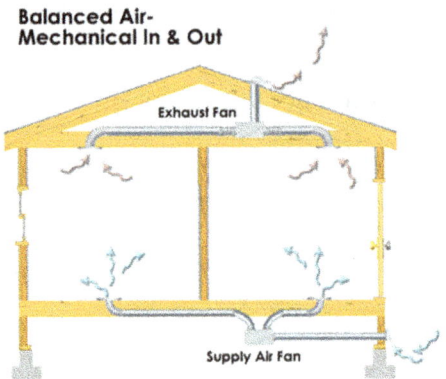

Figure 4.3 Mechanically Balanced Whole Dwelling Ventilation (Panasonic/Morrissey)

IN A COOLING DOMINATED climate when the air inside the house is predominantly cooler and drier than the air outside the house, a primary supply-centered ventilation system will keep the house under slightly positive pressure relative to the outside, keeping unwanted warm, humid air from being drawn into the building structure.

Balanced and Distributed Whole Dwelling Ventilation System

Exhaust-centered and supply-centered systems rely on building leakage to provide the other half of the equation. Negative or positive building pressure balances the mechanical system. Adding a mechanical source of make-up air makes them "balanced systems". Combining a distributed supply system (bringing filtered air into the bedrooms, for example) with a system that exhausts from the bathrooms could be a balanced system if the two flows are at the same volume and running at the same time. This can be accomplished by using one control or wiring both systems to run continuously.

> One of the beautiful features of balanced ventilation is in the name—it's balanced. Unlike exhaust-centered ventilation that pulls the pressure in the house negative or supply-centered ventilation that pushes the house positive, balanced ventilation maintains a neutral pressure on the building structure. When it is perfectly balanced, it can eliminate the natural infiltration and exfiltration forces and lower heating and cooling loads.

Balanced with Heat or Energy Recovery Whole Dwelling Ventilation System - HRVs and ERVs

It may seem counterproductive to spend money to condition air and then blow it to the outside. It would be nice if we could blow the pollutants out and keep the heated or chilled air and use it again. That's essentially what HRVs and ERVs do.

A Heat Recovery Ventilator or HRV[2] uses a heat exchanger to extract the heat or 'coolth' from the outgoing air stream and add it to the incoming stream, pre-conditioning it. An HRV or ERV (Enthalpy Recovery Ventilator) is designed and installed in such a way that the supply stream from the outside and exhaust stream from inside the house pass right beside each other without touching or mixing. The second law of thermodynamics says, "Heat moves toward cold". So if the supply stream from the outside is cooler than the exhaust stream from the house, some of the warmth in the exhaust air transfers to the cooler, supply air. This has to be accomplished without allowing the two air streams to actually mix. If that occurred, of course, the pollutants would just be coming back in and not much ventilation improvement would occur.

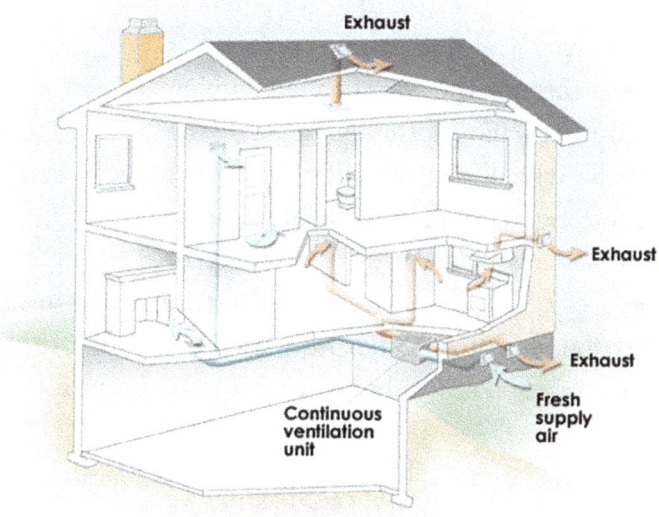

Figure 4.4 Balanced Ventilation with heat recovery (Panasonic/Morrissey)

---

2. See Appendix H for more balanced ventilation information.

Passive House[3] is a building standard that is energy efficient, comfortable, and affordable. Because Passive Houses are so energy efficient (requiring no heating system) they rely heavily on mechanical ventilation to maintain a healthy atmosphere and the use of a heat recovery ventilator (HRV) with at least 75% efficiency is part of the guidelines. Fresh air entering the building must not exceed 30m^3 per hour per person (17.7 cfm). The HRV must have an F7 filter (equivalent to a MERV 12 or 13 filter) (see Chapter 17 for more information about filters).

This temperature conditioning "magic" occurs by offering a lot of temperature touching surface area in a small box. The most common approach is to use a core with a lot of corrugation-like layers, one oriented or turned one way and the next turned the other and so forth, building up a cube. Each face of the cube is open to one air stream and closed to the other. The air streams cross each other (cross flow ventilation), touching thermally through all those corrugations but never mixing.

An alternative approach is to use a heat-exchanging wheel that rotates through both streams. A small motor and belt rotate a wheel designed to carry a heat or heat and moisture absorbing medium around and around through the outgoing and incoming air streams. The wheel absorbs sensible heat (heat that can be "sensed" or "felt") as it moves through the warm stream, which is then given up as it moves slowly through the cool stream. If the wheel is filled with a desiccant or moisture absorbing material as well, latent heat[4] is also transferred, classifying it as an Energy or Enthalpy[5] Recovery Ventilator or ERV. Moisture is captured on the wheel from the air stream, with the higher humidity (either due to the wheel being cooler than the air dew point or because of the desiccant fill). This is another

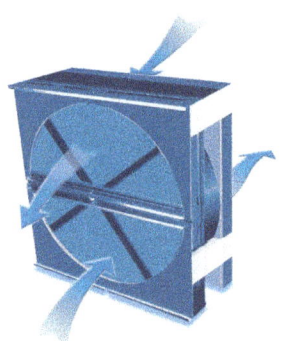

Figure 4.5 Heat exchanger desiccant wheel (Venmar)

---

3. For more information on Passive House go to: https://www.passivehouse-international.org/index.php?page_id=80
4. Latent heat is the energy required to change the state of a substance – a gas to a liquid, for example – without changing the temperature.
5. Enthalpy is the thermodynamic quantity equivalent to the total heat content of a system. The common reference to ERVs as Energy Recovery Systems combines both the heat and moisture recovery functions.

reflection of the Second Law as "wet moves to dry". As the wheel moves through the drier air stream, moisture is released through evaporation. With desiccant filled wheels, this is a "dry" moisture transfer process since the moisture is in the vapor or gas phase. There are no "wet" surfaces and liquid water does not enter the airstream, limiting the possibility for mold growth. The "fill" for the wheel is typically made of aluminum or, for a total heat recovery, a number of different materials treated with a hygroscopic material such as lithium chloride, alumina, or aluminum oxide, each of which has different moisture-absorbing properties.

Seals or gaskets are included to divide the two moving halves of the wheel, but some air is entrained and carried from one stream to the other, which reduces the efficiency. Some transfer occurs because of a difference in pressure between the two sides of the chamber that the wheel is moving through but the negative impact of this can be minimized by balancing the intake and exhaust fans and designing the housing so that any air leakage that occurs moves into the exhausting air stream, carrying it out of the building.

An ERV does not have to have a rotating wheel. "Flat plate" energy recovery exchangers have a special core material that allows the transfer of water vapor and heat between air streams. The moisture passes from the more humid air stream to the drier air stream, so when it is more humid outside, some of the moisture from the incoming air will be transferred to the drier, outgoing air.

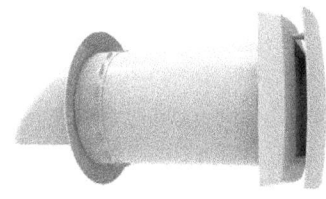

Figure 4.6 Thru-wall ceramic heat exchanger (Holtop)

The efficiencies of the heat and energy exchange products have become quite high, some as high as 80%. Testing of HVI Certified[6] HRV/ERV products is extremely thorough, testing the equipment under a range of operating conditions and durations.[7] Moisture and freezing can be a problem in a winter climate. The incoming air is at outside air temperature initially and any moisture that condenses in the fan system can freeze. Certification testing includes cold temperature tests at freezing and below.

---

6. http://www.hvi.org/resourcelibrary/proddirectory.html
7. See Appendix H for a description of HRV/ERV testing.

There are several efficiency numbers listed in HVI's Certified Products Directory for HRVs and ERVs. All the different information can make it very confusing to choose between systems. The number to look at is the Sensible Recovery Effectiveness (SRE) that defines the "sensible energy recovered minus the supply fan energy and preheat coil energy, divided by the sensible energy exhausted plus the exhaust fan energy. This calculation corrects for the effects of cross-leakage, purchased energy for fan and controls, as well as defrost systems."[8] See Chapter 9 for more information.

Another approach to heat recovery is a *regenerative* or *recuperative* system. These devices have ceramic cores. The system draws air from the room, passes it through this ceramic core that absorbs the heat, and then the air is vented to the outside. After approximately seventy seconds of operation when the core has warmed up, the fan reverses and draws outside air back through the core where it picks up the stored heat, and then the new air is blown into the room. As these units are ERVs, moisture is also transferred during the regenerative process.

The difference between an HRV and an ERV is moisture transfer. In a hot, humid climate, the air moving out of an air-conditioned building is cool and dry. The ventilation air coming in from the outside is warm and humid. Bringing more humidity into the building will increase the work the air conditioning system will have to do to dry the air out. If some of that incoming humidity can be carried out in the exhaust stream, there is an energy saving—a good application for an ERV.

In a heating climate, the incoming air stream may be cold and dry. Transferring some of the moisture from the exhaust or outgoing stream will warm and humidify the incoming air and make it more comfortable. But if the house is tightly constructed and the ventilation strategy relies on the balanced system for exhausting pollutants, it is best to expel the moisture rather than trapping it in the house—a good application for an HRV.

---

8. HVI, "Heat Recovery Ventilators and Energy Recovery Ventilators", http://www.hvi.org/resourcelibrary/proddirectory.html

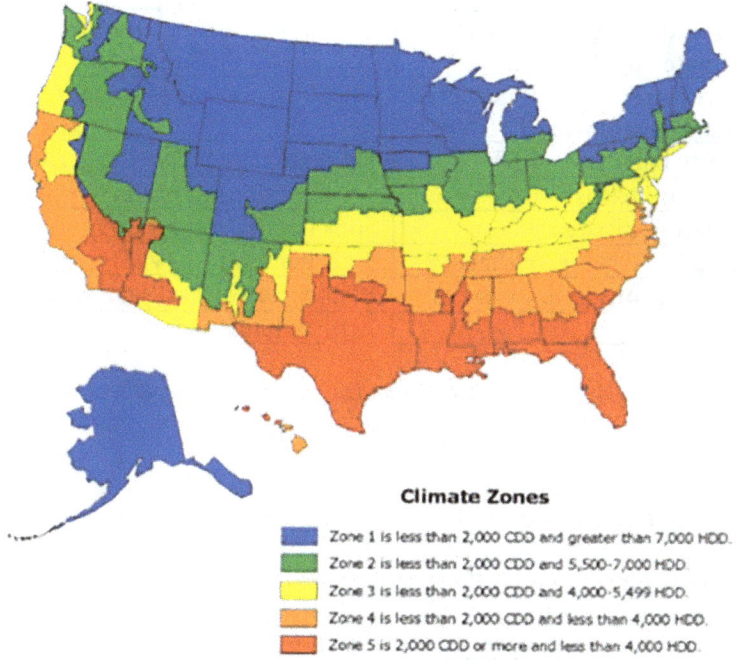

Figure 4.7 U.S. Climate Zones (Energy Information Administration)

Clearly, one type of whole dwelling ventilation system doesn't fit all applications or all climates. In order to keep humidity (RH) from being sucked into the building system, positive pressure ventilation works best for a climate that relies on air conditioning for much of the year. Negative pressure (exhaust-centered) ventilation works well in a climate that is dominated by the heating system. Mechanically balanced ventilation works well in both cases, and again in terms of a starting point, an ERV limits in the infusion of humidity in a cooling climate, while an HRV may be better suited to a heating climate.

Air Conditioning Dominated Climate Hot & Humid	Heating Dominated Climate Cold
Positive pressure—supply-centered (dehumidifying supply)	Negative pressure—exhaust-centered
Mechanically balanced—ERV	Mechanically balanced—HRV
Spot ventilation baths	Spot ventilation baths
Spot ventilation kitchen	Spot ventilation kitchen
Spot ventilation—garage exhaust	Spot ventilation—garage exhaust
Radon/Soil gas mitigation system	Radon/Soil gas mitigation system
Attic Exhaust	Attic exhaust

Table 4.3 System Choices for Different Climate Conditions

Circulation and Distribution Basics

It is certainly a good idea to remove the pollutants near the source with spot ventilation systems like bath fans and range hoods. The make-up air for these devices leaks in randomly around the house through gaps and air leaks, windows and doors, down chimneys and through other exhaust vents that are not being used. Those gaps and leaks and holes are randomly located throughout the house. The air may come from the basement or crawl space, the garage, or the furnace closet, carrying with it pollutants of all sorts. When insulation in the attic or in the wall is removed and it has turned black or there are black streaks on the carpeting or the baseboards, that's the filtering system for incoming air. One of the best things about an engineered ventilation system is that the source of the air is known, and it can be filtered and conditioned before it is supplied to the house.

Residential ventilation system design is more complicated than office ventilation system design, where adults spend most of the day sitting. In an office, fresh air can be introduced at the four-foot level and cover most situations. In a home, babies crawl on the floor, people sit at tables and desks and on sofas and lounge chairs and lie in beds, people stand in the kitchen and walk through the halls. Ventilation air should be mixed, diluted, filtered, and delivered to people at all these heights. Fresh air should be distributed throughout the home, which can be done in several ways.

* * *

DISTRIBUTION *with a central air handler*

If the house is conditioned with heated or chilled air, it already has a distribution system. Unfortunately, most of the time, the HVAC (Heating, Ventilating, and Air Conditioning) contractors ignore the 'V' part. The conditioned air ducting circulates warmed or chilled air to each room and then draws the air back to the air handler to re-warm or re-chill and dehumidify it. Ideally, there will be a supply and a return in each room so that the system will work effectively whether the door to the room is open or closed. Commonly, the small number of central returns will be in the hallways and the system will rely on door under-cuts, transfer grilles, or 'jumper-ducts' to allow the air to flow from the rooms back to the return. (See Chapter 8 for more information on transfer grilles.)

The circulation system should be designed for the climate in which the house is located using computational methods called Manual J and Manual D,[9] developed by the Air Conditioning Contractors of America (ACCA). These approaches analyze the structure of the building to determine how much heat will be gained or lost in each room and match the delivery system to compensate so that the room will be comfortable throughout the year. Since in virtually all the climates in the U.S. a house goes through both heating and cooling seasons and the HVAC system needs to handle both, the design is a compromise in terms of grille locations and sizing. ACCA has a manual for that as well—Manual T.

The grilles in a room, for example, need to 'throw' the air far enough out into the room so that all the air in the room is conditioned and comfortable. But if the grille is too low and the air is chilled, it will cause a 'draft' and be uncomfortable. The 'throw' depends on the location of the grille, the velocity of the air coming out of the grille, and the design of the grille itself. (Smaller grille openings increase the velocity of the air, leaving the grille and "throw" it farther out into the room. Smaller grille openings can also reduce the amount or volume of airflow and increase the noise of the air moving through the grille.)

In a heating climate, the supply grilles are often located under the windows on the outside walls so that the rising, warmed air provides an 'insulation blanket' in front of the glass to keep people warmer. That location will

---

9. Manual J is used to define the heat loads of a house on a room-by-room basis. Manual D is a process for designing the duct layout that will satisfy the design conditions defined by Manual J most efficiently. Manual T is for the grilles or termination fittings. http://www.acca.org/design/

not work as well for chilled air. Carpets or furniture often block grilles that are in the floor or low on the wall. It is important for the designer to think about the complete path of the air from the grille, through the room, and back to the return. Appreciating how the room will be used is critical for having a functional system that satisfies both the engineers and the occupants.

Grille manufacturers use computer simulation tools called Computational Fluid Dynamics (CFD) to visualize how the air moves through the room. Quite often the location of the grille or the face velocity can be too weak to allow the air to sweep through the whole room and back to the return, leaving dead air spots where there is inadequate circulation.

If there is no return in the room, then the air coming in will pressurize the space. It will seek to leak out through gaps and openings and hopefully under the room door when it is closed back to the return grille. If the house has a central return system rather than returns in each room, the rooms must be considered as ducts and the room doors as dampers. If all the air that is supplied to the room can't get back to the return, then the space where the return grille is located will be at a slightly negative pressure as the system tries in vain to suck the air back to the air handler. This slight amount of negative pressure in an air conditioning dominated climate will draw humid air into the building system from the outside through the cracks and leaks just as an exhaust-centered ventilation system would.

It is worth emphasizing that the HVAC system is designed for heating and cooling and not for ventilation. Locating supplies on the floor under windows, for example, is not ideal for introducing cool, winter ventilation air into the room. The air may just lie on the floor and never reach standing or sitting people. If the grilles are near the ceiling in a cooling climate to optimize air conditioning, the warmer outside air may never drop to people's height. Grilles for the HVAC system may be too large to offer adequate "throw" for the lower velocity, ventilation air. The ducts may be too big for the smaller power ventilation fans and the air may just "drop" out of the grilles closest to the system and not move through the whole house. Ventilation air may never reach the rooms at the end of the line. The system designer should consider all these issues when combining the ventilation system with the heating and cooling system.

Many of these problems can be avoided if the two systems run simultaneously, but that means that there is an electrical penalty for running both fans. If high efficiency furnace fans (with ECM or Electronically Commutated or

Controlled motors) are used, the operating cost will be reduced and the penalty minimized.

One other consideration in a cooling climate is that moisture condenses on the cold surface of the cooling coil, drips into the condensation pan, and runs out the drain, drying the air. If the fan is run continuously to improve ventilation, the moisture on the coil can re-evaporate into the air stream and be delivered back to the house, reducing the cooling effectiveness.

* * *

ADDING a fresh air inlet to the air handler

The beauty of adding ventilation to the fully ducted HVAC system is that the full distribution system is there. Adding the 'V', the ventilation, can be relatively easy. Fresh air can be distributed throughout the house, and limiting the number of supply points from the outside limits the difficulties of providing filtered and tempered air.

A duct to the outside can be added to the return side of the air handler. Outside air drawn in through that duct when the air handler is running will be mixed with the air from the house, conditioned, and delivered back to the house. The air handler runs in response to the house thermostat, energizing the system to heat or cool the house. If the weather is mild or if the system has been set back for night or "away" mode, the air handler might not turn on for hours, and there will be no ventilation. Night setback is great for saving energy but not for circulating ventilation air.

> The location of the outside air inlet is important. This is effectively the "nose" of the house. It should not be near bad air sources like behind the garbage cans or in the carport. It needs to be kept clean. If there is a filter on the intake, it must be accessible for servicing.

To compensate for this, controls have been developed that will monitor the runtime of the air handler and compare it to a preset ventilation schedule. If the air handler has not run long enough to meet the ventilation schedule, the control will activate the blower again for ventilation. Some of these controls work with motorized dampers, leaving the intake open only when the blower is running. Others include a connection to a bath fan and if the HVAC blower stops running prior to the completion of the ventilation cycle, the bath fan is activated to finish the job. Some of them have temperature and humidity sensors to override the ventilation schedule if the outside air is too hot, too cold, or too humid. These overrides keep the load on the heating and cooling system down, but it is a trade-off with moving fresh air into the house.

This approach puts the home under slightly positive pressure, relying on leakage and spot ventilation fans to balance out the fresh air that is being drawn into the air handler.

> There can be an occupant issue with this approach. If the efficiency of the house has been improved, but the air handler is cycling on and off for ventilation, the occupants may not understand why and try to defeat the system. Because we have all been sensitized to equate the operation of the HVAC system with heating or cooling, if the house is more efficient, why is the HVAC system running more?

* * *

ADDING an HRV or ERV to the air handler

Another balanced ventilation approach is to tap an HRV or ERV into the HVAC ducting. This approach saves the cost of a separate ducting system for the ventilation system. The HVAC system should be balanced with the same amount of air moving out of its supply registers as is coming back in through its return grilles. It should be a closed loop circulation system, moving the air from the inside through the conditioning system and back to the inside.

An HRV or ERV system is also a closed loop, with the same amount of air being drawn into the house as is being expelled from the house, moving the air from the outside to the inside and back to the outside. If either of these paths is poorly installed, integrating them will affect both of them. Both HRVs and ERVs are self-contained with no impact on other devices such as fireplaces, gas water heaters, clothes dryers or range hoods. Recovery ventilators are NOT make-up air systems for other devices!

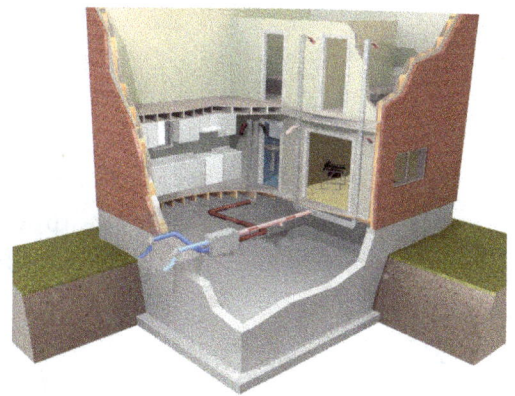

Figure 4.8 Balanced HRV system (Venmar)

Air from the outside is drawn into the HRV or ERV, moves through the heat/energy exchanger core, and is supplied to the return side of the air handler and is distributed throughout the house. Air from the house is either drawn from the return registers or from the polluting points like bathrooms, then moved through the HRV or ERV, and expelled to the outside.

Careful design of these systems is important to limit the impact of unconditioned outside air on the conditioning system. HVAC system manufacturers have specifications on the temperature of the air that directly impacts the conditioning coils. Hitting a heating coil with freezing air can reduce the life of the coil. Even in systems with an attached ERV with latent (moisture) energy recovery, the dew point of the air entering the system can be much higher than the air in the chilled supply ducts resulting in moisture issues and mold when the ERV is running but the central fan isn't. By inserting the supply air on the return side of the air handler far enough upstream, the air has a chance to blend with the house air and will affect the chilled supply ducts at an acceptable temperature and dew point.

Although this approach is frequently used, there are several drawbacks. It is difficult to balance the HRV/ERV because of the ducting and operating variations of the HVAC system. The exhaust side of the HRV/ERV works against the negative pressure in the return plenum as it tries to draw air out of the air stream returning to the air handler. If the negative pressure is sufficiently low, it can severely reduce or even stall the exhaust airflow through the HRV/ERV.

Since the distribution approach is designed for the HRV/ERV to run only when the air handler is running, mechanical ventilation may not be supplied when it is most needed—in the Spring and Fall when the temperatures are moderate enough to not require heating or cooling. Ventilation rates may be excessive during the other seasons when the air handler is running frequently.

If the HRV is coupled to a central system in a cooling dominated climate, the outside air, which will be full of humidity, may cause condensation on the interior surfaces of the HVAC equipment and the supply plenum and ducting. It would not be a positive function for the whole dwelling ventilation system to be the source of indoor mold!

* * *

DISTRIBUTION without a central air handler

Since the HVAC system is a closed and balanced circulation system - taking air from the house, conditioning it, and returning it to the house—it is a bit of a compromise to add ventilation air to the system. It certainly can be considered another form of conditioning of the air like filtering or heating or cooling or humidifying/dehumidifying it. But, as seen from the above discussions, it can also cause issues with humidity and impact on the mechanical equipment. There are many homes that are heated without ducting using hot water, electric heat, or heat pumps, for example, that require stand-alone ventilation systems. Ideally, such a system is fully ducted, purposely and mechanically delivering fresh air and removing stale air to each room and not relying on the rooms, the doorways, and the halls to act as the ducting of the system. Such a system, however, rarely happens. It's a ventilation system engineer's dream.

* * *

"FULLY DUCTED" whole dwelling ventilation

What stands as a "fully ducted" system has both a mechanical supply and exhaust and uses the rooms and halls as ducts to convey the air between the two. It is critical that there is a means to bypass closed doors for this to work either with sufficient door undercuts, jumper ducts, transfer grilles or what some building codes call "return air pathways". A small supply system draws air in from a single outside point, providing the option for pre-conditioning and filtering and delivers the air to the spaces where people spend most of their time, like the bedrooms and living room. The air moves through the rooms toward the exhaust points in bathrooms or kitchen. A supply system may use small two inch or three-inch ducting, allowing it to be run through the wall system. The volume of air to each supply point is low, less than 20 cubic feet per minute, at a velocity that should be barely noticeable in the room.

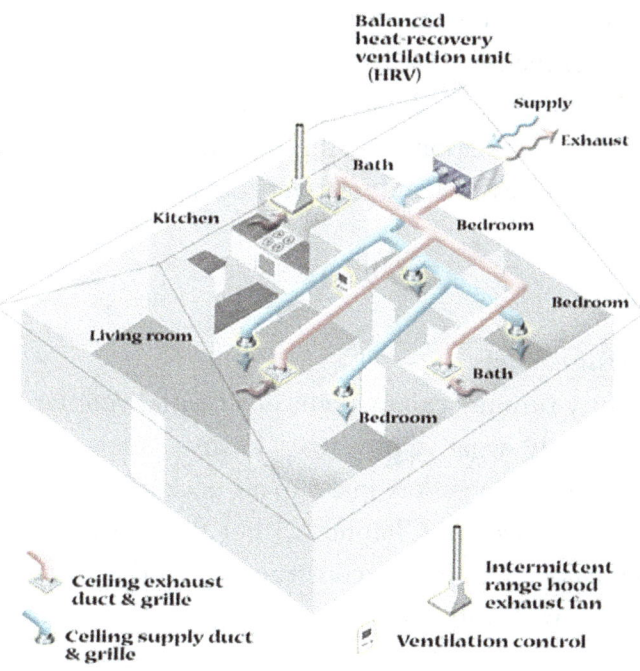

Figure 4.9 Fully Ducted HRV System (Panasonic/Morrissey)

One important note is to recognize the difference between the delivery system for heating and cooling and the delivery system for fresh air ventilation. Air is not very good at holding heat. One cubic foot of air can only hold 0.018 BTU per degree Fahrenheit rise of temperature. To change the temperature of the air in a room, you need to add a lot of "new" air at a higher or lower temperature. That's why HVAC systems use big fans and big ducts. For ventilation, however, a small amount of fresh air has a big effect. A seventy-five hundred square foot house with seven bedrooms only needs 135 cubic feet per minute of ventilation air (according to ASHRAE). A 3,000 square foot, three-bedroom house only needs 60 cfm. The ducting and grilles for a ventilation system can be much smaller since the air will blend with room air at a low velocity. If the grilles are properly designed so that they create a minimal face velocity, just enough to 'throw' the air out gently into the room, and installed so that they are out of the human comfort zone, the flow from them should be hardly noticeable.

Sound level also must be considered as with any air moving system. Smaller grilles and smaller ducts can amplify air noise. The system can use a highly effective filter (MERV 13 rating or higher), but it is difficult to get people to maintain the filters on their primary HVAC system. Maintaining the filter on any ventilation system is perhaps even more critical, since it provides the fresh air that the home's occupants need to breathe and stay healthy. For maintenance reasons, the fan/conditioning/filter housing should be located where it is accessible and relatively obvious.

* * *

Exhaust with passive inlets

Using constantly running exhaust fans or a central ventilation fan can put the house under slightly negative pressure. "Passive" inlets or "smart holes" or "trickle ventilators" can then allow makeup air back into the house. (More on the design of these devices in Chapter 8.) For these systems to work effectively, the house needs to be tightly constructed, tightly enough so that a low volume exhaust fan will pull it to a negative pressure no matter where the inlets are located. Because of the "stack effect" in the house (the rising warm air) and because of the wind loads pushing on different sides of the house at different times, and because of leaks in the HVAC system ducting, the pressures in the house are unpredictable. A passive inlet in the wall of a second-floor bedroom may serve as an outlet.

If the inlet works properly, however, it will provide a simple, non-ducted means for delivering fresh air where it is needed, particularly to bedrooms. Air moves through the room, through the doorway, into the common space where it is vented by the exhaust fan. Note that if the inlets and most of the air is coming into the space from the first floor and exiting through an exhaust fan on the second floor, it is likely to bypass rooms on the second floor, especially if the doors are closed. As simple as this design appears to be, it relies on a thorough knowledge of building pressures by the designer, the installer, and the building occupants to work effectively.

* * *

Stand-alone HRVs and ERVs

HRVs and ERVs are designed as stand-alone systems consequently, they can be used easily without connecting them to a heating or cooling system. They bring in outside air, condition it, deliver it through dedicated ducting, extract stale or 'used' air, and exhaust it to the outside. Like all of these systems, the ducting needs to be well designed and installed so that the system is balanced. There is a level of tolerance in the ducting for these systems, however, because the heat exchanger core and filters often have a much higher resistance to airflow than the ducting. That means that the performance of the system can be effectively pre-engineered simplifying the installer's job (although it does not completely remove the on-site design and balancing that must be done as well).

* * *

Ventilation Distribution Summary

Ventilation air is a critical factor in a home. It is certainly as important as the color of the walls or the tile on the bathroom floor and must be considered as a fundamental issue right from the beginning. The problem is that people can't see what's in the air. They can't see the formaldehyde or the carbon monoxide, and they might not even attribute how they feel in their home to the quality of the air. They know when it is too hot or too cold. They can even feel when it is too dry or too humid. But they don't know when the air quality is bad.

Ideally, the whole dwelling ventilation system would stand on its own with its own ducting, circulation, and distribution system. Anything other than that—integrating it with the HVAC system or using the rooms as ducts - is a compromise. National standards like ASHRAE 62.2 offer a minimum, averaged, national place to start in choosing the ventilation system. Some states and codes mandate local systems, and many green building programs require ventilation as part of their criteria.

There are a lot of options for ventilation system design. No one design will fit all applications.

* * *

System Documentation

Paperwork is a pain, but there are so many times when it would be helpful if the information were written down. And like putting the tools away at the end of a job, it is simplest and least time consuming if the information is recorded immediately. Section 6.2 of the ASHRAE 62.2 Standard requires system documentation, so there is that too! It's not just another exercise in meaningless paperwork, but it is a reference for people who have to work with the system in the future. There have been times when I haven't written something down thinking that it would be impossible to not remember what I had done, only to find that I don't have a clue what I was thinking about when I did it. Not everyone has a perfect, permanent memory, and even if you do, you are not likely to be the person working with the system in ten years.

Chapter 5

Sound

"I wish you could hear this!"

Like the distribution of ventilation air, in the past, the sound or noise of the air-moving device wasn't a major factor in selecting the fan. Bathroom exhaust fans have always been used with the intention of removing excess moisture from the bathroom, even if it was only to control mirror fogging. However, many consumers and even some builders considered the bathroom fan's purpose was odor control. People joked bath fan noise was a benefit because it covered up the rude noises in the bathroom. With tighter houses and fans being used as the whole dwelling ventilation system required to run all the time, reducing the sound level of the fan became a serious concern. As houses become tighter, outside background noises are hushed. Internal noises become much more noticeable—the drip in the sink, the running toilet, the refrigerator, the HVAC system running in the basement, or the bathroom fan running for ventilation. The occupant of the home notices these things, and if they don't have a good understanding why they are running, will seek ways to shut them off. The interrelationship between a quieter home and the need for a quieter ventilation system emphasizes the obvious system's nature of a building and, particularly, a house. A house (and its occupants) are a system.

Unfortunately, you can't listen to an installed fan before you buy it, and the contractor that installs it doesn't have to live with it. Therefore, sound ratings must be numeric values that enable the person making the selection to rank products in the same order that average people would rank them if they heard them running. That means the ratings must be comparable. It also means that the ratings must be in terms of the human response to sound. And last, the sound test must be repeatable. If a fan is tested several times at long intervals of time, the measurements must be the same within reasonable tolerances.

General Sound Considerations

The most common engineering approach to describe a sound level is to talk about 'decibels'. But to the average mortal, decibels make little sense. The decibel scale is logarithmic. It rises in an increasingly steep curve. Decibels are the ratio of a sound unit to a base unit, expressed logarithmically; a decibel is an exponent of 10.

Twenty decibels are 10^{20} or 100,000,000,000,000,000,000 times louder than the base unit. Something that is 100 decibels is not twice as loud as something that is 50 decibels. It is much, much, much louder than that. Fifty decibels might be a couple having a quiet conversation. A hundred decibels is the sound of a jackhammer or a noisy rock concert. It is just not intuitive that forty decibels are twice as loud as thirty decibels, for example. The useful thing about the decibel scale is that it is relatively simple to measure, and it makes it possible to work with fewer zeros.

Many activities are measured in decibels and, even for sound, there are different kinds of decibels, e.g. dB(A), which means the decibels are weighted for some type of response to the character of the sound. (In the "A weighting" scale, the sound pressure levels are "weighted" to more accurately reflect the human ear by reducing the lower frequency and higher frequency bands before they are combined to give a single sound pressure level value.)

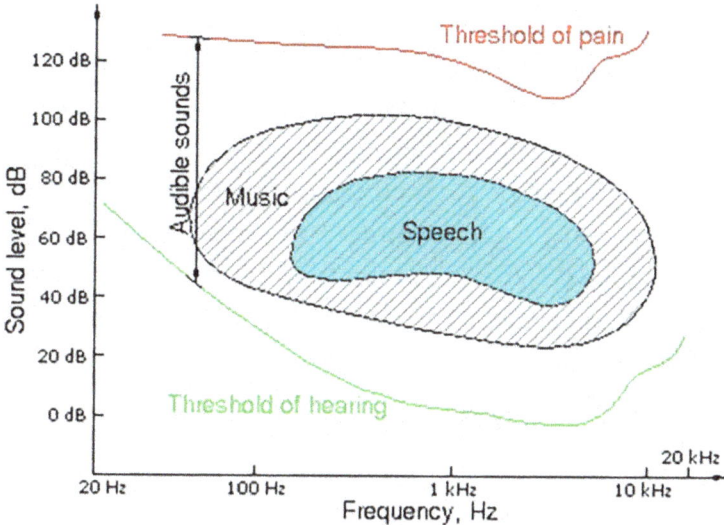

Figure 5.1 Measurement of audible sound (dbx Consulting)

To sell quiet fans and to be able to compare one to the other, a more understandable means of measuring sound needed to be developed. A metric was needed that increased linearly. Along came the **sone**.

According to the Oxford English Dictionary, one of the first uses of the word sone in English literature was from a poem in 1616, where the poet (J. Lane) was waxing eloquently about the "music of the spheres" and needed something to rhyme with "tone". Much later, in 1936, Dr. S. Smith Stevens, while he was head of the Harvard Psychoacoustic Laboratory, proposed the sone scale as a linear indication of perceived loudness. People, unfortunately, perceive noise or loudness in different ways that are difficult to quantify. By measuring the decibel level at different frequencies or pitches and combining them, a linear scale for sones was developed that is simpler to understand. A fan that is rated at 4 sones is twice as loud as a fan that is rated at 2 sones!

The problem is that without some sophisticated equipment, measuring sones is a lot more complex than measuring decibels and converting one to the other is, to say the least, difficult. Rather than pulling out a relatively inexpensive decibel meter and pointing it at the fan, measurement has to be done in a sophisticated sound chamber with a clearly prescribed location for the microphone and a lot of other elements. Human beings are pretty good at pinpointing a sound and mentally filtering out all the background components and sound reflections in the room, etc., but what you hear and what your neighbor hears are very different, not something you can put on the end of bath fan packaging as an official rating. To get a repeatable and comparable sound or sone rating the product needs to be tested in a laboratory that has been constructed to standardized criteria such as the Texas A & M Environmental Systems Laboratory[1] in College Station, Texas which is where the Home Ventilating Institute (HVI) certifies home ventilating products.

This measurement process becomes even more difficult as fan products get quieter and quieter. When the sound level is down to one third of a sone or less, the smallest of background noises becomes much more critical. Even in the carefully constructed acoustic chamber (where you can hear your heart beating) at the remote location of the Energy Systems Laboratory (ESL) of Texas A&M, they have to wait until late at night when trucks stop passing on the highway three miles away, before they can get accurate information! Even in this sophisticated laboratory, the quietest reliable, repeatable sound rating measurement is 0.3 sones! Fans rated at "Less than 0.3 sones" have gone beyond that level.

After the fan is tested for airflow, it is installed in the "diffuse, reverberation chamber" at the ESL lab making no modifications to the product. The chamber is constructed with heavy, multi-layered, insulated, non-parallel, reasonably airtight walls with hard (reverberant) interior surfaces. It is approximately 25 feet long, 20 feet wide, and 12 feet high. It is supplied with makeup air through an insulated, labyrinthine inlet duct with a throttling device to control the rate of flow. The outlet from the chamber is through a rectangular isolation duct, into an anechoic muffler that opens out into the atmosphere, avoiding the entry of environmental sound. The chamber is built on a resilient base that minimizes the transmission of ground-borne (sound) vibration. A single personnel opening is equipped with two heavy, insulated doors with seals and positive latches. A microphone is mounted in the chamber on a rotating boom that can move the microphone through approximately 180 degrees during the thirty-second data collection period. As fans get even quieter, the sound of the motor rotating the microphone has become the greatest noise source and has been replaced with a series of fixed-point microphones.

---

1. https://esl.tamu.edu/reel/facilities/

Sound 71

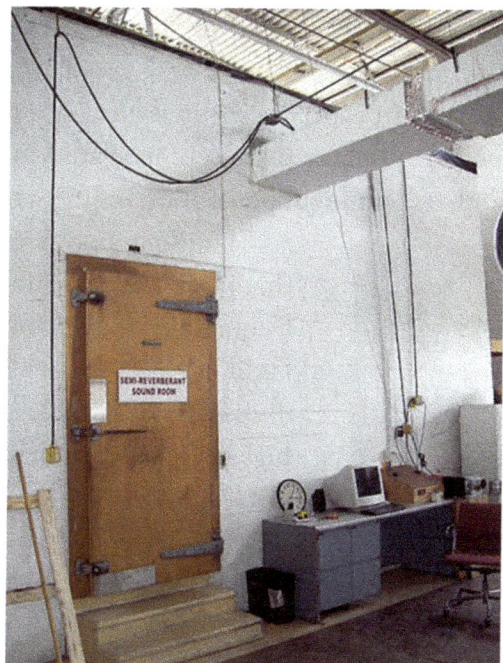

Figure 5.2 Sound Testing Chamber (ESL)

The only meaningful basis for rating a fan's sound is its sound power, but there is no single instrument for measuring that. The rotating microphone or microphone array measures sound pressure on their diaphragms.

Four sound pressure measurements are conducted in twenty-four, one-third-octave bands. The first measures the fan and the background noise so that the background noise can be subtracted. The second measures just the background noise. The third test measures the background noise plus the sound from a precisely calibrated reference sound source (RSS) without the test fan running. (The RSS is an expensive, noise generator that is regularly sent to a standards laboratory for calibration.) And the fourth measures the test unit, background noise, and reference sound source running simultaneously to check for background steadiness.

Each sound measurement chamber has its own peculiar characteristics. By running both the fan and the RSS in the same chamber in quick succession, the two can be compared without regard to the room's character because the room will behave the same for both devices. The sound power (or noise level) of the test unit is determined by mathematically comparing sound pressure measurements in the chamber to sound pressure measurements of the reference sound source. For this to be consistent, the chamber must meet specific requirements, especially related to standing waves and background quality.

The sound power the fan is producing in the twenty-four bands produces twenty-four sound power numbers that are not related to human perception. Converting those numbers to human perception requires two steps.

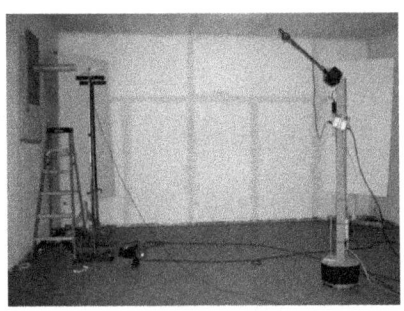

Figure 5.3 *Sound Chamber Interior (ESL)*

The first step is to recognize the fact that humans do not perceive various frequencies in the same way. The human auditory system is most sensitive in the middle ranges and less so at the lower and higher frequencies. There are also differences between people. Dr. Stevens measured a vast number of research subjects comparatively. He started in the frequencies where people have great sensitivity, 1000 Hz at 40dB, and asked people to tell him when another frequency was equally loud. He also asked when two tones were twice or half each other. This provided a reliable set of data representing the response of normal humans to a variety of frequencies and sound levels. These data were next reduced to mathematical curves and applied to all twenty-four of the frequency bands. The result is the 'Equal Loudness Indices' table where the computer looks up each single-band sone number.

The second step is two steps in one. The twenty-four bands are combined for total loudness, and the human response to dominant tones is factored into the equation used for totaling. When a sound spectrum has dominant tones, it is perceived as being louder than a 'white noise' spectrum that an instrument might measure as being the same. The twenty-four bands are simply added, and the dominant band is added after being reduced by the penalty for dominance.

Since the sone is a measurement of how the human ear perceives "noise" and since our ears hear noise differently at different frequencies, the sone measuring process "listens" to the twenty-four frequency bands and then assembles all that information to arrive at the certified single fan loudness number weighted for human dominant tone sensitivity in sones[2] for the fan under test.

Source	Sone level
Low cost range hood	7.5
Low cost, noise masking bath fan	4.5
TV set at normal living room level	4
Max level for intermittently operating ventilation fans in ASHRAE 62.2-2007	3
Washington State Ventilation Code bath fan sound level	1.5
Continuously operating ventilation fans in ASHRAE 62.2-2007	1
Quiet Refrigerator in a quiet kitchen	1
Very quiet computer fan	0.6
Really quiet bath fan	0.3

Table 5.1 Relative Sound Levels of Various Devices

It's strange that people like to ride around in their cars with the stereo blasting and the entire car shaking, but they complain about bath fan noise. There are so many annoying abrupt sources of sound in our world, like cell phones and motorcycles (and even the impact of titanium golf clubs!). Tightly constructed, quiet homes are havens where the occupants can control the environment to their heart's desire. Combining sound with air pollutants (Indoor Air Quality or IAQ) results in the level of Indoor Environmental Quality (IEQ), which is critically important in a tight house.

It is important to recognize the extent fan manufacturers go to verify the 'noise' levels of their product. Buying a HVI certified fan product that has a sound level of < 0.3 sones means it is truly scientifically quiet. Not just because the manufacturer says it is.

Sound Considerations for the Whole Dwelling Ventilation System

The Whole Dwelling Ventilation System should run constantly, changing the air throughout the day, and if not acoustically invisible, the homeowner will defeat it. If the product used for this purpose is in the room, it should operate

---

2. HVI Publication 915, "HVI Loudness and Rating Procedure"

at one sone or less. If it is remotely mounted, the installed system should operate in the same way, effectively at one sone or less. To test this, the refrigerator might have to be unplugged to hear the fan running or it may mask the sound.

The simplest way to achieve a one-sone level in the space, if the fan is installed in the ceiling, is to use a fan that is rated at one sone or less. To achieve the one sone operating level once the fan is installed, it is important to follow the manufacturer's installation instructions. If a quiet fan is noisy after installation, there is a problem with the installation. Sounds generated by the fan motor can be transferred to the building structure through the mounting. Building surfaces can act as large sounding boards that will amplify minor fan noises. Fans with DC or ECM (Electronically Commutated Motors) will change their speed if the ducting is restricted, resulting in greater noise. If a fan that is sound rated at 1 sone or less and seems excessively noisy, the ducting is restricted. The air gets ANGRY. The more restricted, the louder the fan will be. Because of the extraordinary engineering, the fan may still move an adequate amount of air even if it is noisy, but in a tight house since sound is a component of Indoor Environmental Quality (IEQ), it will be become annoying enough for the occupant to turn it off. And a fan that isn't running is no use at all.

If the fan can move more air than is required for continuous operation, the fan speed can be reduced with a speed control if the fan is rated for variable speed. The method used for speed control sometimes induces a 'hum' in the fan motor that is disturbing. This may be from a single operating point in the control, and can be reduced by adjusting the fan speed above or below that point to remove or reduce the 'hum'. This may also be the case with a remote mounted fan.

Occasionally with a remote mounted fan, the air moving through the ceiling grille can produce objectionable noises. Changing the grille to a different configuration may help to solve or reduce the problem.

Mounting is also important for HRV/ERV primary ventilation systems. Their motor noise can also be transferred to the building structure and amplified. Some HRV/ERV manufacturers supply mounting straps that "hang" the unit away from building components to isolate operational hum. (Remote mounted fans (in-line fans) and HRV/ERVs are not rated by HVI for sound level because they are mounted remotely from the living space and every installation will be different, making a prescribed, laboratory mounting configuration unrepresentative.)

In some cases, the fan will be too quiet and the occupants won't even know that it is on or off. If the air quality in the home and the health of the occupants depends on that fan running all the time, it is extremely important that it keeps running. It is vital that the occupants know what it is and what it is doing, and it may be advisable to add an indicator light, labeling, or fan-proving indicator that provides a clear sign that the system is working. If the house changes hands, a new occupant may have no idea why there is an exhaust fan running all the time.

Sound Considerations for bath fans

There are times when a bath fan that creates some background noise would be advantageous. Such fans are available and are not well suited for whole dwelling ventilation systems. They make too much noise. Turn 'em on. Get the job done. Turn 'em off. Often, little or no thought was put into the installation of these fans. Just because they are making noise doesn't mean they are moving any air. Try holding a piece of tissue paper up to the grille and see if the air draws it up. Noise does not equal air motion!

In order to minimize cost and size, the noisier fans generally use a small "blower" wheel and spin it fast. The air squeezes in through the grille and is pushed out through a small, often a 3" diameter, duct. All of those components make the fan noisy. It is like a lot of water moving through a river and reaching the rapids. Banging around the rocks and through the narrow passages, tumbling and falling it makes a lot of noise. When it reaches the unencumbered, wide open stretch, it quiets down and flows smoothly.

To quiet the fan, manufacturers began making the system more efficient, removing the sharp edges, widening the openings, using a larger blower wheel and spinning it more slowly. All the components of the products contribute to their efficiency and performance. The fan is a system. The number of blades on the wheel and the size of the air inlet openings in the grille contribute to the efficiency and the noise the fan makes. Fan designers are trying to make products attractive both aesthetically and economically. And that forces compromise. When the sound level of the product gets below one half sone, however, everything has been done to keep the fan quiet. As we age, even the 1.5-sone fans are a stretch to hear!

If an existing bathroom has a noisy, annoying fan, there isn't a great deal that can be done in terms of the installation to make it quieter. Often it will be poorly installed, making the noise worse. If the ducting is kinked and twisted and has many sharp, ninety degree turns, increasing the diameter of the ducting and straightening it out will make the air flow more easily and take a small amount of the fan noise out. Replacing small diameter ducting with a larger diameter will also quiet the fan down, making it easier for the air to move through the system and out of the building.

Replacing a noisy fan with a quieter one is the best way to keep the system noise down. A straight, smooth, reasonably large diameter duct will certainly help. Following the manufacturer's installation instructions helps a great deal.

Another alternative is to use a remotely mounted fan or an in-line fan. By removing the fan from the room, most of the noise is also removed. Kits are available to retrofit a remote mounted, in-line fan to an existing ceiling mounted fan box. Disconnecting or removing the existing fan wheel and motor will ease the flow of air through the housing, improve the operating efficiency, and keep the noise level down. Most of the in-line fans can be operated with a speed controller (Check the product manual. If it doesn't say "Not for use with a solid state speed control", then it probably is okay). The advantage there is that the fan can be slowed down. If it is operating more slowly, the air will move more slowly and making less noise. The speed of the fan can be manually adjusted for an acceptable sound and airflow level.

> Some fan motors will develop a 'hum' when operated with a speed control. The full AC power that comes directly to the fan is a sine wave, alternating smoothly from full positive to full negative and back again, 60 times per second in the U.S. (60 cycles or 60 Hz). Solid-state speed controls 'chop' that sine wave, using an electronic switch like a transistor to turn on and off, providing part of each wave to the fan motor. The more the switch is off, the slower the fan runs. It is sort of like switching the room lights on and off and on and off, slowly or rapidly. It will make it dimmer in the room than just leaving them on. There are some versions of these devices that are more sophisticated, using microprocessors to carefully adjust the fan speed for minimum motor impact and hum generation.
>
> There are other fan speed control approaches, such as variable reactance transformers, that will provide the full sine wave at lower amplitude. Some motor speeds can be adjusted by using matching capacitors for different oper-

ating points, and some motors are specifically made to operate at different speeds that have several 'windings' on their motors. These are generally the bigger motors, like the furnace blower motors or some of the large attic fans. There are also "electronically commutated" or EC motors that are specifically designed to be used with their own matching speed control. These motors use only the power necessary to perform the required task and almost always include the control. Make sure that any speed control you use has been safety tested by an agency like UL or ETL or CSA or a similar laboratory, and make sure that the fan manufacturer has approved their use since the control may overheat the motor or burn it out in a short time.

Besides adjusting the speed, there are other new technologies coming along that will quiet the operating noise of the fan. Manufacturing a fan to be really quiet requires compromises sometimes in the "strength" of the fan: its ability to aggressively push or pull the air through the ducting. Ventilation has become so important to healthy buildings that manufacturers are working hard to develop new technologies and approaches and provide better and more versatile products.

For a new installation, all the options are open. Starting with a quiet product, designing and employing a good ducting design (at least as good as the manufacturer's instructions), making it easy for the air to move smoothly from the inside of the house to the outside will all make the system quieter.

Note that manufacturers want these products to operate as they conceived them. They think about how they work every day. They test them. They poke them. They prod them. They are required to put a great deal of information in product manuals warning about health and safety, but there is also a great deal of good information about how to install them so they work correctly. Failing to read the product manual is a common mistake. After all, how hard could it be to put in a bath fan? But like everything else about the product, from the backdraft damper to the packaging, the product is a system. By ignoring the installation manual, the product is not likely to work as described.

Sound considerations for kitchen fans

A kitchen range hood is designed to remove the airborne cooking effluents, carrying the smoke and grease and odors out of the working space. In a commercial application, that process is required by code to be at a high enough velocity to prevent the grease particles from settling where they might cause a fire hazard. Grease spatters and droplets fall rapidly downward without being captured. Grease leaves the cooking zone as a vapor and cools quickly into tiny (aerosol) particles that remain airborne for hours. It generally takes a lot of air movement to remove them and a lot of air movement means a lot of noise, especially if the fan or blower is located right there in front of you in the range hood.

The fan in the range hood has to be powerful enough to move a large amount of air from the area around the stove, draw it through grease filters, push it through a length of ductwork, to exit the building through a vent or hood. Range hoods are available that are rated at 1.5 sones, although their flow rates at those sound levels are relatively low.

Mounting the fan remotely, such as on the exterior of the building, helps, and you will almost always see commercial exhaust fans remotely mounted on the roof or sidewall of restaurants. This is both for noise and for size constraints. Since the ducting for a range hood needs to be smooth and made of metal, the sound will echo back into the room. Sound mufflers that work like a car muffler are available to install in the exhaust duct.

Most range hoods have speed controls as well, although slowing them down will obviously reduce their airflow and their sound level.

If it is an existing fan mounted right there in front of you in the kitchen, there isn't a great deal you can do to quiet it down except slow it down. It is possible to leave the filters and remove the blowers from the fan and install a new external fan on the outside of the house.

If the hood has no ducting and instead simply recycles the room air through a filter, it is not a ventilating device and doesn't accomplish much by way of air quality improvement. They will collect some particulates, but they need to be maintained regularly.

For a new installation, selecting a hood with a low sone rating is a good place to start. To help compare hoods with high airflow to those with less flow, HVI provides a "Working Speed"[3] sound rating; often a high quality, 500 cfm hood is several times quieter at working speed than a 150 cfm hood. Alterna-

---

3. HVI Publication 915: "Range hood working speed testing provides an optional opportunity for a member to obtain a second HVI rating at 'working speed', for range hoods with multiple speeds." The procedure relies upon a second airflow test at or above 100 cfm.

tively, there are fans designed to be installed remotely from the hood and even mounted on the exterior of the house. Quiet hoods have sound insulation and anti-vibration mounts so that their motor noise does not get transferred to the building structure and amplified. As with all fans, keeping the air moving smoothly through the path to the outside will help to keep the sound level down. The effect of a convoluted ducting path is less with a range hood than with a bath fan because of the volume of air is so much greater, but all the elements make up the system and by optimizing each of them, the total noise produced by the system will be reduced.

Work is being done at Lawrence Berkeley National Laboratory to optimize the "capture efficiency" of range hoods. The purpose, after all, is to remove the cooking effluents, not move a lot of air. Optimizing the design of the hood for capture efficiency should be able to reduce the fan noise. Look for a Capture Efficiency rating.

It should also be noted that a central kitchen open to most of the house is an ideal place to locate the whole dwelling ventilation system. Fan products are available that have additional settings that allow them to run continuously at very low background levels that meet ventilation requirements. It is hard to tell if these fans are running, which can make whole building leakage or blower door testing a challenge.

Sound Considerations for Radon/Soil Gas Exhaust Fans

A soil gas or radon mitigation system is designed to draw the air up from the ground surrounding the foundation of the house. Commonly, these systems run inside the house with the fan mounted either in the basement or the attic, outside the pressure boundary. The primary consideration is that the fan mounting be isolated as much as possible from the structure of the house to minimize vibration. Airflow noise should be completely contained within the ducting.

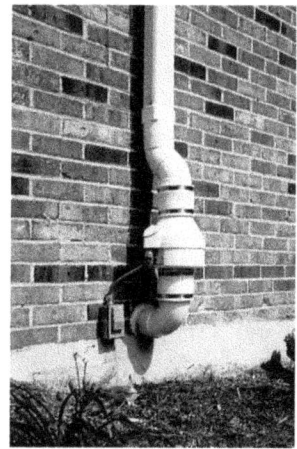

Figure 5.4 Exterior Soil Gas/radon fan (Infiltec)

If it is a retrofit application, however, and the fan is mounted on the outside of the house, it will be important to locate and mount the fan in such a way that operating sounds are not transmitted back into the house through open windows. The exhaust opening from the ducting should extend all the way to the roof from the standpoint of removing the pollutant and also the fan and airflow exhaust noise above the level of the house.

Chapter 6

Installation Details

System Design Overview

Having chosen the type of system to be used, it is vital that it be installed so that it works well and that it is serviceable. Remember that air is lazy and doesn't enjoy working too hard. Duct runs should be as straight and smooth as possible. Flexible ducting is twice as resistant to airflow as smooth, metal ducting. Think about sucking your drink through a straw: the smaller and more twisted the straw, the more suction it takes. Abrupt, ninety-degree elbows slow the airflow and make it more turbulent. Changing those ninety-degree turns to a pair of forty-five degree fittings will ease the turn and ease the flow. Transitioning from small diameter ducting to larger ducting will also improve the flow. Use fittings that match the system and transition to a larger size, never a smaller one. Use a 4" duct with at least a 4" hood, for example. Flex duct should be pulled out to as close to its full, extended length as possible and not left bunched up in a tight corner or worse yet, bunched up in the box. If oval duct runs are needed to move air through a small wall cavity, the run should be kept as short as possible.

Keeping the air moving through the system by using larger ducting and fittings at a low velocity of 500 fpm or less (2.5 m/s) will keep the resistance lower and keep the noise level down. "The resistance of any system of ducts, grilles, filters, etc. is proportional to the square of the air velocity through it—keep velocities down by using recommended duct, grille, and filter size."[1]

To CALCULATE the resistance of 100 feet of flexible duct, use the formula:[2]

$$Friction_{loss} = 2.74 \times (V/1000)^{1.9}/Diameter^{1.22}$$

Where:
$Friction_{loss}$ is in inches of water gauge;
V = the velocity of the air flow in feet per minute;
$Diameter$ = diameter of the duct in inches.

FOR EXAMPLE, consider a clothes dryer trying to move 140 cfm through a hundred feet (effective length) of 4 inch duct would result in a velocity or fpm of 400 and a resistance of 0.089 iwg or 22 Pascals. Increasing the duct diameter to 5" would reduce the flow rate to 256 fpm and the resistance to 0.029 iwg or 7.22 Pascals. Because of the elbows and the external hood with its damper, clothes dryers commonly have effective lengths of over 100 feet. It's no wonder that clothes take so long to dry!

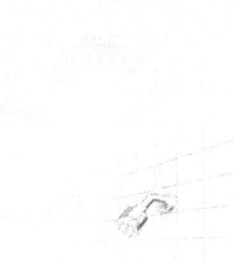

Figure 6.1 Exhaust Vent in the Shower (Panasonic/Morriessey)

The first turn out of the ceiling mounted bath fan is the most important. Making a ninety-degree turn right out of the fan will have a significant impact on the flow through the system because it is the highest pressure point in the system. Try to ease the first direction change using 45° turns instead of a 90° or move the first turn at least four feet away from the fan. (Fan and ducting manufacturers' instructions have good installation details. Reading them will help you install the system correctly.)

Wall cavities in the United States are commonly framed with 2 x 4 wood,

---

1. Vent-Axia has extremely detailed and useful ventilation information: https://www.scribd.com/document/25144576/VENT-AXIA-Ventilation-Handbook
2. See the tables later in this chapter for equivalent duct fitting lengths.

which provides only a 3 1/2" wide cavity which is not conducive to using 4" ducting. "Ovalizing" or crushing four inch flex ducting is very resistive to airflow. Try using hard metal, oval ducting instead. Oval, plastic ducting is available although not common. Runs made with any of these approaches should be kept as short as possible because, despite the extended area of the oval duct, it is surprisingly resistive to airflow.

Every mechanical system, no matter how beautifully engineered and manufactured, will need to be serviced at some point in its life. Homes should have a very long life—one hundred or two hundred years or more. It should not require tearing out the 100 year parts to get to a ten or fifteen-year-old component that has failed. Design and install the system so that it is serviceable. Don't bury an in-line fan in a ceiling without providing a maintenance cover. If the fan vents a first floor bathroom, think about using an externally mounted fan, remote in-line fan, or through-wall fan. Or put a grille in the bathroom and run the ducting down to the basement and out of the building from there. Duct runs don't always have to go up.

Hoods or termination fittings and backdraft dampers also resist the flow of air. A backdraft damper (flapper or valve) prevents outside air from coming back down the duct into the room. They are pushed open by the airflow and close by gravity. Although they are lightweight, they still take energy away from the fan flow. They are often designed not to close completely so that a small flow of air can slide around the edge and start the damper moving when the air starts pushing in the desired direction. Without that slight opening, there would be no air movement and the damper wouldn't open.

It may not be necessary to have dampers in both the fan and the external hood. Stopping the incoming flow of air at the external wall surface means that the duct won't be full of freezing air in the cold weather months, but if the damper in the hood is not effective and the damper in the fan is removed, cold drafts will be felt in the bathroom. Because there are variables in every system, it is unfortunately impossible to state categorically that one damper or the other can be removed.

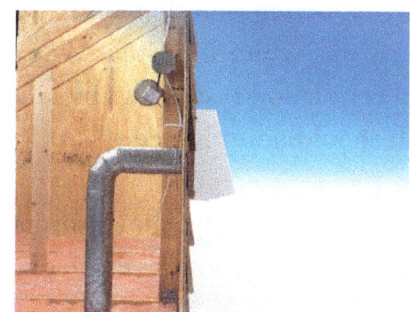

Figure 6.2 Remote Mounted Fan (Fantech)

It is not often that the ideal ducting path can be accomplished, so compromises will have to be made along the way. The goal is to keep the number of compromises as low as possible. Some fan designs are more tolerant than others to installation variations. In-line fans, for example, are specifically designed to move air through ducting and overcome resistance and since they are mounted remotely from the space they vent, they can be noisier. Through-wall fans don't have any extra resistance to deal with and so their designers can engineer the performance characteristics in the laboratory. Fans with EC motors vary their speed (and their noise) automatically as the pressure increases. A fan that is rated for quiet operation (less than 1 sone) that is noisy when it is installed means that there is high resistance in the installation details—a crushed or blocked duct, for example.

Air moving through a duct is larger, slower, lazier, and has less energy than electrons moving through a wire. If there is a design decision to be made about whether the path for the ducting or the path for the electrical wire should be shorter or straighter, the ducting should always win out. A few extra feet of wire may cost a few extra pennies, but the electrons rarely care (on the scale of a house). Air, on the other hand, does care. Keep the runs as short, straight, and smooth as possible. And never, ever vent a bath fan into an attic. It will deposit excessive moisture in the attic and cause problems. Ventilation systems must be vented all the way to the outside, not just close to it!

Ducting

Types of ducting

Ducting is available in a variety of styles for a variety of purposes. Never use that white, uninsulated flexible ducting that is sold as a dryer vent duct for a ventilation system of any kind or purpose. It's like using duct tape on ducts! It should never happen.

> Note: ducting for ventilation systems should be installed with as much thought and care as ducting for other conditioned air systems.

Smooth Round Duct Diameter	Free Area (Square inches)
2"	3.14
3"	4.71
4"	6.28
5"	7.85
6"	9.42
7"	11
8"	12.57

Table 6.1 Duct Areas

Round, galvanized, 24 gauge sheet metal ducting comes in standard, four-foot lengths 'un-locked' so that it can be cut to length. One end is crimped so that it will fit into the next section of ducting. The crimped ends should be oriented away from the source of pressure (the fan) otherwise, it is like installing a roof from the bottom up! There are all sorts of fittings—elbows, 'Y's (or Wyes), 'increasers', 'de-creasers', etc.

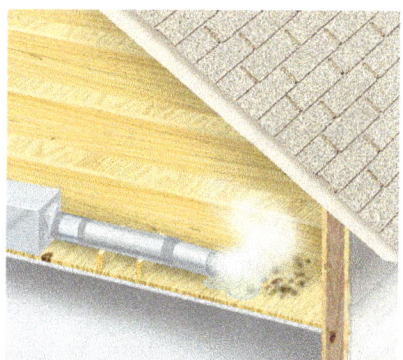

Figure 6.3 Fan Venting Into Attic Space (Panasonic/Morrissey)

It's smooth and ventilation air moves easily through it with little resistance. There are a lot of joints, however, each of which needs to be carefully sealed with duct mastic to prevent losses. It's also un-insulated so that warm moist air moving through it will condense in it when the duct passes through cold, ambient conditions such as a cold winter attic. Insulating ducting blankets are available and can be wrapped around the pipe. (Metal building insulation comes in rolls that can be wrapped around the ducting.) The blanket has a vapor diffusion retarder, which should be kept on the outside and sealed tightly along the seam and at the joints to make it continuous. Ducting in an attic can be covered by the attic insulation or foamed over. Just bear in mind any service issues that may need to be dealt with in the future. Don't make mechanical devices inaccessible.

Duct Material	Roughness Category	Absolute Roughnesss, foot
PVC plastic pipe (Swim, 1982)	Smooth	0.00003 to 0.00015
Galvanized steel, longitudinal seams, 4 ft joints (Griggs, et al. 1987)	Medium smooth	0.00016 to 0.00032
Semi-flexible duct, metallic, when fully extended	Medium Rough	0.0003 to 0.003
Flexible duct, all types of fabric and wire	Rough	0.004 to 0.007

Table 6.2 Duct Roughness

White, Schedule 40, PVC sewer pipe[3] comes in much longer lengths, which reduces the number of joints that have to be made and sealed, and, as can be seen from the above table, it is more than 100 times smoother than flexible ducting. Limiting the joints makes it even smoother. It too will need to be wrapped or covered in insulation, however, when it passes through a space outside the thermal envelope of the house.

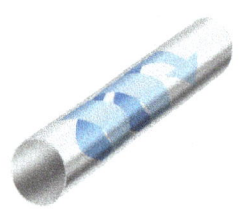

Figure 6.4 Flow in round sheet metal duct (Panasonic/Morrissey)

Oval, galvanized pipe is commonly used for heating or air conditioning system risers or stacks, passing up through wall cavities. Although it is considerably less resistive to airflow than ovalizing round, flexible ducting, it is still much more resistive than round ducting of a similar cross-sectional area. For the equivalent of a 4" diameter, galvanized duct, you would need to use a 3" by 6" oval to achieve the same area.

Metal semi-flexible ducting is smoother than the fabric type because the joints have a lower profile. It needs to be extended out to its full length for optimum performance, and it too needs to be insulated. This ducting has a tendency to get damaged easily as well and should not be in a vulnerable spot. When it is dented, it will not recover on its own.

Non-insulated flexible duct has the same flexibility as the insulated variety, but it does not include the insulation blanket. It comes in a variety of styles and qualities. The white vinyl stuff that is supplied for dryer vents is at

---

3. Table excerpted from ASHRAE Handbook of Fundamentals 2021, p21.7

the low end of the quality scale. Smaller diameters (less than 4") are often qualified as "hose" rather than ducting. Underwriter Laboratories (UL) has test procedures for flexible ducting that qualify it as either "air duct" or "air connector", suitable only for shorter runs. When flexible ducting is used in commercial applications where there is a significant amount of pressure in the duct, a large amount of air is forced into a small diameter space. Ventilation air velocities and pressures (particularly in residential applications) are not high pressure, and the air is moving at low speeds. Therefore, it is unnecessary to use "high pressure" ducting. Increasing the volume and increasing the velocity of air movement will increase the noise of the system.

> Pressure is listed in "inches of water gauge" (iwg) on the Inch/Pounds scale and in Pascals (Pa) on the metric scale. The two are getting blended in the building science business. Most residential ventilation systems experience pressures of much less than 1 iwg or 249 Pa. Most bath fans are rated at 0.1 iwg (24.9 Pa) and some ventilation codes require a performance rating at 0.25 iwg (62.2 Pa). As fabric duct gets larger in diameter, its ability to handle higher pressures is reduced, and requires tougher material to achieve the same rating. Lower pressure handling ducting is rated by UL as "Connector", applicable only for short runs. Higher-pressure capable materials get defined as "Duct". Ventilation systems can use the "Connector" grade because of the low pressures involved.

Figure 6.5 Unsupported Ducting (Panasonic/Morrissey)

Flex duct manufacturers make ducting of a trilaminate of aluminum foil, fiberglass and aluminized polyester or PVC coated fiberglass cloth or chlorinated polyethylene (CPE) materials. Air duct rated flex duct can handle as much as 10 iwg through 12" diameter ducting. They are rated for velocities in the range of 5,500 feet per minute (fpm). (Remember, for ventilation, the velocities should be below 500 fpm to keep the sound level down.) Just to confuse things more, the UL ratings between "air duct" rating and "air connector" rating depend on the number of tests that the manufacturer has put the product through. Air Duct must pass all the tests of the UL 181 Standard. Air Connector must pass only a few tests and is limited to "installation in lengths not over 14 feet". Maybe the manufacturer doesn't think the air connector product will pass the full range of tests or maybe the manufacturer simply doesn't want to invest in all that testing. For residential ventilation systems, however, it doesn't matter whether it is Air Duct or Air Connector, because unless something strange is being installed (see your qualified engineer), the velocities and the pressures will not get high enough to be a concern.

Insulated flex duct is flexible duct wrapped up in an insulating blanket. Typical insulation levels are R4.2, R6, and R8. The insulation is commonly fiberglass held in place with a vapor diffusion retarder of metallized polyester (if it is the silver version), a black polyethylene covering, or a scrim reinforced polyester jacket. To make the vapor diffusion retarder work as designed, both the ducting and the vapor diffusion retarder need to be sealed at the ends. If only the ducting is sealed and the vapor diffusion retarder is left open, the cooler or hotter ambient air will successfully penetrate under the vapor diffusion retarder, and it will lose its effectiveness. Fiberglass insulation is not good at blocking airflow that sneaks into the open ends of the of vapor diffusion retarder. If moisture gets under the vapor diffusion retarder and condenses on the ducting, it will eventually saturate the fiberglass, eliminating the insulating properties, and pooling in the vapor diffusion retarder with the ensuing potential disasters.

The Air Diffusion Council has some excellent installation details, much of which are included by manufacturers in their installation instructions.[4] Their installation details include how to attach the ducting to fittings, making splices, and what tapes, duct mastic, and connectors to use. The details are primarily for HVAC or higher-pressure ducting but should apply to good ventilation system installations as well.

Flexible ducting needs to be supported along its length. Sags and dips increase flow resistance (each one is a series of turns), and each dip is a potential moisture reservoir where water can collect and increase the dip.

Duct Joints and Mastics and Duct Tapes

Elbows, 'Y's (Wyes), 'T's, are all places where the air is forced to change direction. Making direction changes with hard pipe fittings is less resistive than making similar direction changes with flexible ducting. Keeping the air

---

4. Air Diffusion Council, Schaumburg, IL http://flexibleduct.org/ADC_Inst.asp

moving in a straight line is the best way to keep it moving with the least resistance. A straight line from the outlet of the fan to the outside is not a reality, however, but achieving the straightest, smoothest path—minimizing dips and sharp bends and crushed ducts — will provide the best performance.

Joints that are factory made are considerably tighter than those that are made in the field. Ideally the seam in a four-foot length of galvanized pipe should be sealed with mastic, but if it comes down to what to seal and what not to seal, in-field-made rather than factory-made joints should be addressed first, working out from the highest pressure points near the fan, HRV/ERV, or air handler.

In an HVAC system, there are numerous bends and turns as the air moves from the central air handler, commonly through a "trunk duct" with "take-offs" or branches out to the individual rooms. Those take-offs leave the main trunk at an angle, commonly 45°, as the branches of a tree. Turning vanes may be used to guide the fast moving air around corners, all ways to help the air move smoothly and quietly from its source to its destination.

The installation of a stand-alone HRV or ERV system requires many of the same design considerations. Air is moving from the outside to the HRV or ERV, from there to the rooms, from the rooms back to the HRV or ERV, and from there back to the outside. To keep the system operating smoothly, care needs to be taken in the design and installation of the ducting. Slamming air into a right-angle turn will create internal turmoil in the flow and slow it down far more than if the air is coaxed into changing direction through a series of forty-five degree turns.

* * *

Fittings

Metal duct elbows come segmented so that they can be adjusted from a ninety-degree turn to a straight line. One end is crimped to fit into the next section.

> The crimped end of any duct section or fitting should be at the low-pressure end, away from the fan to lessen the leakage.

Many fittings are more commonly used for HAC (Heating and Air Conditioning) applications where the air is moving out from the air handler to the rooms so the crimping may be on the wrong end for ventilation, which moves the air from the rooms to the outside.

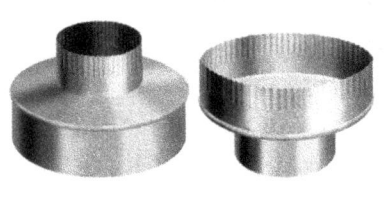

Figure 6.6 Untapered Increaser/Reducer (Morrissey)

Increasers increase the diameter of the ducting, which will reduce the pressure and improve the airflow. They can increase the diameter by one or two inches. When they are tapered, the air flows easily from one size to the other. Un-tapered increasers save on size, but the transition is an abrupt 'T' so they will increase turbulence at the fitting. Although these un-tapered "increasers" can also be used to decrease the duct size, the friction losses will be very high.

'Y' (or Wye) fittings can bring two duct runs together, blending them into a single and larger duct. 'Y' fittings can look just like the letter or they can be "Tee-Wyes" that look like a straight duct with a branch entering at the side. There are also "Tri-Wye" fittings that have three connections in and one connection out. If it is desirable for the airflow from the inlets to be equal, then the duct diameters going into the 'Y' should be equal and the duct diameter going out should be greater—4" x 4" x 6" for example. Reducing the size of one of the inlets will reduce the flow through that inlet. This might be desirable in tapping off a primary bath and a powder room or the middle of the bathroom and a toilet space.

Collector boxes can join the ducts from several rooms together into a box with a single outlet that is then vented to the outside. This allows for several rooms to be vented to the outside through a single fan and a single opening in the building envelope. All the rooms will be vented simultaneously unless a controllable, dampering arrangement is added to the system.

* * *

Mastics

Mastics are flexible sealants that vary in consistency from yogurt to mashed potatoes. They remain flexible over an extended period, shrinking and expanding with the changes in duct temperature. It is sold in tubs or buckets or cartridges, like caulk. They are either solvent or water based. To work in confined spaces, the water-based caulks are preferable for the health of the installer. Mastic can be applied with a putty knife or stiff brush or even fingers.

THERE ARE a number of elements to seek in good mastic:

- *High solids content* - Solids content listed in the product literature should be at least 50 percent. Some have as much as 70 percent. Higher solids means less shrinkage as the material cures.
- *Excellent adhesion* - The mastic must stick to metal, wood, drywall, plastic, concrete and just about any other material that might be found in a house. Since these surfaces are seldom clean, look for mastics that hold well to dirty or oily surfaces.
- *Excellent cohesion* - The mastic must also stick to itself so it doesn't crack as the surface moves or "blow out" under the air pressure inside the duct.
- *Water resistant* - Condensation may collect on ducts during cooling, so the mastic must hold even when exposed to water.
- *Non-toxic* - Check the Material Safety Data Sheet for warnings. If you choose to spread the material with your hands, you may need to wear gloves. Water-based mastics are less irritating than petroleum-based ones.
- *Surface burning characteristics* - Duct mastics should be tested for flame spread and smoke developed (UL723 and ASTME-84). National Fire Protection Association Standard 90A requires duct mastics to have a flame spread rating no higher than 25 and a maximum smoke developed rating of 50.
- *Viscosity* - Some installers like thicker mastic that they can apply with a trowel or gloved hand. Others like it thinner, so it brushes on easily. Viscosity is measured in units called centipoise (cps). Higher numbers mean thicker mastic. Viscosity around 100,000

cps indicates a consistency similar to mashed potatoes, while 60,000 - 75,000 cps suggests something closer to yogurt.
- *Storage* - numerous manufacturers emphasize that their products have a limited shelf life, usually about one year. Most mastics should not be allowed to freeze during storage or shipping.
- *Color* - If ducts will be visible, you may want to select a pleasing color.
- *UL Listing*—Mastics are tested by Underwriter Laboratories to Standard 181-B and may be marked as 181B-M on the container.

BECAUSE THERE IS no standardization of these products, not all of this information will be comparatively available. To reinforce the air sealing, fiberglass mesh tape should be applied to the cleaned joint before the mastic is applied.

*　*　*

TAPES

"Duck" tape, the cloth kind with the adhesive backing, is good for just about everything except for ducting. It was originally made of a duck fabric and used as a weatherproof joiner in the military. (The 'duck' name came both from the fabric and from its waterproof qualities.) It wasn't until after World War II that it changed to grey or silver and was attached to duct work. Now it comes in an enormous variety of colors, has dozens of books and myths surrounding it, but it is only mentioned here in passing because it shouldn't be used for sealing ducts. It dries out quickly and falls off.

There are, however, many other tapes that are effective and long-lived for sealing the joints between ducts, connectors, equipment, and each other. It should be noted that tapes and mastics are not designed to mechanically attach or support duct connections. Their purpose is to stop leakage.[5]

Underwriter Laboratories (UL) has several tests for tapes: UL-181A for rigid ducting, UL-181B for flexible air ducts, and connectors and UL-181B-

---

5. LBNL-41434. "CAN DUCT-TAPE TAKE THE HEAT?" Max Sherman & Iain Walker
https://eta-publications.lbl.gov/sites/default/files/lbnl-41434.pdf

FX for adhesive tapes on flexible ducting. UL-723 is used for surface burning of building materials. Manufacturers have many "grade" designations such as Economy, Utility, General Purpose, Contractor, Industrial, Professional, and Premium, but even with these tests and labeling, it is difficult to know what tapes will function effectively over an extended period. If the ducting is to be "buried" in a wall or building component that will be inaccessible without extensive destruction, mastic is a much better choice for sealing the joint. Ventilation ducting is not subjected to the same variations in heating and cooling that conditioned air ducting is exposed to. Nevertheless, it is important that the air not leak into or out of ventilation ducting. Ventilation air is the air that the occupants are relying on to breathe.

The color of the duct tape is not an important component of its ability to do its job. It may be more attractive to join pieces of silver ducting together with silver tape, but using clear tape will allow the installer or inspector to see the joint and determine if the gaps have been completely covered. Clear, UL-181B tape is available.

Installation details are as, or perhaps, more, important than the tape itself. Understandably, in an attic, basement, or crawlspace, it is virtually impossible to make the joint clean and free of dust, but the closer the installer can get to that, the better. From a duct sealing standpoint, the UL rated tapes don't have an advantage, but local codes may require their use.

* * *

DUCTING *Routes and Layout*

The airflow through the ventilation system depends on the layout and installation of the ducting and fittings. When an air stream changes direction, a dynamic loss occurs. Unlike friction losses in straight ducting, fitting losses are due to turbulence rather than skin friction. It is not always easy to calculate or measure the static pressure of the system. The resistance to the airflow can be estimated by using the actual length, the equivalent length, and the effective length as stand-ins for static pressure.

- the actual, physical length of the duct run (double the actual length to estimate the resistance of flex duct run);
- *Equivalent length*: the equivalent of resistance to airflow for a specific fitting;

- *Effective length*: the total of the actual length and the equivalent length of all the fittings in a run

Installing a ventilation product and attaching ducting without understanding how much resistance there is in the ducting and fittings guarantees that the airflow will be severely diminished. The common industry rule-of-thumb is that the flow will be about half of a fan's certified flow-rate. What is surprising about going through these steps is how much resistance is generated by the fittings and how quickly most ventilation products will reach their performance limit. The best way to know how the installed product is working is to test it or measure it.

The airflow of a fan or ventilation product is certified at a specific static pressure (0.1 iwg for ducted fans like bathroom exhaust fans or whole house comfort ventilators, 0.03 iwg for direct discharge products without ductwork, in-line fans 0.2 iwg, 0.1 iwg for kitchen range hoods) although in the process of being tested, the performance is measured at a variety of pressures from zero to the maximum resistance the fan can handle when the flow goes to zero cfm, generating a "flow curve". To accomplish that flow once it is installed in the house, the ventilation product has to be installed so that the static pressure point or flow resistance at which it was rated is not exceeded. If it is exceeded, the installed flow will be less. Because most installations are not carefully done and do not consider the laziness of the air motion, it is common to find most ventilation installations are operating at about one half or less the rated flow.

The exceptions to this are the products that use DC motors. These motors naturally adjust their speed based on the pressure so their performance is tolerant of bad installations. They will, however, use more power and become noisier as the resistance increases.

An ERV or HRV layout is similar to the layout of an HVAC system. Both the fresh air supply and the stale air return have to go out to the rooms and back to the heat exchanger. The resistance to the flow through each of those paths should be equal so that the same amount of air moves in both directions. For an HVAC system, balancing the ducting design means that when the conditioned air reaches the grille in the room, it will move at a velocity that will satisfy the needs of the room for conditioning the air, and it will move quickly enough through the grille to be 'thrown' out into the room to stir up the air throughout the room. The velocity of the airflow through the grilles of an HRV/ERV installation or a supply-only ventilation system should be equally carefully considered so that the occupants are not subjected to drafts.

Note: The complexity of ERV/HRV system design is detailed in Appendix H —Manual BV.

Calculating the Effect on Performance

For an exhaust fan, the ducting layout must go directly to the outside through the smoothest, straightest possible path. This is true for a bath fan, kitchen fan, or range hood. Minimizing the resistance will maximize the performance.

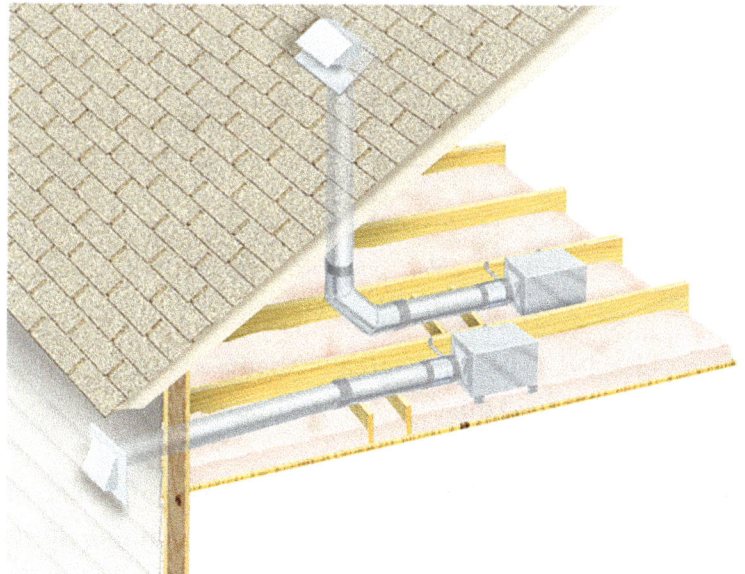

Figure 6.7 *Attic Venting System to Outside (Panasonic/Morrissey)*

1. Select the desired flow rate or cfm for the fan. (For example 60 cfm)
2. Determine the location of the fan.
3. Orient the fan so that the fan's outlet is pointing toward the outside of the building, whether that means exiting through a wall or through the roof.
4. Choose the starting type and size of ducting to be used from Table 6.3. (For example, 4" insulated flex duct for a duct run in an attic

to the roof for a 60 cfm fan will move that much air up to a total *effective length* (the total of the *actual length* of the duct and the *equivalent length* of the fittings) of 20 feet. If rigid ducting were used, the *effective length* could be increased to 40 feet.)

Table 6.3 Maximum Effective Flexible Duct Length at 0.1" w.g.							
	3 inch dia.	4 inch dia.	5 inch dia.	6 inch dia.	8 inch dia.	10 inch	12 inch
30 cfm	17 feet	75 feet	225 feet	NL	NL	NL	NL
45 cfm	8 feet	35 feet	100 feet	250 feet	NL	NL	NL
60 cfm	DU	20 feet	60 feet	150 feet	NL	NL	NL
75 cfm	DU	13 feet	40 feet	100 feet	400 feet	NL	NL
90 cfm	DU	9 feet	28 feet	65 feet	300 feet	NL	NL
105 cfm	DU	DU	20 feet	50 feet	225 feet	NL	NL
120 cfm	DU	DU	15 feet	40 feet	175 feet	NL	NL
135 cfm	DU	DU	12 feet	30 feet	130 feet	400 feet	NL
150 cfm	DU	DU	10 feet	25 feet	110 feet	350 feet	NL
165 cfm	DU	DU	DU	20 feet	95 feet	275 feet	NL

Table 6.3 Maximum Duct Lengths.

DU = Don't Use, NL = No limit (greater than 400 feet)
Effective lengths for rigid ducting can be double these numbers.

5. Determine the path or "outside duct run" between the fan outlet and the vent or hood (termination fitting), determining the number of 90° and 45° elbows. (Use Table 6.4 for the equivalent length of the fittings.) (For example, the 60 cfm fan installed in the bathroom's ceiling. The flexible ducting will run for 2 feet before being turned up 90° headed straight up 4 feet to the roof where it will attach to a low profile roof cap with a backdraft damper and bird screen. If the 90° turn was made with two, 45° metal, adjustable elbows, each elbow will have the equivalent length of 5 feet (a total of 10 feet). If the 90° turn is made using the insulated flex without the metal elbows, it will have the equivalent length of 20 feet (doubling the 90° metal fitting length from Table 6.4).

6. Select an exterior vent or hood and note the *equivalent length*. (Use Table 6.5 for the equivalent length of ducting for the vent.) (For example, a low profile roof cap with a backdraft damper and bird screen will be used for this installation because that's what the owner wants, with an *equivalent length* of 60 feet.)

Total *equivalent length* of this installation:
Flex duct 90° elbow = 20 feet
Vent = 60 feet
Total *equivalent length* = 80 feet

7. Calculate (or measure) the actual length of ductwork to be used. In this example, 2 feet plus 4 feet or 6 feet of rigid duct, doubled to 12 feet for flexible ducting.
8. Add the actual length to the total equivalent length for the elbows and the vent to determine the overall effective length and use Table 1 to determine the duct size to be used for the required airflow rate.

Image	Description	Equivalent Length (Ft) for rigid ducting
	45° adjustable elbow, 2-piece	5
	90° adjustable elbow, 4-piece	10
	Wye, equal sizes	10

	Tee, take-off	50
	Tapered increaser/reducer	4
	Hard increaser/reducer	8

Table 6.4 Equivalent lengths of duct fittings. (Rigid ducting)

Image	Description	Equivalent Length (Ft)
	Triangular wall cap for round duct with backdraft damper & bird screen	60
	Triangular wall cap for round duct with bird screen, without backdraft damper	35
	Rounded wall cap for round duct with backdraft damper & bird screen	40

	Louvered wall cap	40
	Low-profile soffit vent with backdraft damper and bird screen	60
	Roof cap, low-profile for round duct with backdraft damper & bird screen	60
	Roof cap, 'goose-neck', for round duct with backdraft damper & bird screen	35

Table 6.5 Equivalent Lengths for Termination Fittings

Equivalent Lengths (Rigid ducting)[6]

The equivalent lengths of all the fittings for this example plus the the actual length will be the total effective length - the resistance that the airflow 'sees' as it moves through the ducts to the outside.

TOTAL *EFFECTIVE LENGTH* in this example:
  Total *equivalent length* = 80 feet
  Total *actual length* = 12 feet
  Total *effective length* = 92 feet

---

6. Adapted from HRAI "Residential Mechanical Ventilation"

9. To move 60 cfm through 92 feet effective length of ducting at 0.1 inches of static pressure would require using 6" diameter flexible duct (150 feet in Table 1). 4" ducting would be too small, allowing only 20 feet of *effective length*.
10. If the resistance exceeds the capability of the fan, use the next larger size duct, reduce the number of elbows, select a better exterior vent or a fan with a higher performance. The fan's rated performance is measured at 0.1 iwg. Some fan performance curves are also certified at 0.25 iwg. Will the fan be able to deliver the required flow for the installation?

FROM THIS EXERCISE, it is easy to see why most installations do not deliver the rated amount of flow. Flexible ducting less than 6" in diameter is too resistive for almost any length of duct run with a fan that is rated at 0.1"[7].

* * *

CONTINUOUS OPERATION *of the HVAC or furnace*

> NB. The term *furnace* is used here to refer to a forced air heating system and HVAC to refer to a forced air heating and cooling system. In climates where no air conditioning is required, it is possible to exhaust from and supply to the furnace return and operate the furnace blower continuously. (Although there may be a significant electrical penalty for the continuous operation of the furnace blower 24 hours/day.)

Continuous operation of the HVAC blower is strongly discouraged in climates with warm summers and high humidity, where fresh air is introduced to the system. If the blower continues to run for extended times after the cooling thermostat is satisfied, the moisture remaining on the coil and in the drain pan re-evaporates. During this time, the air continues to be cooled by the cold AC coil and by the evaporation of moisture, so the space temperature continues to decrease, while the relative humidity increases. In the next cooling cycle, this humidity has to be condensed again, so any efficiency gain

---

7. Spiral Manufacturing has very useful engineering information at: http://www.spiralmfg.com/wp-content/uploads/2015/09/engineering_data-1.pdf

in evaporating this moisture is offset by the next cycle and by the loss of comfort at higher relative humidity.

More importantly, with air conditioning, do not duct the supply air from the HRV to the ducting of the HVAC. (During summer months, the outdoor humidity supplied through the HRV may cause condensation on interior surfaces of the HVAC equipment and the supply plenum and ducting. These surfaces will be around 60° F, and outdoor air dew points in the summer in much of the US are well above this temperature. These are the very conditions that promote mold growth. How ironic it would be that the system tasked to provide good indoor air quality by ventilation can be the means of promoting mold growth, by lack of attention to basic psychrometric principles.

Termination Fittings

Exterior Hoods and Vents

The termination fitting or exterior vent or hood is one of the most overlooked and taken-for-granted components of the ventilation system. The air from the ventilation system has to pass through the building envelope and leave (or enter) the building. That penetration must not allow water or creatures to enter, and it should only allow air to enter or leave when the ventilation system is running. And it must accomplish all that with as little resistance to the desired air movement as possible.

To keep the water out, roof and wall vents make a sharp, ninety-degree turn at the wall surface or roof. The sharper that turn is, the more the resistance that the vent creates. Vents that have a rounded turn ease the air into the new direction and are less resistant to the flow.

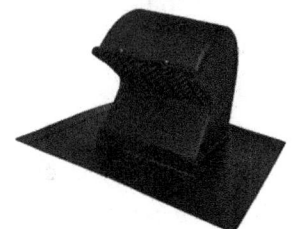

Figure 6.8 Roof Mounted Exhaust Hood (Primex)

Most exterior vents include an airflow operated backdraft damper or flap that blows open and closes with gravity. (On some vents, the damper is removable so that the vent can be used as an intake.) Although the damper material is light, it takes energy to push it open. That energy is subtracted from the airflow. Some flaps can reduce the flow by as much as 50%! If there isn't much airflow by the time it reaches the vent, there won't be much energy to push the flap open at all.

The outside surface of the home is the ideal place to block the incoming flow of outside air, keeping the interior ducting at room temperature. Most ceiling mounted bath fans have built in backdraft dampers. If there is a damper in the fan, the second damper in the exterior vent can be removed and the damper in the fan will block flows of outside air into the room, but as mentioned previously, since all installations are different a decision needs to be made at the installation site. Airflow performance will be improved.

For a remote mounted or in-line fan that does not include a backdraft damper, the damper in the exterior vent serves the purpose reasonably well. If greater protection is required, a separate backdraft damper in the line can replace the exterior flap.

For an HRV or ERV, there can be no airflow-operated flap in the intake side to prevent air from coming in. A motorized damper can be used if it is desirable to seal the system off when it is not running—something of particular concern in location with forest fire risk.

Low airflows or no airflows through the vent (particularly wall vents) will provide an ideal spot for nesting birds. They quickly learn to flip open the damper and climb inside, where it is warm and dry and make a nest. And when the baby birds grow up and leave, the mites that live in their feathers may seek other homes farther into the house. It is a good idea to use an exterior vent or termination fitting that has a creature screen. These are too broad to cause much resistance to flow and serve their protective purpose well. (Insect screens, on the other hand, are extremely resistant to airflow and should only be used with powerful fans and in conditions where insects are a major problem. Running the fan frequently or constantly solves the problem better.)

Grilles, registers, and diffusers

Ceiling mounted bath fans include a grille. The certification process requires that they be tested with the grille installed, so the grille is engineered to match the product and is figured into the airflow specification.

In-line or remote mounted exhaust fans, however, do not come with grilles, and a variety of options are available. Most fan manufacturers will offer grilles to match their fans. In calculating the equivalent length of duct for the resistance of the grille, use 10 feet for a relatively open, round grille and 15 feet for a stamped metal louvered grille.[8]

If the rate of airflow is low relative to the size of the opening, the grille will have less resistance and make less noise. At higher velocities, grilles create

---

8. See Chapter 9 for more information on grille resistance

noise in the room as the air rushes through the opening. An open, low resistance, well-designed grille will make the system operate more quietly.

If an HRV/ERV or supply-only ventilation system is integrated with the home's HVAC system, the supply grilles will be installed to meet that system's requirements. Supply diffusers for dedicated ducting HRV/ERVs and supply-only systems must be designed so that the air leaving them is moving at a high enough velocity to "throw" the air out into the room and satisfactorily mix with the room air. Discharge velocities between 500 and 800 fpm are a reasonable compromise between air mixing, noise, and pressure drop. In a cold climate, the air leaving these diffusers will be at a cooler temperature than the room air, so they need to be installed high enough so that they are not creating drafts that the occupants feel are uncomfortable. If the diffuser is on the floor, the incoming air temperature should not be less than 60°F (16°C). If the diffuser is located high on the wall or on the ceiling, the incoming air temperature should not be less than 54°F (12 °C). Many grille manufacturers have performance data on their products.

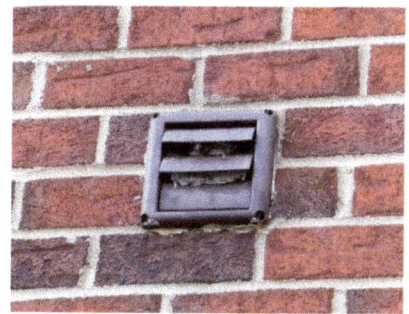

Figure 6.9 Lint Clogged Louver Fitting (PHR)

Dampers

Balancing Dampers

HRV and ERV systems need to be balanced—equal amounts of air supplied and exhausted to and from the house. (More on HRV/ERV dampers and balancing in Appendix H.) A carefully designed and installed ducting system will do most of that work, but balancing dampers should be included to finish the task. A typical balancing damper is an adjustable vane in the air stream that can be manually adjusted to block some portion of the flow by rotating the damper to be parallel or perpendicular to the flow with a small handle on the outside of the ducting. An alternative balancing damper is constructed like an iris that can be manually opened or closed to vary the amount of air passing through it. An increasing number of HRV/ERV units include built-in balancing adjustments.

A manometer is used to measure the flow in the two air streams while the adjustments are made. Then the balancing dampers can be locked in position to maintain that consistent air flow.

BACKDRAFT DAMPERS

Most of the time, air should flow through a duct system in only one direction. Exhaust ducts should only exhaust. Supply ducts should only supply. Backdraft dampers like the flap on an exterior hood blow open with the flow and fall back to the closed position when the flow stops. They are generally flat, like pieces of metal or plastic that don't take a great deal of force to push open but have enough weight to close. Some fan manufacturers counterbalance their dampers to make them more rigid and to close more positively.

The duct attached to an exhaust fan is purposefully designed to provide a low resistance "hole" to the outside of the building. If it has been properly designed and installed to optimize the performance of the fan, it is akin to cutting a four, five, or six-inch hole in the side of the house. The damper is the only thing that blocks the flow of cold air in winter or hot, humid air in summer from coming back down into the house. Although its conductive insulation value is so low it is not worth considering, its convective resistance (its ability to block air movement) should be high.

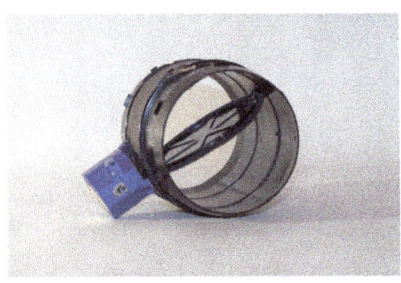

Figure 6.10 Motorized Damper (PHR)

Most backdraft dampers installed in fans work well at blocking the backflow of air when they are new. When a fan is labeled "For ceiling installation" it primarily means that the damper has been balanced to be installed in the ceiling. When it is closed, the damper rests on a surface in the "nozzle" of the fan. There is often a "bumper" or rest on that surface that keeps the damper slightly open at all times so that airflow can be established when the fan starts so that damper will open, but even with that designed opening, backflow leakage is tight.

When the fans are performance certified to the HVI 916 Standard, their flow is measured with their integral backdraft dampers in place. Additional backflow prevention in the duct or in the hood itself will add considerable resistance to the flow.

A motorized damper can be much tighter when it is closed and does little to resist the desired flow because a motor pushes the damper open and holds it there rather than using the moving air for that purpose. Motorized dampers need to have a control interlock with the fan so that both devices turn on and off at the same time. Motorized dampers may work against an internal spring, so they only use power when they are opening and use the spring to push them back into the closed position. This arrangement means that shutting off the power to the damper will make it close. Without the spring, the damper will need a constant source of power—power to open and power to close. It will be a small amount of power, but it complicates wiring.

Although more common in commercial applications, some dampers are operated by pneumatic pressure, a small pump providing air pressure to move the damper blade.

VENTILATION CONTROLS

Without a means to turn it on or off, a fan is just a pile of metal and plastic parts. It can be installed so that it is "hard-wired" or permanently connected to a power source so that it is never shut off, running twenty-four hours per day, seven days per week. This eliminates the need for a control and for any backdraft protection. If the fan is quiet enough and energy efficient enough, this can be the optimum strategy.

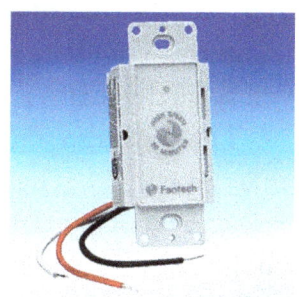

Figure 6.11 Adjustable Flow Rate and Cycling Controller (Fantech)

Generally, homeowners like to have some control over how their house is operating. It has been a common practice to wire the exhaust fan in the bathroom to the light switch, an "occupancy" sensor of sorts—when the bathroom is occupied the fan and the light is on. Moisture stays in the bathroom, however, for a much longer time than that. It runs down the walls after a shower. It stays in the towels, and it hangs in the air. In most bathrooms, the relative humidity can remain above ninety percent for two or more hours after a shower. Turning off the fan when turning off the light means that fan flow has little to no effect on the conditions in the bathroom.

A delayed off timer is a more effective approach to the spot ventilation needs of a bathroom application, particularly if the delay can be extended to an hour or two and the fan is quiet and energy efficient. Some light switches are available that allow the light to be turned off while the fan continues to run.

Another approach to controlling the ventilation with time is to install a cycle timer, a control that can be programmed either mechanically with "pins" or electronically to turn the fan on and off periodically throughout the day. These can be set up to cycle the fan to run for ten, twenty, thirty, or more minutes per hour. Some of them have multi-speed capability so that they run continuously at a low speed and are boosted to a higher flow rate during times of occupancy. This strategy allows the fan to serve multiple purposes—as the continuous, low volume primary ventilation system and the higher volume the occupant may feel is necessary to clear the air.

It would seem that running the fan on relative humidity with a dehumidistat would be an acceptable approach. Relative humidity is not as familiar as temperature, and people have a tendency to equate the two, thinking seventy percent relative humidity is comparable to seventy degrees Fahrenheit. The ideal living conditions are between thirty percent and fifty-five percent relative humidity, varying by the time of year and the climate, factors that also make it difficult for a dehumidistatic control to work effectively. Small changes in the humidity settings will cause significant changes in fan run time, from minutes to hours. Without microprocessor technology, the control will operate the fan when the ambient humidity is high, sometimes causing the fan to run all the time in summer. Controls exist that respond to rapid changes in humidity rather than a natural, steady rise. A shower is a humidity event that will spike the sensor and activate the fan.

There are also sophisticated controls that operate on what is characterized as "air quality"[9]. These are "mixed gas" sensor controls to sense a variety of gases, particularly those found in cigarette smoke such as hydrogen, ethanol, iso-butane, carbon monoxide, and methane. The difficulty with these controls is that they operate when the level of invisible gases is high, even when the occupant can't smell or sense the contaminant. That can be a good thing, but it is difficult to know why the ventilation system is running or if it should be.

"Demand controlled ventilation" generally uses a CO_2 sensor. Carbon dioxide is a good indicator of human occupancy of a space. Higher levels of CO_2 are a reasonable indicator of higher occupancy and the need for higher

---

9. A company like Sendal, for example, has sophisticated cloud based solutions that are capable of integrating a number of aspects of indoor air quality.

ventilation rates. CO_2 levels under 800 parts per million (ppm) are common in outdoor air conditions. These levels inside may mean the house is being over-ventilated. Between 800 ppm and 1200 ppm is normal. If the air contains over 5000 ppm, there are probably other nasty gases in the air and the space should be cleared of people until the air is cleared.

"Smart" control technologies are becoming increasingly available. After all, if we can ask a sound system to play Beethoven, why can't we ask the ventilation system to change the air in the house or even to know when it is necessary to change the air in the house? We can do almost anything with electronic control, but is it necessary? The important thing is to live in an environment with the best air possible. If the ventilation system is tasked for that purpose, it has to run.

* * *

System Commissioning and Documentation

Does it work as designed? Will someone be able to service the system in five years if it needs to be brought back to its original effectiveness? In the rush to get a project completed, the simple step of making sure that the system works is often overlooked. Once the fan has been wired and installation has been completed:

1. Make sure that all the set-up steps outlined in the installation manual have been followed;
2. Refer to the design documentation details for system operation and programming details;
3. Turn on the power;
4. Listen to the fan - give it a moment or two to come up to steady state operating speed;
5. Go outside and look at the termination fitting and see if the damper is being pushed open;
6. If the fan is being controlled by a timer, program it to meet the whole dwelling ventilation requirements;
7. If the controls are inside the fan, set them up to meet the requirements;
8. Measure the airflow.

Section 8.1.2 of the ASHRAE 62.2 Standard requires installed system documentation as described previously (See System Documentation in Chapter 4 of this book). This can be as simple as a compilation of :

- The brands and models of devices;
- Who they were purchased from;
- Who designed the system;
- Who should be contacted for service in the future;
- The purpose of the system;
- When it was installed.

If the system is an HRV/ERV, commissioning must include balancing. The supply air should move freely into the system through the intake and exhaust vents on the outside of the house. (These sometimes are installed backwards!)

How hard could it be just to make sure the system actually works?

* * *

Replacing an existing bathroom fan

The first step in replacing a bathroom fan is to determine the ductwork path to the outside of the house. Is there ducting? (Installers have been known to install a fan in the ceiling but not connect it to anything.) Is ducting that runs through an attic insulated? Is the path as straight and smooth as possible? How about the exterior vent? Does that need to be replaced as well? (Check the vent for old bird nests.)

Determine how much airflow is required. If the fan is to be used as the whole dwelling ventilation system, running continuously at a low flow, use the table from ASHRAE Standard 62.2 found in Chapter 3 of this book or use RedCalc.

Kits are available that can be added to an existing, ceiling mounted bath fan that can use the existing grille and housing or add an in-line fan to upgrade the old product to provide better performance. These products require removing the existing fan blade and motor and adding the new, in-line fan remotely. The advantage of this approach is that there is no impact to the bathroom ceiling. The wiring will need to be moved so that the switch in the bath will be connected to the new fan. In-line fan designs are generally powerful enough to be able to handle the resistance of the existing housing.

Alternatively, removing the housing in the bathroom ceiling and adding a new grille and a remote fan will work equally well. (It will just require repairing the ceiling.) There are also exterior vents that include a fan, taking all the fan noise out of the building. The ducting from the bathroom to the exterior of the building still needs to be checked for insulation and a direct and smooth path to the exterior.

There are a wide variety of choices for replacing an existing ceiling mounted fan with another ceiling mounted fan. There are fans alone, fans with lights, fans with heating elements, and fans with lights and heating elements. Many of them have the Environmental Protection Agency's (EPA) ENERGY STAR® label, so they will be relatively quiet (under 2 sones) and energy efficient. ENERGY STAR evaluates bath fans by comparing their airflow (cfm) per power consumption (watts). To be ENERGY STAR rated, a bath fan needs to deliver at least 1.4 cfm/watt if the flow is between 10 and 89 cfm and 2.8 cfm/watt if the flow is between 90 and 500 cfm. In choosing the replacement fan and knowing how much air needs to be moved, you can compare the sound level and cfm/watt of the fans that meet your certified flow rate.

* * *

Replacing an existing range hood

If the existing range hood doesn't vent to the outside but just recirculates the air, it is the same as starting from scratch. A path to the outside is required, either straight out through the wall, up through the ceiling, or down through the floor.

If the existing range hood already vents to the outside, there are a number of options. The hood itself can be left in place and an exterior mounted, in-line fan can be installed on the outside of the building. The fan motor in the hood should be disabled so that it is not working against the new fan, and the existing grease filters, which will protect the fan motor, should be replaced with new ones.

An in-line fan in the ducting can also be used with the existing hood and filters. And to keep the sound level to a minimum, a "muffler" can be added to the duct line.

The ducting should be carefully examined, and if necessary, cleaned, before pursuing either of these options. As in any duct installation, the path should be a short and smooth as possible. If there is a damper in the exterior hood, it should be checked to make sure that it will open and close easily and seals effectively when it is closed.

Unless the kitchen is being remodeled, it is likely that there will be limitations on the size of a replacement hood. ENERGY STAR rates range hoods up to 500 cfm, requiring an efficiency of 2.8 cfm/watt and a sound level of no more than 2 sones. The performance must be third party certified by an organization like HVI. Refer to Section 3.4.1 for sizing, but the hood should exhaust no more than 100 cfm per linear foot of cook-top if it is located against a wall or 150 cfm per linear foot of cook-top if it is an island installation.

* * *

Installing a Radon/Soil Gas Mitigation System

Radon/soil gas mitigation systems need to be sized by the needs of the specific application. If the system piping has been installed during construction, it will be relatively easy to add a fan to the system. In most cases, a 100 cfm, in-line fan can get the job done. It would be advisable to have your home checked for radon levels and to communicate with a certified radon mitigation contractor for the right system. One installation note: since these fans run constantly, make sure that the fan is not located where its operating noise will be offensive (such as near a commonly open window).

Installation Details 111

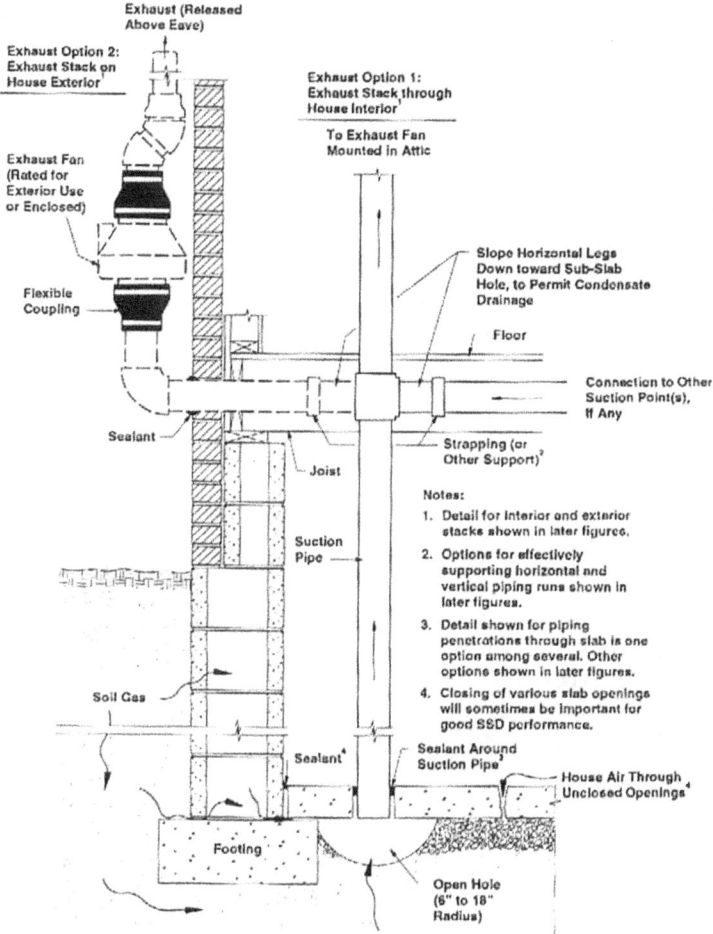

Figure 6.12 Radon/Soil Gas Mitigation System (EPA)

Chapter 7

House Pressures

Building Pressures

The role pressure plays in the movement of air throughout a house cannot be overemphasized.

Ventilation Rule #4: For air to move, there have to be three components: air, a hole, and a force.

AIR, a hole, and a force. Since this entire book is about air movement, the presence of air is a given. Holes and forces can take all sorts of different shapes and features. Holes could be as simple as the gap around the edge of a window or a poorly connected, large return register in a hallway. Forces could be mechanical devices like fans or simple variations in pressure like the wind pushing on the side of the house. Where the holes are and how big they are makes a major difference in how air much air moves through them. The strength of the force—the height of the building or the size of the fan—also impacts the amount of air that moves through the hole.

Understanding the role pressure plays in moving air around a house will provide an understanding of one of the largest components of comfort and of energy consumption.

Ventilation Rule #5: High pressure always moves toward lower pressure.

Think of a balloon. Make a hole in it, and the pressurized air comes rushing out. The pressures are seeking equilibrium. When the wind blows on one side of a house, it puts that side of the house under a higher pressure. The opposite side of the house will be at a lower pressure. The air will be pushed in through holes on the high-pressure side of the house and be sucked out through holes on the low-pressure side of the house. Air flows into a powered vacuum cleaner because the fan in the vacuum puts the end of the hose under low or negative pressure. Air is pushed out of the supply registers by the high pressure created by the supply side of the blower. On the other side of the blower, the pressure is lower, and air is sucked back into the system through the return vents.

Air is constantly moving due to pressure differences in small, convective flows in wall cavities and large flows through heating and cooling and ventilation equipment, and it all has to do with pressure and holes.

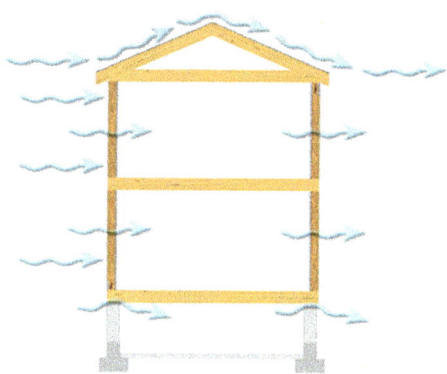

Figure 7.1 Wind Pressures (Panasonic/Morrissey)

Stack Effect[1]

Warm air rises. Warm air is lighter than cold air and so it rises. On a still day, with no mechanical equipment running and the house out in the middle

---

1. The Energy Conservatory has a tool called See Stack for simulating the stack effect under a wide variety of conditions.

of a plain, the pressure will be higher at the top of the house than at the bottom. Holes near the bottom of the house let air in. Holes near the top let air out. And holes in the middle have no air moving through them in either direction. These middle holes are in the "neutral pressure plain". This distribution of pressures is known as "the stack effect". A chimney relies on the stack effect to draw combustion gases in at the bottom, transport them up, and exhaust them out of the top. Until the chimney warms up, the effect is weak, which is why fires smoke until the temperature differences have been established. Once the draft has been established, the smoke (and even the fire) can roar up the chimney.

The "stack effect" is generated from the difference in weight of the warm air column within the building and the cooler air outside. The stack effect can be calculated with the following formula:

$$Q = 9.4 \times A \times \sqrt{(h \times (t - t_o))}$$

Where Q = airflow in cubic feet per minute
A = free area of inlets or outlets (assumed equal) in square feet
h = height from inlets to outlets in feet
t = average temperature of indoor air at height h in °F
t_o = temperature of outdoor air in °F
9.4 = constant of proportionality, including a value of 65 percent for effectiveness of openings. (This should be reduced to 50 percent (constant = 7.2) if conditions are not favorable.)[2]

So, if the house is 18 feet tall and there is a one foot hole at the top and a one foot hole at the bottom and it is 70°F inside and 45°F outside, an airflow of about 200 cfm will be generated without a fan!

When the wind blows against the side of the house, the design of the house affects the shape of the flow. For a simple shape, the side of the house that the airflow impacts will experience an increase in pressure. The air stream moves up and over the roof and down the other side, creating a nega-

---

2. Audel HVAC Fundamentals Volume 3, James E. Brumbaugh, Wiley Publishing, 2004

tive pressure or vacuum condition on the back and sides of the house as the air moves away. These pressure conditions affect the flows due to the stack effect in the house.

The wind is a variable force. Averaging the winds over the course of the year may show that there is adequate natural airflow to eliminate the need for mechanical ventilation. But the need for ventilation in the home is <u>constant</u>. In the seasons when the heating system isn't running or the windows are closed or the temperature inside is close to the temperature outside, the natural air movement forces just can't get the job done.

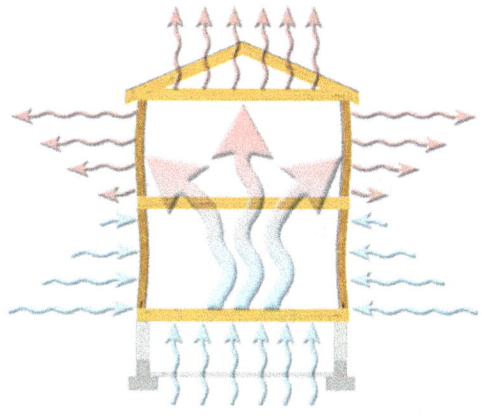

Figure 7.2 Stack Effect (Panasonic/Morrissey)

Ventilation Rule #6: A constant need cannot be satisfied by a variable, average force.

Diffusion

A high concentration of a gas will move toward a lower concentration, seeking to balance out the two, seeking equilibrium. This is the process of diffusion or vapor pressure. Cooking bacon in the kitchen will eventually diffuse the fragrant molecules throughout the house. The room deodorants or "air fresheners" move their fragrances throughout the room by diffusion and airflows. Gases and water vapor can diffuse through solid materials like walls, moving slowly from molecule to molecule.

Diffusion is a much slower process than the movement of air mechanically or naturally with the other pressure forces of winds and stack effect. It is a force that should be recognized and appreciated, but on the scale of air movement in the house, diffusion is not a major ventilation factor.

Leaky Ducts and Air Handling Equipment

Leaky ducts, on the other hand, can have a major impact on the movement of air in the house. The heating or cooling system that uses conditioned air is a closed system. House air moves into the return or low-pressure side of the air handler, and is pushed out through the ducts into the house on the high-pressure side. It moves through the rooms and back into the returns and back to the air handler. By design, the same amount of air that is pushed out is drawn in.

If the ducts are tightly connected (all the joints sealed with mastic for minimal leakage) or if they are all within the conditioned space, the system should work as designed. But if there are leaky ducts that are located outside the conditioned space, there will be an impact on the pressures in the house that will drive airflows.

The air handler doesn't care where it gets its air from, it will continue to push air out and suck air back in regardless of the ducting. Leaks in ducting on the return side, drawing a portion of their air in from outside of the conditioned space, put the conditioned space under positive pressure because the system draws less air back to the air handler than it is putting into the conditioned space.

Leaks in the ducting on the supply side can have the opposite effect. If the supply ducting leaks to the outside, those leaks put the building under negative pressure because the air handler will add less air to the conditioned space than it is taking out through the return ducts. Of course, at the same time, the leaky supply ducting is conditioning the outdoor world.

In a cold or heating dominated climate, putting the house under positive pressure, even if it is very slight, will force the warm, potentially moist air in the house to leak out through any cracks or gaps or holes that it can find. When that warm, moist air strikes a cold surface below the dew point, the moisture in the air will condense out. That cold surface may be somewhere in the wall or roof system of the house. That moisture will encourage the growth of mold and degradation of the building materials. The same effect will occur in the opposite direction in a cooling climate when the house is under negative pressure from leaky supply ducting. The warm, moist air will be sucked in from the outside.

These air leaks and the associated flows may be very small, but small "drips" can accumulate. Nature is very patient.

It would be highly unusual for the duct installation to be completely airtight on only one side of the system. It is likely that there will be pressure leaks on both sides. The question is which side has more leaks? It is difficult to determine that, and it doesn't really matter. It is more important to seal <u>all</u> the duct joints or install all the ductwork within the conditioned envelope.

It is common practice (and required by code in my places) that the HVAC ducting be pressure tested for leaks for determining the amount of conditioned air that is lost. There are two versions of this testing: Total Duct Leakage testing, tests for all the leaks both inside and outside the pressure boundary. And Leakage to Outside testing, which measures only those duct leaks that are outside the pressure boundary.

Unfortunately, ventilation ductwork is rarely pressure tested for leaks, the reasoning being that the air in the ventilation ducting is not conditioned. But the same care should be exercised for the installation of ventilation ducting.

Effects of Pressure on Backdrafting

Chimneys are designed to guide polluted, unwanted air, gas, smoke, and particulates from combustion appliances to the outside of the house. They work by carrying the pollutants in the air stream. The chimney is the "hole". The "force" is assumed to be there by the "stack" effect of the warm, rising column of air. However, just because there is a chimney or vent pipe doesn't guarantee that the air will move up and out through it.

The venting system should be designed and installed according to the local building code. All the factors like the length of the horizontal run, the number of elbows, and the height of the vertical rise should be figured in. (Notice the similarity in other ducting resistance issues?) The National Fuel Gas Code (NFGC) or ANSI Z223.1 or NFPA 54 sets the venting requirements for all natural draft, Category 1 gas-fired appliances. Category 1 vent systems work by allowing the heated pollutants to rise vertically. The longer the horizontal run relative to the vertical rise, the more work the pressure has to do to get the air to flow up and out through the vent.

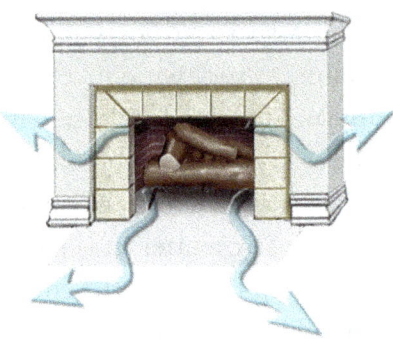

Figure 7.3 Fireplace Backdrafting (Panasonic/Morrissey)

Note that a gas exhaust vent is not sealed to the gas appliance (unless it is a Category IV or "sealed combustion system"). There is an opening between the vent and the boiler or furnace that is protected by a "flue hat" or "draft diverter". As the exhaust air moves out of the combustion appliance, room air is drawn in around the edges of the "hat". Air can also be exhausted out of the vent and appliance into the room if the air pressure in the room is lower than the air pressure in the vent: that pressure can be as little as a fraction of a Pascal, a very, very small amount.

> A Pascal is a tiny amount of pressure, something akin to a dust mite's sneeze. (1 Pascal = 0.00401865 iwg) It is important to recognize the major effects such a minor force can have on an object as large as a house.

For the health and safety of the house's occupants, the appliance venting must be installed to code and the manufacturer's instructions, and there must be an adequate pressure difference (higher in the space and lower in the vent pipe) to compel the combustion gases to move up the chimney and out of the building.

Using a sealed combustion system, a system that mechanically draws its combustion air in from the outside and power vents the flue gases back to the outside independently from the house air, assures that pressure variations in the house will not affect the performance of the combustion system. Power assisted combustion appliances, appliances that use a fan on the exhaust side, are the next best step to insure adequate venting.

Of all the pressure issues in a house, venting of combustion appliances is the most immediate and critical. Small changes have a big impact. The effects of very low-level carbon monoxide poisoning are still being studied. The effects of moderate levels of carbon monoxide poisoning can be deadly. The flow through a basic bathroom fan can backdraft a water heater!

Attached Garages

Garage doors are large holes. Even when they are closed, most garage doors are not well sealed around the edges. And they are at the lowest level in the house. (It's difficult to put the garage in the middle of the building!) As such, most of the time the air pressure is pushing in on the doors. Unfortunately, garages are commonly just like another room in the house, separated from the outside by a door, but not well air sealed from the house. So if the pressure in the garage is higher than the pressure in the house, all the pollutants that are in the garage will flow into the house.

This may be corrected by adding an exhaust fan to the garage (the International Mechanical Code says 0.75 cfm/square foot),[3] but if there is a combustion appliance in the garage (like a water heater), an exhaust fan may cause backdrafting as mentioned above.

If there is ducting in a garage, it is particularly important that all the joints be air sealed with mastic, otherwise those holes can suck in all the pollutants in the garage and distribute them throughout the house. ASHRAE's ventilation standard (62.2) allows "no more than 6% leakage of the total fan flow when measured at 0.1 iwg (25 Pa)"[4] in the garage.

If the air handler itself is in the garage, it is almost a sure thing that the garage pollutants will be distributed to the house. Appliance manufacturers will not allow the air handler's housing to be completely air sealed. The air handler could be boxed off from the garage and provided with an access door to the exterior to allow for service. The joints in the walls of the air handler closet must be carefully air sealed.

Ideally, the garage should be physically separated from the house. If that is not the case, keeping the mechanical equipment including the ducting (for both conditioned air and ventilation) out of the garage, air sealing the barrier

---

3. IMC, Table 403.3.1.1
4. ASHRAE Standard 62.2-2007 p6

between the house and the garage, and installing an exhaust fan in the garage are the next best steps. If the combustion appliance has to be in the garage, using sealed combustion eliminates the problem of venting the garage and putting it under negative pressure.

House Tightness or Building Tightness Limits (BTL)

Can a house be too tight? If the house will not allow the occupants to live comfortable and healthy lives and pursue their personal activities, yes, it can. The house is a place to shelter and protect the occupants. It must allow them to live comfortably and safely.

These calculations are listed here for historical purposes. Most energy efficiency programs no longer use them, but they are an interesting way to look at the pressure performance of a building.

Building tightness limit (BTL) (or Building Airflow Standard (BAS) or Minimum Ventilation Level (MVL) or Minimum Ventilation Rate (MVR)) is a general term for a house-tightening limit that was used for ensuring adequate air quality for the occupants of the house.[5] Weatherizing or reducing the energy consumption of a house requires tightening it up, closing up the air leaks and holes where pressure forces the air in and out of the building. Many homes, particularly manufactured homes, get much of their air from the air leaks and once those have been carefully sealed, the requirement for mechanical ventilation increases because the natural air changes have decreased. The Building Tightness Limit was developed as a benchmark, a limit beyond which the health of the occupants may be jeopardized. Most homes can use a whole dwelling ventilation system. The BTL threshold calculation has been eliminated from most weatherization programs because if the house has adequate leakage "on average" means that half the time it is under-ventilated and half the time it is over-ventilated.

THE BTL CAN BE CALCULATED USING three formulae:

---

5. Survey of Tightness Limits for Residential Buildings – July, 2001, Rick Karg for the Chicago Regional Diagnostics Working Group – available at
http://www.karg.com/pdf/Survey_of_BTL.pdf

Formula #1: 15 cfm x the number of occupants x n = CFM_{50} BTL. This formula estimates a tightness level based on the number of occupants.

Formula #2: 15 cfm x number of bedrooms + 15 x n = CFM_{50} BTL. This formula calculates the tightness level based on the number of occupants as estimated by the number of bedrooms.

Formula #3: Volume of the conditioned space x 0.35 x n/60 = CFM_{50} BTL. This formula calculates the tightness level based on 0.35 air changes per hour of the volume of the building.

The BTL equals the highest number calculated using formulas 1, 2, or 3. The number recorded would be the minimum allowable CFM_{50} of the conditioned living space. For example, a 1 story, 1,200 square foot, 2 bedroom house in Massachusetts with 3 occupants is tested with a blower door to 960 CFM_{50}. (For this house in this location n = 14.8 from the LBL tables.)

Formula #1: 15 cfm x 3 x 14.8 = 666 CFM_{50} BTL

Formula #2: 15 cfm x 2 + 15 x 14.8 = 666 CFM_{50} BTL

Formula #3: 1200 x 8 (ceiling height) x .35 x 14.8/60 = 828 CFM_{50} BTL

All of these calculations are less than 960, showing that this house would be loose enough not to require mechanical ventilation. A better alternative would be to tighten up the house further, dropping it below 650 CFM_{50} and then adding mechanical ventilation.

* * *

THE TIGHTNESS of the house can be measured using instrumentation such as a "blower door". Many green building and weatherization programs have criteria for how tight a home should be before mechanical ventilation must be added. This may be a reference to a BTL or to a Minimum Ventilation Rate (MVR). Indiana, for example, sets their MVR at 1,200CFM@50 Pa. (This is the "CFM_{50}" level.) That means that a blower door must be used to exhaust air from the house until the house reaches a negative pressure relative to the outside (with respect to or WRT) of 50 Pascals. If the amount of air flowing through the test fan to accomplish this exceeds 1200 cfm, then, by their criteria, the house is leaky enough not to need additional mechanical ventilation (in their program). Luckily, homes are not being continuously exhausted to this artificially high level, which is used to exaggerate the conditions and to reach a standardized, comparative level. The CFM_{50} level can be converted to a more realistic $CFM_{Natural}$ or CFM_{Nat} level by dividing it by a factor that considers the location or wind conditions and the height of the building known as the "N" or "n" factor. These vary from a low of 9.8 for an exposed three-story house in a cold climate like North Dakota to 29.4 for a well shielded, one-story house in a warm climate like Miami. Dividing the CFM_{50} number by the "n" factor provides CFM_{Nat} or approximately how the air will move through the home under average natural conditions.

For example, a two-story 1,200 CFM_{50} house in Massachusetts that would be considered "normal" in terms of wind exposure would use an "n" factor of 14.8. Its CFM_{Nat} would be 1,200/14.8 or 81, meaning that under average conditions, this house would be leaking 81 cubic feet of air per minute. If the house were tightened up to 900 CFM_{50}, its CFM_{Nat} would be reduced to 900/14.8 or 60 cubic feet per minute. This is under "average" conditions. Much of the time, it would be leaking less than this.

Because it takes such a small amount of pressure to potentially backdraft a combustion appliance, caution should be taken in aggressively tightening up the house and employing mechanical ventilation. It is highly recommended that combustion safety testing be done before, during and after the air sealing/tightening process. The calculated CFM_{Nat} number is an approximation under "average" conditions, meaning that half the time the natural ventilation will be greater than this and half the time it will be less than this. Using a continuous, whole dwelling mechanical ventilation system ensures that some ventilation will happen all the time and is an advisable approach unless the house is obviously too leaky to warrant it.

Chapter 8

Passive Inlets, Outlets, Transfer Grilles and Makeup Air

A wise man once said, "People are systems. They have specific openings for specific purposes. Air for breathing goes in and out of specific, controlled openings not randomly all over the body." Houses are systems and they should have specific openings for specific purposes as well.

Ventilation means exchanging air between the inside and the outside of the house and circulating it around the living spaces. Mechanical equipment only provides part of the solution. Exhaust fans, range hoods, central vacuums, and clothes dryers mechanically exhaust from the house. Fireplaces, water heaters, and furnaces passively exhaust air and pollutants from the house through their chimneys. It is common practice to consider that there will be more than enough leaks and holes in the house to provide an adequate amount of "make-up" air. As homes become tighter, that is not always true.

Getting air in from the outside to the inside and back out to the outside is only part of the challenge. Circulation, moving the air throughout the living spaces, is required to keep the building and the occupants healthy. Ideally, every room would have a correctly placed supply and return for heating and cooling and a second pair for ventilation. That way, adequate circulation could be assured. However, since the object is to circulate fresh air through the rooms, using the rooms as the conduit is a reasonable approach. After all, people don't live in ducting.

Rooms have doors, however, and doors serve as dampers, manually operated blockages to airflow. Doors that are sealed well enough to block the transfer of sound and provide privacy also block the flow of air. The crack under the door is usually only enough to allow the bottom of the door to clear the carpeting and open and close properly. That crack is often relied upon for transferring conditioned air, balancing the pressure between the room and the rest of the house. To do that effectively, the crack needs to be more than a crack.

Over, Under and Through-wall Circulation

Like the ducting design, the circulation issues for ventilation differ from the circulation issues for the HAC system (dropping the 'V' from HVAC). The airflows and pressures created by the HAC system are considerably greater than for ventilation alone. If ventilation has been integrated with the HAC system, then, of course, they have become one and the same. But if the ventilation strategy is to use a separately ducted, positive pressure system or a non-integrated HRV or ERV or some other dedicated ventilation ducted approach, circulation solutions can be different. If the HAC system has a dedicated supply and return in each room, then bypassing the closed door may be limited to ventilation issues. But, as is typical of many HVAC systems, each room has a supply and the return is in the hallway, then the bypass must serve for both ventilation and conditioned air.

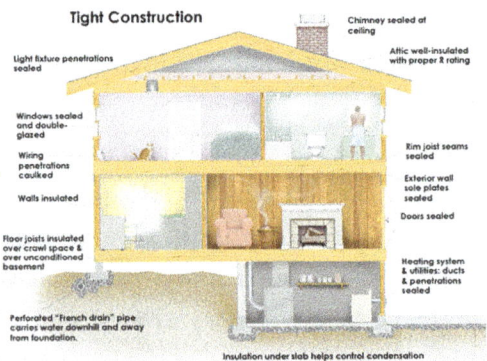

Figure 8.1 Tight Construction Details (Panasonic/Morrissey)

For ventilation alone, the opening between the hall and the room can be fairly small. If the room is being supplied with 30 cubic feet per minute or less, the typical half-inch crack under the door will suffice. A 30-inch wide door with a ½ inch undercut would provide a 15 square inch opening, which would be adequate to keep the pressure in the room below 2 pascals relative to the rest of the house. A door insert (a grille that mounts in the door and blocks the transfer of light or sound) works for just ventilation air pressure relief. The resistance of the grille in a door insert, however, offers much too much resistance for HVAC pressure relief, and since both ventilation air and conditioned air must be circulated, the higher-pressure requirement of the conditioned air must determine the dimensions of the pressure relief.

Both conditioned air and ventilation air will need to bypass the door. The object is to allow the air to flow from the room under, through, over or around the closed door and keep the pressure from one side of the door to the other at 2.5 pascals or less. Ideally, there would be no pressure differential, but that is difficult to achieve.

For flexible "jumper" duct: $diameter = \sqrt{airflow_{delivered}}$

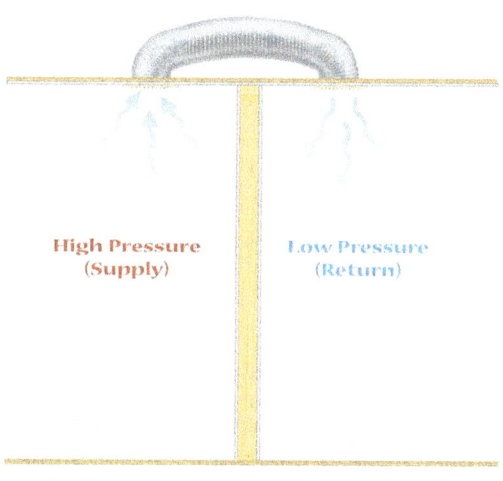

Figure 8.2 Jumper Duct (Morrissey)

To go over the door, from one side of the wall to the other, a "jumper" duct can be used. A jumper duct is simply a piece of ducting that is attached to a "collection box" or boot in the ceiling covered by a grille on one side of the wall to a box in the ceiling also covered by a grille on the other side of the wall. This allows the air to flow, pushed by the pressure imbalance from one side to the other. It also reduces the flow of light and sound, affording some privacy. The simplest approach is to use flexible ducting for this, which, with its rough interior surface, is resistive to easy airflow. The grilles are also barriers to the small pressures referred to here. If just 30 cfm of ventilation air is being delivered to the room, the jumper duct could be constructed of 6" diameter, flexible ducting. If 100 cfm of conditioned air is being delivered to the room as well as 30 cfm of ventilation air, the duct diameter should increase to 12". Tests at the Florida Solar Energy Center have shown that the diameter of the jumper duct should be approximately equivalent to the square root of the delivered airflow to keep the pressure differential below 2.5 Pascals. This takes into account the other components of the system, including the duct boxes and the grilles.

For slot under door: $Area_{slot} = 1/2 \times Airflow_{delivered}$

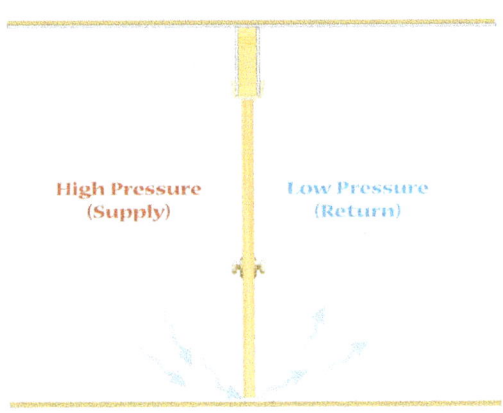

Figure 8.3 Door Undercut (Morrissey)

The slot under the door is simple and doesn't need to be concerned about grille resistance. A one-inch slot under a 30-inch wide door will allow approximately 60 cfm to be delivered to the room and maintain the 2.5 pascal pressure difference. (The same FSEC tests showed that doubling the area of the slot would allow for doubling the airflow.) For 130 cfm, the slot would have to be cut to approximately 2 inches. A slot that large will certainly infringe on privacy and reduce the purpose of closing the door in the first place.

For grille covered opening through-wall: $Area_{opening} = airflow_{delivered}/0.83$

Passive Inlets, Outlets, Transfer Grilles and Makeup Air

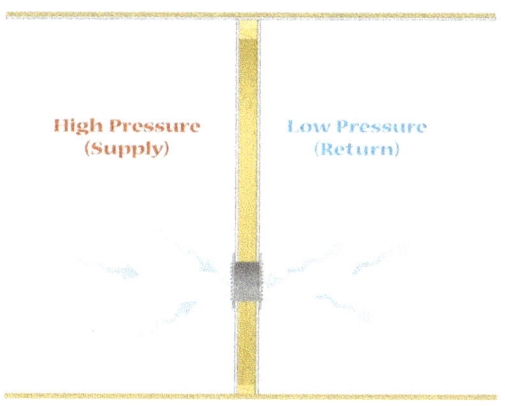

Figure 8.4 Straight Through Pressure Relief (Morrissey)

Going straight through the wall is another approach that provides limited privacy. It is also important for through-wall approaches to have a sleeve that completes the passage from one wall surface to the other otherwise air from the wall cavity will be drawn into the system. Most of the air resistance for the straight-through-the-wall approach will come from the grilles covering the opening. Dividing the airflow by 0.83 provides the area of the opening. Using 130 cfm again, the opening would need to be 156 square inches, perhaps 10" by 15" or 10" by 16" - a large opening.

OFFSET GRILLES ARE an approach that affords some privacy since the hole does not go straight through the wall. The flow, however, will draw cavity air into the system and the maximum flow to keep the pressures below 2.5 pascals is limited to 72 cfm if it is a standard 2 x 4 constructed wall. No matter how big the openings are on either side of the wall, the limiting factor for the flow is the thickness of the cavity. In fact, increasing the openings beyond 112 square inches has negligible impact on the flows in an offset grille arrangement.

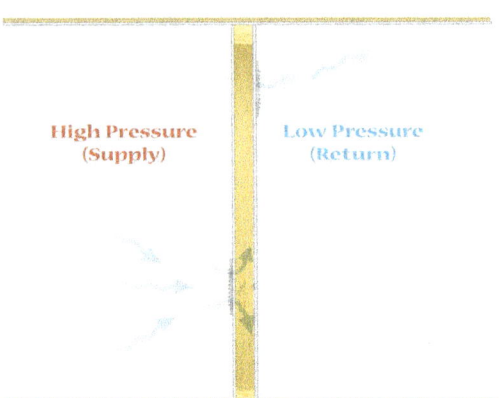

Figure 8.5 Offset Grilles (Morrissey)

Of course, these transfer methods are additive. It is likely that there will be some space under the door. That opening can reduce the size of other approaches that are used. And as stated previously, the smaller airflows and lower pressures involved with ventilation mean smaller relief "holes" can be employed IF ventilation circulation is the only concern.

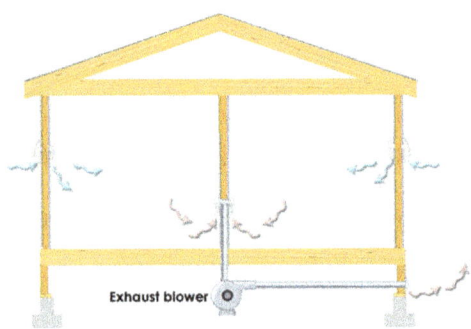

Figure 8.6 Central Exhaust with Passive Inlets (Morrissey)

Inlets and Outlets

Okay. So you go to all this effort to seal up every crack, hole, gap, and chink in the house's envelope and now you need to intentionally make holes in that envelope to let air in. Why not just save all that sealing up time and effort and leave the existing holes? Mainly because all the inadvertent holes and gaps are in uncontrollable places, many in the wrong places, and there are too many of them adding up to a much larger "hole" than is needed for ventilation air.

What you need are affectionately called "smart holes" or trickle vents or devices that are designed to allow a specific amount of air to pass through them no matter what the weather. They often include filters, which will remove the large particles that might be floating around in the outside air.

The performance of trickle vents or passive inlets is affected by unintentional building leakage to the exterior and between living units, the ventilation rates, the control of heating and cooling in the bedrooms, the acoustic performance requirements to minimize outside noise infiltration, the location of the inlet to minimize the perception of drafts, and the design of the inlet itself. Trickle vents and inlets are not stand-alone components and won't function effectively without the rest of the system, particularly in relation to resolving indoor air quality problems.

Bear in mind that these small holes are not designed as make-up air sources for major air sucking appliances and other devices like clothes dryers, range hoods, fireplaces, or wood-stoves. If those devices are activated, they will draw air from any place that is an opening to the outside, but these "smart" holes should <u>not</u> be their primary source of air.

TRICKLE VENT/SMART *Hole Design*

Trickle vents are not simply holes with grilles on either side. They are fairly complex products that have been used for many years in Europe and other parts of the world.

Through-the-wall "passive inlets" include an exterior hood to keep the weather out with critter and insect protection, a through-wall fitting or short duct length that is round or rectangular, an air filter, possibly sound abatement padding, and an interior cover that sometimes includes a means to close the system completely. Some of them have

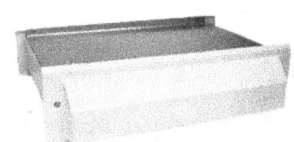

Figure 8.7 Trickle Vent (American Aldes)

humidity-controlled dampers that shut down as the level of relative humidity increases. The systems regulate the amount of air that can pass through them, which can be as low as 10 cfm to not more than 20 cfm.

For trickle vents to work effectively as inlets, the air pressure in the room must be lower than the air pressure outside. The building needs to be tight so that the vents comprise most of the building's leakage. When the building is leaky, the inlets have to be made larger to assure that the airflow through the dedicated inlet supplies most of the air to the room. If the inlets are made too large, the building is much more subject to the vagaries of the wind and stack effect. This becomes less of a problem if the vents are not intended to be associated with a mechanical ventilation system, but are simply a means for adding additional leakage at the windows, allowing the air to flow either way across the openings.

LOCATION

Where the "smart holes" are located will affect how they perform as inlets. Just because a "hole" is supposed to serve as an inlet doesn't mean it will work that way. It will depend on the building pressures described in Chapter 7. These devices are smarter than using a hammer to smash an opening in the wall, but they're still just holes. The laws of stack effect and wind loads still apply.

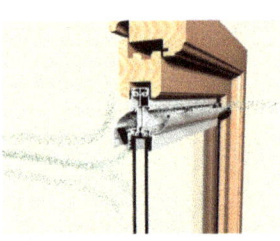

Figure 8.8 Tricke Vent in a Window Frame (Titon)

Ideally, the trickle vents are located in bedrooms where people spend the most time. Air is drawn in from the outside, flowing through the bedroom to the primary ventilation system located near the center of the house. If the "holes" are located high on the walls, the incoming, untempered air enters at a very low flow rate that is barely perceptible by the occupants. It mixes with the room air and enters above their heads.

On a single story home, however, openings in the walls near the ceiling may serve as outlets because of the stack effect.

If the inlets are located on the side of the building facing the prevailing wind, they are more likely to serve their purpose. Air pressing on that side of the house will be forced through the vents, and the internal mechanisms will limit the amount of air that enters.

When trickle vents allow the air to flow out of the building, it is not a disastrous situation since the amount of air that moves through them is limited. It is just another air leak, and it won't be providing the fresh, make-up air that the design requires.

Design and Tempering the Make-up Air

When introducing outside air into the living space, the temperatures will not be the same. When the outside air is warm and humid, it will add to the load of an air conditioning system, but tempering is less critical for comfort than when the outside air is frigid. Make-up air that is added directly to the return side of an air handler will be tempered as it passes through the conditioning elements.

Small amounts of make-up air (20 cfm or less for bedrooms, for example) introduced into the living space at a low velocity and out of the occupied space, will blend with the room air and cold drafts will be avoided.

> HRV/ERVs as whole dwelling ventilation systems temper their own air, but they should not be relied on to provide extra make-up air to the living space. They are designed as "balanced" systems, bringing in the same amount of air as they exhaust. They will not provide "extra" air for other appliances such as range hoods or fireplaces.

Even if the air is tempered, a large volume of outside air flowing into the house will manifest itself as a draft. It is not always easy to find places to locate the openings. Kick spaces in the kitchen may cool occupants' feet. An opening behind a refrigerator will pick up the appliance's heat and may improve its operation.

Maintenance should also be a concern for any mechanical system. If the make-up air system has a filter or a heating element, it must be located in a place where those features can be maintained.

If a large amount of make-up air is required (for range hoods, for example), fan forced tempering will definitely be needed.[1] For commercial applications, several companies manufacture make-up air units, particularly for kitchens. These can have heating or cooling components to temper the thousands of cubic feet per minute flowing back into the building. The following table describes the amount of electric heat required to raise the outdoor temperature for different airflows at different temperature differentials. For example,

---

1. There are a number of companies that make tempered make-up air systems that can be found in Appendix F.

if it is 20°F outside and you want to raise the temperature to 60°F, 1,000 watts is needed for an 80 cfm system. A 400 cfm would require 5,000 watts (5kW).

Watts	50 deg. difference	40 deg. difference	30 deg. difference
1,000	60 cfm	80 cfm	100 cfm
2,500	160 cfm	200 cfm	260 cfm
5,000	320 cfm	400 cfm	525 cfm
10,000	630 cfm	785 cfm	1050 cfm
15,000	945 cfm	1185 cfm	1580 cfm

Table 8.1 Electric Heat for Conditioning Make-up Air

An air duct bringing combustion air to a fireplace is generally not fan forced, relying solely on the stack effect to draw air through the ducting and through the combustion chamber and up the chimney. When the fire is burning, the tempering of the incoming air is occurring. When the fire is not burning, that duct is a conduit from the outside; air will leak into it and out of it depending on the pressures in the house. The flow may be small enough to be unnoticeable. (But in terms of energy efficiency of the building, these make-up air ducts can be a significant part of the total leakage component of the house.)

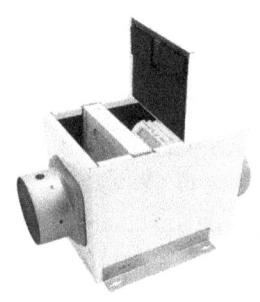

Figure 8.9 Make-up Air System with Filter and Heating Element (Air King)

Clothes dryers draw a significant amount of air out of the house (commonly between 100 and 200 cfm). Gas dryers also need air for combustion. A make-up air vent near the dryer (even underneath it), can improve the efficiency of the drying cycle. A pressure switch controlling a motorized damper can close off that intake line when the dryer is not operating.

Note that the International Mechanical Code (IMC 504.6) regarding clothes dryer exhaust states that "Installations exhausting more than 200 cfm (0.09 m³/s) shall be provided with make-up air. Where a closet is designed for the installation of a clothes dryer, an opening having an area of not less than 100 square inches (0.645 m²) shall be provided in the closet enclosure or make-up air shall be provided by other approved means." And for range hoods (IMC 505.2), "Exhaust hood systems capable of exhausting in excess of 400 cfm (0.19 m³/s) shall be provided with make-up air at a rate approximately equal to the exhaust air rate. Such make-up air systems shall be equipped with a means of closure and shall be automatically controlled to start and operate simultaneously with the exhaust system." Dampers on these systems must be motorized and not rely solely on pressure differentials to operate because those differentials are too small.

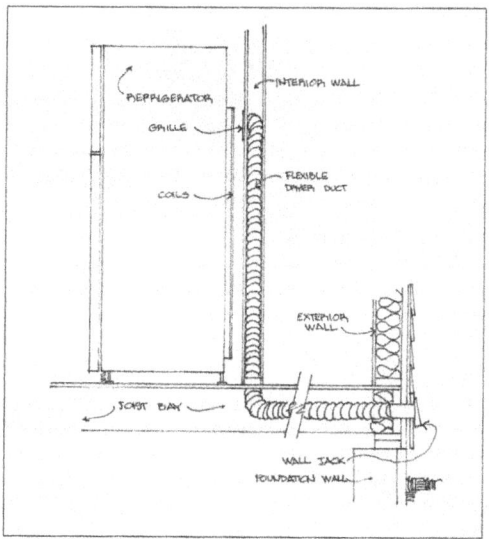

Figure 8.11 Make-up Air Behind Refrigerator (Ben Nickerson/Fine Homebuilding)

If the makeup air comes in behind the refrigerator, the waste heat from the coils will preheat it and if the occupant feels cold air around the base of the refrigerator, they might think that it's a good thing! You would want to use something better than dryer ducting and think about how much airflow you need. Four-inch ducting will be restrictive. Remember too, that this duct will be open all the time unless there is a motorized damper.

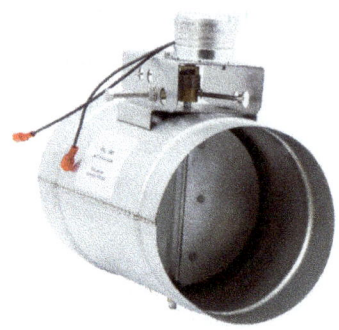

Figure 8.12 Motorized Damper (Air King)

Chapter 9

Commissioning and Testing

Flow Testing Processes and Equipment

The only way to be sure an installed system is operating the way it was conceived and designed on paper or computer is to test it. Anything else is just a guess. All of the estimates of equivalent duct length and laboratory testing are just estimates and only approximate the actual installed conditions. The fact is that in a real house, construction elements are not always in exactly the spots that they were called out to be on the plans (if there are plans). There will inevitably be places where the ducting has to make additional twists and turns to get to the outside of the building. There will be places where someone just may have stepped on a piece of flexible ducting in the attic or could not make a connection air tight.

Measuring *Airflow*

The most important element to test in any ventilation system is the airflow. Because residential flow testing is not a requirement in the United States, the equipment has been adapted from commercial equipment, designed for higher rates of airflow than are seen in most residential applications. Flows in homes as low as 30 cfm are difficult to measure partially because the flow measuring device has to be in the air stream and anything that gets in the way of the airflow will affect the airflow.

Processes can be as simple as holding up a hand and feeling the flow of air or the use of "particle streak-velocimetry" or tracer gas to actually "see" the movement of air. In measuring the performance of a ventilation system, we are concerned with the flow of air through the grille or fan that is in the room. Flow measurements can certainly be made in the ducting and should be for heat or energy recovery ventilators in order to balance them. Measuring the flow in the ducting requires making a hole for the probe or adding a small section of ducting in which to install a "flow grid".

<u>Pieces of paper</u> - Paper works as a gross indicator of airflow through an exhaust fan. As the air flows up to the fan opening, it can draw paper up to the grille. If it is strong enough, it will hold the paper over the grille opening. Different weights of paper can indicate different airflows. At least you'll know if air is moving through the fan. You won't know if it is flowing out of the building.

Material	Flow that draws it up to the grille
Single ply toilet paper	> 30 cfm
Double ply toilet papers	> 60 cfm
"20 pound" copier paper	> 110 cfm

Table 9.1 Fundamental Airflow Measurement

NOTE that this is a gross approach, only slightly more accurate than a "calibrated hand", and should not be used for anything more than a relative measurement of airflow. However, if the fan can't lift any of these papers, it is pretty clear that something needs to be done to improve the flow.

<u>Garbage bags</u>[1] – The Canadian Mortgage and Housing Corporation (CMHC) determined that air moving-out or evacuating a space could deflate a pliable bag, like a garbage bag (for example a "Glad" 66 x 91 cm). The time that it takes to accomplish that is parallel to the amount of air that the ventilation device is moving air out of the space. The opposite is true for a supply

---

1. http://www.home-inspectors.com/Testing_Airflow.pdf

ventilation system, where the air will inflate the bag. Tape the opening of the garbage bag to an expanded wire hanger, scoop up the air, hold the opening over the grille of the fan, and time the deflation. The deflation time is an indicator of the airflow rate: 1 second = 50 cfm, 5 seconds = 30 cfm, 12–13 seconds = 10 cfm. Higher flow rates happen in a fraction of a second and are very difficult to time. Although this approach sounds crude, it is surprisingly accurate and certainly inexpensive.

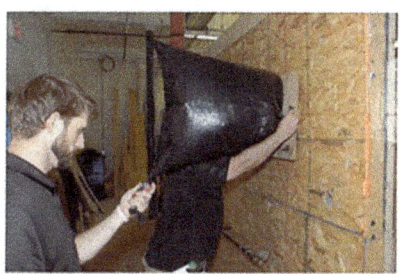

Figure 9.1 Capture Bag (PHR)

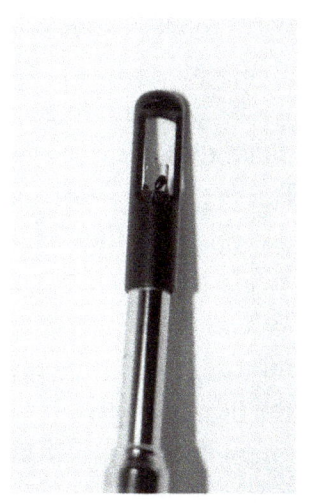

Figure 9.2 Hot Wire Anemometer Tip (PHR)

Hot-wire anemometers – When air moves across a heated wire (commonly tungsten), the wire seeks to maintain its temperature at a rate that is relative to the airflow. The heated wire is extremely small, so the flow is a measurement at that point. To get the total flow across a fan opening or duct, multiple measurements need to be made and averaged out. The result is a measurement of the velocity of airflow (feet per minute (fpm)) not volume of airflow (cubic feet per minute (cfm)), which is calculated from the average velocity multiplied by the area of the opening. The area of the opening must be calculated carefully, removing the area blocked by the ribs of a grille, for example, which can be as much as 50% of the opening. Some of these devices can accept a vent area and calculate the volume of flow. Hot-wire anemometers can sense flows from 0 to 10,000 feet per minute

Vane anemometers – A vane anemometer is a small fan blade that spins when it is positioned in an airstream. The more air that moves across it, the faster the fan spins. Mini-vane anemometers can be as small as ½ in diameter. Measurements with these devices are like measurements with a hot-wire anemometer - a single point. Multiple measurements need to be made and averaged and multiplied by the area of the opening to convert from feet per minute to cubic feet per minute.

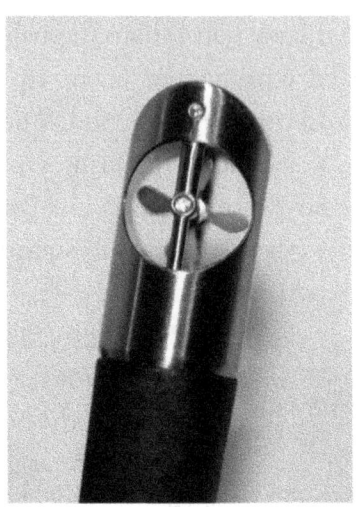

Figure 9.3 Mini-vane Anemometer (PHR)

Large vane anemometer that can typically measure flows from 50 to 6,000 fpm can be purchased with hoods that will cover the fan opening and internally convert from velocity to volume. They are not dependent on the density of the air or compensation because of air temperature, humidity, or atmospheric pressure to generate an accurate measurement. Every effort is made to make these devices as low resistant as possible to spinning in the air stream. But it takes at least some energy away from the flow being measured to make the blade of the measuring device spin. At the same time, the body of the measuring device is in the air stream and that also affects the flow of air. When there is a need to measure flows as small as 5 or 10 cubic feet per minute, these impediments have more impact than in an application where the flows can vary by 100 or 200 cfm and be acceptable. The accuracy of vane anemometers is also affected by the angle they are held to the direction of the flow. At these low flows, it is important to hold the device as close to perpendicular to the flow as possible so that the vanes will spin with the greatest accuracy.

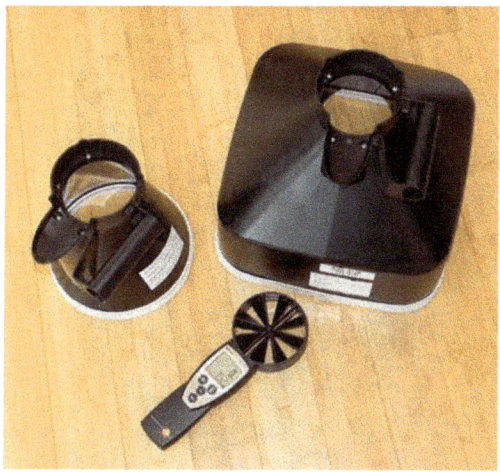

Figure 9.4 Large Vane Anemometer (PHR)

<u>Flow hoods</u>[2] – Flow hoods are collapsible, fabric hoods which serve as a flow capture device that are large enough to cover the grille with an internal flow measurement grid, hot-wire, pressure drop, plate deflection, or vane design and generally include a built-in digital meter. Small residential grilles often cause enough turbulence that reduces the accuracy of these devices. There is a wide range of issues that affect the performance of these devices on residential applications, including the placement of the hood over the grille being measured. It is important to center the grille in the hood opening and use as short a capture hood as possible.

---

2. "Evaluation of flow hood measurements for residential register flows", Walker, Wray, et al, LBNL, September, 2001

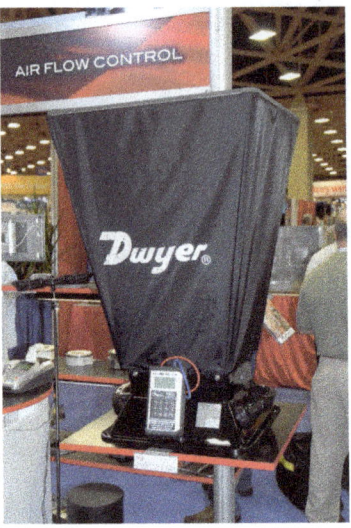

Figure 9.5 Flow Capture Hood (PHR)

Exhaust Fan Flow Hood[3] – Standard *pressure pans* are primarily used to cover openings and measure pressure drop or losses through the ducting and do not allow any flow of air through them.

An exhaust fan flow hood is different. It is a box with an adjustable or calibrated opening can measure the flow through a fan. The airflow through a known sized hole can be calculated if the pressure differences are known using the formula:

$$Q = 1.07 \times A \times \sqrt{\Delta P}$$

where
Q = airflow in cfm
A = the area of the hole in square inches
= the difference in pressure in Pascals

---

3. Note that this does not refer to the "pressure pan" sold by the Energy Conservatory used to measure duct leakage and cannot be used to measure flow.

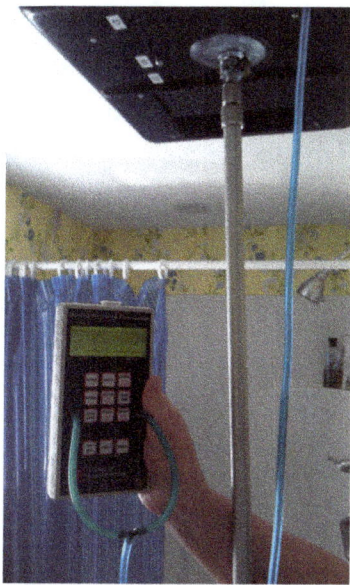

Figure 9.6 Exhaust Fan Flow Box with Manometer (PHR)

Devices that are specifically made for this purpose include a fabricated box with an adjustable, calibrated opening, and an attachment for a hose that is connected to a digital manometer. They can measure flows between 10 and 125 cfm and often include a pole to hold the box up on the ceiling, covering an exhaust fan opening. A dual channel manometer should be connected to monitor both the pressure and the flow simultaneously. If the pressure is too high, the accuracy of the reading will be degraded.

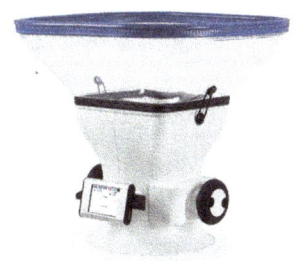

Figure 9.7 Powered Flow Hood (Retrotec)

Duct testers (powered flow hood) – Duct testers are calibrated fans that can pressurize a duct system to measure how leaky it is. The same system can be used to accurately measure the flow through a ventilation fan. The ducting from the calibrated fan is installed over the grille or opening to the fan being tested. The flow through the calibrated fan is increased until there is no pressure difference between the two fans. At that point, the flow through the calibrated fan will be equal to the fan under test, and the flow reading can be read directly on the digital manometer or pressure gauge. This eliminates all the effects of the testing device and is a very accurate means of getting an accurate flow measurement, even at very low flows. Stand-alone powered flow hoods[4] can also be extremely effective and accurate devices and do not require the bulky, umbilical duct connection.

Installed System Testing and Balancing

Although they are known as "exhaust only" or "supply only" ventilation systems, that obviously doesn't work based on the fundamental principle of "one cubic foot in equals one cubic foot out". Even though the mechanical system is only on one side of the equation, the air is dragged in or forced out from somewhere to make up the balance. So if you are testing an exhaust-centered system, for example, and you don't get the flow you expected, you might try opening a window and testing again, (although it is far more likely that the ductwork, grilles, and the rest of the system itself is the culprit). Although it would be a remarkably tight house, you might notice a difference in airflow, in which case you might have to consider adding a second mechanical system to balance things out. Building codes that require very low air change rates create tight houses, and tight houses restrict the amount of air that flows in or flows out of them.

For an existing ventilation system, the first step is to review the installation to determine what sort of system it is—supply-centered, exhaust-centered, Heat Recovery Ventilator (HRV), Energy Recovery Ventilator (ERV)—and perform some common sense, visual checks to make sure that the system has been installed in such a way that it will function as designed and as required for the application. It would be a true waste of time to do a series of performance checks, only to find that the outlet vent had been stuffed full of socks! A physical inspection of the system will tell you a lot before you start measuring airflow, and you need to know how the system was supposed to work and how to turn it on and off before you can test it.

---

4. https://retrotec.com/flow-finder-mk2.html

How is it ducted? Is it integrated with the HVAC system or does it stand-alone? If it is an outside feed to the return side of the HVAC system, is there a motorized damper in the line to the outside? Is there a flow regulator that will allow only a defined amount of air into the system? (A feed into the return side will make the system essentially a positive pressure ventilation system.)

If it is an HRV or ERV, does it have its own fully ducted distribution system or is it integrated with the air handler? Check the ducts to and from the outside and make sure that they are open and clear of debris. Make sure that they are not blocked on the outside or clogged up on the inside. Make sure that during the original installation, the openings into the HRV or ERV device were properly opened (these devices sometimes allow for a variety of installation configurations and a variety of openings through their housings). Make sure that the ducting from a bath fan runs all the way to the outside and that birds have not nested in the vent or that the uninsulated ducting in the attic is not full of water from condensation. Make sure that ducting running across joists is fully supported, not sagging down in an undulating wave across the attic floor. Check to see if all the duct connections or joints are tightly sealed with mastic or tape (UL DC181B-FX) and not hanging off.

How is the system controlled? Is it designed to run on occupancy like a bathroom light switch or is it designed to turn on periodically throughout the day, or is it designed to run continuously? If it is coupled to the air handler, there may be a control that monitors the operating time of the air handler to periodically open the outside vent and run the air handler. HRVs and ERVs are sometimes "hard-wired" to run continuously, with no control switch or they may have a power switch that is near the fan unit. They may also have indoor air quality or humidity controls that will boost their airflow if the humidity or gases in the house increase.

Exhaust-centered or supply-centered systems may have associated "pin" timers that would be set up to operate the fan at particular times during the day.

After performing a visual inspection of the system and determining its desired operating configuration, flow measuring and system balancing can be done. Note that in measuring the flow through an exhaust-centered or supply-centered system, the measurements are being made on only one side of the system. These systems rely on leakage either in or out. Their effectiveness at accomplishing their purpose will be affected by other devices operating in the house. Making flow measurements of an exhaust fan in a tight house with the clothes dryer running will reduce the flow through the exhaust fan because both devices will be competing for the same make-up air. To get a reasonable estimate of a particular device, other ventilation related devices should be turned off while the testing is taking place. That means shutting off the dryer, air handler, and combustion appliances that rely on house air for moving the air up the chimney. If you do shut off or subjugate such devices, be sure to liberate them by turning them back on before leaving the house being tested. You might consider leaving your car or truck keys on the kitchen table or on top of the water heater so you can't leave without turning things back on.

* * *

Setting up the House for Testing

The house is designed and built to affect the flow of air into and out of it, therefore before measuring the flow through a ventilation system, the house needs to be set up so measurements are standardized and repeatable. No matter what the type of ventilation system is or whether it is purposed to be a whole dwelling or local exhaust ventilation system, the house must be set up the same way prior to testing.

1. Open all interior doors in the house;
2. Doors and windows to the exterior must be closed;
3. Fireplace dampers must be closed;
4. The air handlers and all exhaust fans, including the clothes dryer and central vacuum (any device that will affect the pressure inside the house with respect to the outside) must be turned off.

Flow testing an exhaust-centered system

Some sort of measuring device will be required to ascertain a numerical rate of flow through a fan or grille attached to a remotely mounted fan. Determining whether air is moving at all can be as simple as using a tissue, smoke pencil, or back of the hand.

Hot-wire or mini-vane measurement

If the measurement is made with a single point device like a mini-vane or hot-wire anemometer, the reading will be in feet per minute (fpm) which must then be converted to cubic feet per minute (cfm) by multiplying the velocity by the area of the opening.

$$Q = V \times A$$

where:

Q = the airflow in cubic feet per minute (cfm)

V = average velocity of the airflow in feet per minute (fpm)

A = cross sectional area of the duct in square feet (ft^2)

To determine the average velocity, divide the opening into equal areas and sample the velocity in each area. If the velocity profile is relatively flat, only a few areas need to be sampled. A traverse across the duct in two dimensions will define the uniformity of the airflow. If there are significant variations, use the mean velocity between the two extreme points. The velocity profile is generally more uniform on suction (exhaust) openings.

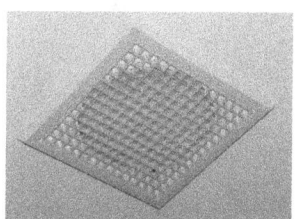

Figure 9.8 "Egg Crate" Ventilation Grille (PHR)

The air will move into the grille or fan at different rates at different points across the face of the grille, so multiple measurement need to be taken, averaged, and then multiplied by the area to come up with a reasonable flow measurement. For a surface mounted grille taking nine measurements will give a good approximation of the flow: the middle, the edge at four opposed compass points, and four points halfway between the middle and the four compass points.[5]

Calculating the actual open area of the grille is not always easy. It can vary between 40% and 90% of their face area.

APPROXIMATE FREE AREAS of different grille designs:

- "Egg Crate" (similar to the grilles in fluorescent light fixtures) - up to 90% open
- Pressed steel (metal grilles with straight vanes) - up to 75% open

---

5. A good discussion of measuring the airflow in ducts, pipes, hoods and stacks can be found at https://www.omega.com/en-us/resources/how-precise-and-accurate-are-air-flow-measurement-instruments

- Fixed Louvre (these can be metal or plastic with angled vanes, the plastic vanes are thicker and more restrictive) - 30-70% open
- Double deflection (vanes pointing in both directions) - up to 60% open

Although these are reasonable approximations, actual measurement of the particular grille in question would be required to get an accurate opening area to refine the accuracy of the measurement and calculation. Calculate the face area of the grille (length times width or area of the circle) and multiply by the opening percentage (for example–pressed steel at 75%) to get the "clear" area (net free area or nfa). Multiply that times the average velocity of flow reading to arrive at a cfm measurement through the fan.

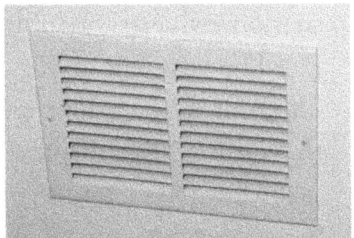

Figure 9.9 Presse Metal Grille (PHR)

Inputting the area into a digital mini vane or hot-wire anemometer can provide a remarkably accurate measurement of flow without transverse measurements, averaging or carefully calculating the open area of the grille. Simply inputting the area of the ducting behind the fan or grille may be enough. In some tests, entering the actual open area of the grille, which was approximately one half the area of the duct, provided flow measurements that were one half the actual flows as measured with a powered anemometer. The problem, of course, is knowing when to enter the open area and when to use the ducting dimensions. If high accuracy is required, taking several measurements with several devices will provide the best information.

If laboratory flow for the model of the fan can be checked against this tested reading, a level of reasonability can be achieved. For example, if the fan is rated to move 120 cfm at 0.1 iwg and the reading is 150 cfm, the calculations need to be rechecked. Installed system performance for most bath fans (because of the resistance of the ducting, etc.) is commonly about one half of their rated performance, so a 60 cfm measurement of a 120 cfm fan would not be out of line.

Flow measuring devices with capture hoods

Devices like large vane anemometers that have capture hoods can provide a more accurate reading because the need for multiple measurements is removed, the capture hood allows all the air flowing through the fan to flow through the hood, and the conversion from velocity (fpm) to volume (cfm) can be automatic. Determining the actual open area of the grille, however, may still affect the accuracy of the calculation.

Using a powered flow-testing device will provide the most accurate flow measurement. The powered flow hood completely covers the fan opening. The flow through the powered flow hood is increased until there is no pressure difference between the air going into the fan under test and the room. At that point, the flow through the powered flow hood will equal the flow through the fan under test. This approach removes any impact that the flow-measuring device might have from the equation.[6]

Exhaust-centered systems summary

The primary purpose for a large majority of exhaust systems has been to ventilate a bathroom or kitchen, serving as a local exhaust system, removing pollutants close to the source. These systems can also be used for whole dwelling ventilation. When they are used for whole dwelling ventilation, they need to have clear access to the rest of the volume in the house. But when they are only used for local exhaust, it is common (particularly in a bathroom) to keep the bathroom door closed.

Testing bathroom-type or single port or multi-port in-line fans for whole dwelling ventilation:

1. Open all interior doors in the house;
2. Doors and windows to the exterior must be closed;

---

6. The Energy Conservatory's Duct Blaster® can be used for this process very effectively. Refer to the Duct Blaster Manual, Chapter 13, Section 13.2. https://energyconservatory.com/support/minneapolis-duct-blaster-user-guide/

3. Fireplace dampers must be closed;
4. The air handlers and all exhaust fans, including the clothes dryer and central vacuum (any device that will affect the pressure inside the house with respect to the outside) must be turned off.
5. The door to the room under test must be open[7];
6. Measure the flow with the appropriate tool.

* * *

TESTING BATHROOM-TYPE *or single port or multi-port in-line fans for local exhaust ventilation*:

1. Doors and windows to the exterior in the room being tested must be closed;
2. The door to the room under test must be closed;
3. Measure the flow with the appropriate tool.

Flow testing supply-centered systems

Supply-centered systems pressurize the building. They can be stand-alone devices delivering air to single or multiple points or they can be ducts from the outside that supply air directly into the air handler, using that system to circulate the air throughout the house.

If the system supplies air to the air handler through a duct from the outside, the flow could be measured from the outside of the house. Passive supply-centered systems don't have their own fans, so the flow is started by turning on the air handler. Make sure that if there is a motorized damper in the inlet pipe, it is open and measure the flow at the hood on the outside of the house. It may be difficult to get an accurate reading from the outside of the house if the inlet is near the top of the house and the siding does not allow a good seal around the edges of the flow hood because of the ridges in the clapboard or shingles. Readings on the outside of the house will also be affected by wind and weather.

---

7. It is common to close the bathroom door while the bathroom is occupied. However, if the bathroom fan has been designated as the whole-dwelling exhaust fan, then the bathroom door must be open for testing. The position of the bathroom door (as well as the rest of the house) must be done consistently to provide consistent results.

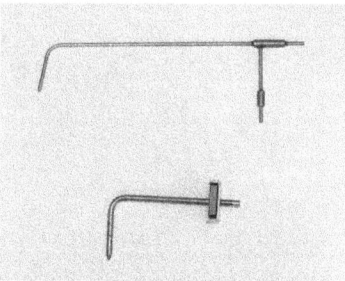

Figure 9.10 Pitot Tube and Static Pressure Probe (PHR)

A second approach is to drill a hole in the ducting that leads from the outside and use a hot wire or mini-vane anemometer to take a series of readings across the duct, averaged and multiplied by the area to come up with a cfm volume measurement. The hole should be drilled away from any sources of turbulence, like elbows or dampers (four feet if possible). At least five measurements should be made across the duct—against the wall, halfway between the wall and the middle, in the middle, halfway between the middle and the opposite wall, and at the opposite wall. Be sure that the hot-wire or mini vane is as perpendicular to the flow as possible. New mini-vane anemometers, however, are fairly tolerant of yaw and pitch in facing the flow. Angle changes of up to 10% will result in less than 1% error, which is certainly acceptable in residential ventilation measurements.

A third approach would be to use a pitot tube or averaging flow station and a digital or analog manometer. A pitot tube is an 'L' shaped pipe that has a small hole at the end of the 'L' for measuring *total* pressure and small holes on the sides of the 'L' for measuring *static* pressure. At the top of the 'L' there is a connection for reading the *total* pressure, and near the top of the 'L' at the side there is a connection for reading the *static* pressure of the air moving through the duct.[8] The two connections are made to the two ports on the manometer, and the result is a measurement of the "velocity pressure".

Digital manometers like the Energy Conservatory's DG-700 or DG1000 or Retrotec's DM32X can be connected directly to the Pitot tube or Averaging Flow Station and will calculate the velocity (fpm) of airflow directly using the equation:

---

8. Note that velocity pressure cannot be measured directly. It can be calculated from the equation: Velocity pressure = Total Pressure – Static Pressure

$$V = 1096.2 \times \left(V_p / 0.075\right)^{0.50}$$

where:
V = velocity of the airflow in feet per minute (fpm)
V_p = the velocity pressure in inches of water gauge
0.075 is in pounds per cubic foot (density of air at sea level)

THE RESULTING velocity measurement is then multiplied by the area of the duct to arrive at a flow measurement.

Refer to the RedCalc tool for pitot tubes, plugging in the necessary factors from the pitot tube manufacturer.[9]

* * *

A FOURTH APPROACH and perhaps the most accurate way is to drill a hole in the duct as you would for the hot wire or pitot tube testing, and measure the "operating static pressure" in the duct. This is like measuring the pressure in a room by pushing the hose under the door. Once this pressure measurement has been made and recorded, the duct should be disconnected from the return plenum and connected to a calibrated fan or duct-testing device. Increase the flow through the duct tester until the same pressure with respect to the room pressure is achieved. At that point, the flow through the calibrated fan will be the same as the flow through the duct when it is attached to the air handler. And don't forget to reconnect the duct to the air handler.

Supply-centered systems summary

Supply-centered systems pressurize the house. They primarily apply to cooling dominated climates. These systems put the house under positive pressure and force the air out through cracks in the structure. A low volume of mechanically driven supply air is provided to spaces where people spend the most time, such as bedrooms.

. . .

---

9. https://www.redcalc.com/pitot-tube-airflow/

TESTING an in-line supply-only fan for whole dwelling ventilation:

1. Open all interior doors in the house;
2. Doors and windows to the exterior must be closed;
3. Fireplace dampers must be closed;
4. The air handlers and all exhaust fans, including the clothes dryer and central vacuum (any device that will affect the pressure inside the house with respect to the outside) must be turned off;
5. Prepare a hole in the supply duct on the low pressure side of the fan;
6. Using a pitot tube or averaging flow station inserted into the intake duct on the low pressure side of the fan, measure the pressure and calculate the airflow.

AN ALTERNATIVE (same house setup as above). The following process uses a calibrated fan/flow measuring device to temporarily simulate the flow:

1. Prepare a hole in the duct on the low pressure side of the supply fan;
2. Turn on the supply fan;
3. Insert a static pressure probe into the duct and measure and record the static pressure;
4. Disconnect the outside air duct where it connects to the fan;
5. Connect the outside air duct to a calibrated fan such as a duct tester so that the duct can be depressurized;
6. Use the duct tester to bring the pressure in the outside air duct back to the same pressure measured in Step 3;
7. Record the measured flow through the duct tester. This is equivalent to the flow through the supply fan and would equal the whole dwelling supply ventilation;
8. Restore the connections when the measurement is complete.

An outside air connection to the return side of an air handler can provide fresh air through the air handler when the air handler blower is running. Some of these systems include a control that will cycle the air handler on periodically to meet the ventilation requirement. Some of these systems also include a motorized damper to keep the outside air supply closed when ventilation air is not required.

TESTING a supply-only system connected to the return side of an air handler:

1. Open all interior doors in the house;
2. Doors and windows to the exterior must be closed;
3. Fireplace dampers must be closed;
4. The air handlers and all exhaust fans, including the clothes dryer and central vacuum (any device that will affect the pressure inside the house with respect to the outside) must be turned off.
5. Motorized dampers in the outdoor air supply duct must be open;
6. Prepare a hole in the outside air supply duct on the low pressure side of the fan;
7. Turn on the air handler and using a pitot tube or averaging flow station inserted into the intake duct on the low-pressure side of the fan, measure the pressure and calculate the airflow.

An alternative (same house setup as above). The following process uses a calibrated fan/flow measuring device to temporarily simulate the flow:

1. Prepare a hole in the outside air supply duct on the low pressure side of the fan;
2. Turn on the air handler;
3. Insert a static pressure probe into the duct and measure and record the static pressure;
4. Disconnect the outside air duct where it connects to the return duct;
5. Connect the outside air duct to a calibrated fan such as a duct tester so that the duct can be depressurized;
6. Use the duct tester to bring the pressure in the outside air duct back to the same pressure measured in Step 3;
7. Record the measured flow through the duct tester. This is equivalent to the flow through the supply fan.
8. Restore the connections when the measurement is complete.

Flow testing balanced systems

Balanced systems must be tested for both the air coming in and the air going out. They rely on mechanical devices to move the air in both directions so both mechanical devices must be doing the same work: they must be balanced!

Appendix H details testing and balancing HRV and ERV systems.

Note that a "balanced system" does not just have to be a single package system like an HRV or ERV. A supply-centered system, like a controlled supply into an air handler, can be combined with an exhaust-centered system like a central exhaust fan to operate as a balanced mechanical ventilation system. It is important to match the flows on the two systems so that they work in harmony. It is also important to use a control strategy so that the two systems will work together.

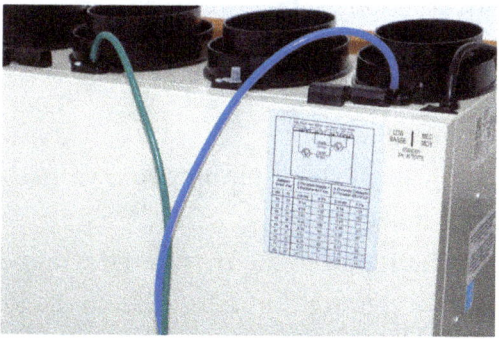

Figure 9.11 HRV Flow Measuring Taps (Fantech)

Using an Averaging Flow Station (AFS) to measure airflow

An averaging flow sensor is a type of pitot tube. It has taps for two pressure hoses. The upstream port (H) senses *total pressure*. The downstream port (L) senses *static pressure*. The difference between these is the *velocity pressure*. The sensor inside the duct has openings on both the upstream and the downstream sides. The velocity pressure can determine the airflow velocity in feet per minute (fpm) and converted to provide airflow volume (cfm). The square root of the velocity pressure times the constant (253.29) equals the velocity of

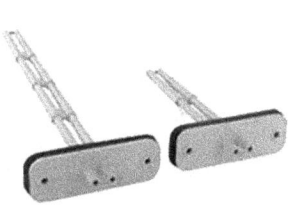

the airflow in feet per minute and multiplying that by the area of the duct provides the cubic feet per minute (cfm).

Note: Refer to https://www.redcalc.com/pitot-tube-airflow/ 4" Sensor K factor = 1.32, 6" sensor K factor = 1.39

Figure 9.12 Averaging Flow Stations (Dwyer)

INSTALLATION:

1. If possible, install the AFS horizontally to assure accurate velocity reading;
2. Install in a duct section that will provide a smooth flow of air - at least 2x duct diameters downstream from a hard elbow (8" for a 4" AFS, 12" for a 6" AFS);
3. Drill a 7/8" hole in the duct;
4. Attach the AFS using (2) self-tapping screws inserted into the 3/16" mounting holes;
5. Attach the H (High) port to the Input on the manometer;
6. Attach the L (Low) port to the Reference on the manometer;
7. Reading will be the VP (velocity pressure).

Air movement through the duct measured with the AFS:

- VP = TP - SP (ΔP in Pascals)
- FPM (velocity) = VP x 253.29
- CFM (volume) = A x FPM

Where:
VP = velocity pressure in Pascals
TP = total pressure in Pascals
SP = static pressure in Pascals
FPM = feet per minute

CFM = cubic feet per minute
A = area of the duct in square feet
4" diameter duct = 0.087 ft2
6" diameter duct = 0.196 ft2

Commissioning and owner education

Ventilation systems in homes can make a great deal of difference to health and comfort of the occupants and the durability of the building itself, but only if they are running and only if they are operating effectively. There is absolutely no point in a beautifully designed and installed ventilation system if it shut off or defeated because the occupant of the house doesn't understand it.

Commissioning is the process that is used in commercial applications to make sure that installed systems work as they are supposed to work when the building is completed. The same process can be used for a residential application. With a new home, there are two steps. One is making sure the systems work, and the second is getting the owner to understand what they are doing, how they work, and how to maintain them. Good car dealers will carefully go over the systems in a new car when they transfer ownership. It is amazing how little new homeowners know about the systems in their homes.

As noted repeatedly in this book, the home should be reviewed as a system because everything should work effectively together and not interfere with each other. This is a book about residential ventilation systems, however. Commissioning the ventilation system essentially means making sure that it will work as it has been designed and installed.

Ideally, all elements of the ventilation system should be documented from the concept and design to the installation and commissioning. That document should list the designer and installer names and contact information and the equipment that was used, when it was installed, how much air it should move, the system's performance on installation, and all the information necessary to effectively maintain it. If that documentation exists, it is simple to review the components.

Reviewing the system as described previously is the first step. Simply making sure that the fans run and move air and the air moves from the inside to the outside of the house (and is not vented into the attic) is essential. The controls should work as they have been designed to work, boosting the flow, or activating the flow on motion, humidity, pressure, gases, or time. Timers should be programmed. If they have backup batteries, they should be fresh. (It is not uncommon during the construction process to activate and program timers and then shut the power off to the building for an extended time, longer than the backup batteries can handle.)

For HRV/ERVs, the connections to and from the outside should be checked to make sure they are not blocked. (It is not uncommon for the connections inside the exchanger box to be blocked.) The filters should be in place and clean. The core should be in place and clean. The controls should all be functional. (The installation manuals for these products have a great deal of helpful information on installation and testing. If there are questions, contact the installer or the manufacturer. They want their systems to work well, and they want the owners to be satisfied. They know how important word-of-mouth advertising is.)

A room-by-room check of air flowing into and out of the grilles can be done with a tissue or a smoke pencil or even a sensitive hand. Supply air should not be delivered at a rate that will cause uncomfortable drafts on the room occupants if it is cold. If necessary, redirect the flows.

Check the condensation drain and the drain tubing.

After making sure the systems are running correctly, a walk-through with the homeowner will assist them in understanding what the systems are, how they work, and how to maintain them. There are so many systems in a house that the care and feeding of the ventilation system may play a very minor role in the homeowner's mind and memory, and they may not even know that something has gone wrong. It is the out-of-sight out-of-mind scenario. They want it to work, and they don't want to think about it.

> Take, for example, setting a *dehumidistat*. Relative humidity is a difficult concept to begin with. Understanding that 75% RH is not the same as 75° F is not intuitive. Raising the set point on a *dehumidistat* will allow the humidity in the house to increase before the controlled device is activated. Raising the set point on a *humidistat* will allow the controlled device to run longer before it is deactivated, adding more humidity to the air. The ideal relative humidity levels in house are between 35% and 55% RH. They can be a bit lower during the winter and higher in the warmer weather.

An exhaust-only system like a bathroom fan, either runs or it doesn't. Pretty simple. But the fans are so quiet now that it is difficult to tell even in a quiet house whether they are working. The homeowner needs to understand how important it is that the exhaust-centered fan is for the air quality in their home and periodically check with a tissue or some other means that it is still running. Removing the grille to clean it is a reasonable way to accomplish this as well.

Sometimes a more dramatic demonstration of the relationship of the ventilation system to the air quality is required. A theatrical smoke generator in the garage is a dramatic way to show how the air flows from the garage into the house, through the duct systems, and is fully distributed.

A small humidity recording data logger (like the Hobo)[10] with the ventilation system off for a few days can provide a clear printout of the effect of air movement on humidity build-up. These devices are quite small and can be left in several places in the home, downloaded, and graphically printed out.

There are also companies like AirAdvice[11] or Aircuity[12] or HomeAirCheck[13] that will provide a multi-contaminant logger that will provide a complete analysis of the pollutants in the home.

Sometimes it takes more than just knowing that the ventilation system is running to convince the occupant of its importance. And what about the next owner of the house? Leaving documentation that can be passed along that can also serve as a maintenance log will serve as an ongoing reminder.

Product Testing and Laboratories

It is simple enough to know whether a fan is moving any air. It is a different thing to know how much air it is moving and how much air it will move when it is on the job, pushing or pulling air through ducting. People have a sense of how much light a 40-watt bulb will produce because they can see it. How much air is 40 cubic feet per minute? As the importance of residential ventilation grows, as homes get tighter, the importance of knowing how the system will work when it comes out of the box and gets installed also grows. Without standardized, third party testing, a manufacturer can say anything they want about the product, and it may or it may not move any air or exchange any heat and the homeowner wouldn't know because the moving air can't be seen.

---

10. https://www.onsetcomp.com/
11. https://www.airadviceforhomes.com/
12. https://www.aircuity.com/
13. https://www.homeaircheck.com/

To address this issue, the ventilation industry submits their products to a number of third party laboratories to test the products under standardized procedures for air movement, sound level, power consumption, and heat exchange efficiency.

Residential ventilation product manufacturers addressed these issues by forming the Home Ventilating Institute (HVI)[14] as a nonprofit trade association in 1955. HVI developed a series of standards and criteria for fan performance that could be repeated so that products could be directly compared to one another and so that consumers would have a scale to evaluate product A and product B. As of this writing, HVI has about 50 members and the Certified Product Directory is the place to find information on the performance of residential fans.

HVI uses the Texas Energy and Environmental Systems Laboratory (TEES) at Texas A&M University as the third party testing facility for residential fans and static vents and Bodycote[15] for testing heat and energy recovery ventilators. The product performance program has four elements: certification, verification, challenge, and presentation of product performance ratings in the marketplace. Certification goes beyond just an initial test of the performance of the product. Every two years, sample products are purchased in the marketplace by HVI and sent back to the laboratory for retesting to verify that the product is still performing as it was initially defined. And the performance of a certified product can be challenged, requiring a series of steps to confirm the performance or compel the manufacturer to make adjustments to bring it into compliance. To further assure the public of the quality of the HVI label, there are strict rules on the use of the logo on products and literature. Airflow testing is done under HVI Publication 916, sound testing under HVI Publication 915, Publication 920 defines the Certification Procedure, and HVI Publication 925 regulates labels and logos.

---

14. https://www.hvi.org/
15. Bodycote Testing Group www.bodycotetesting.com

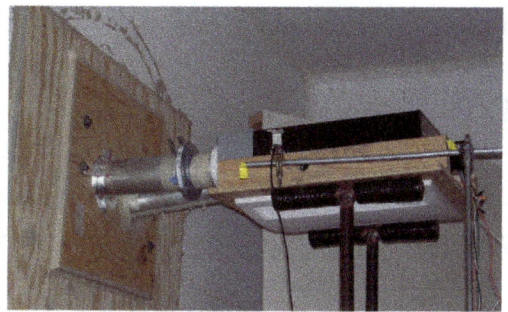

Figure 9.13 TEES Test Laboratory (ESL)

Airflow testing at TEES[16] varies depending on the product being tested, whether it's a ceiling mounted bath fan, remote mounted in-line fan, whole house comfort ventilator, through the wall fan, static vent, etc. All product testing is done in accordance with the American National Standards Institute (ANSI) and Standards Council of Canada (SCC) consensus standards. It should be noted that HVI lists ratings in steps of 10 cfm. A fan that has a flow of 81 cfm and another fan that has a flow of 89 cfm are both rated at 80 cfm in the certified directory. From that standpoint, ratings will always be on the conservative side.

> HVI does not certify the sound levels of exterior mounted or in-line fans or heat/energy recovery ventilators. The sound level experienced by owners of these products will depend on how they have been installed, the length and type of ducting, and the distance of the air mover from the interior grilles.

The Certification process requires having the fan safety tested (UL, ETL, CSA, Met Lab, etc.) and having the fan tested under the requisite airflow measurement setup. Sound testing is performed promptly after airflow testing with no modification to the product. Sound testing is performed in a prescribed, diffuse, reverberation chamber using a reference sound source (RSS), and an extremely low background sound level. Four sound pressure measurements in 24, one-third-octave bands are conducted. "Sound power of the test unit is determined by mathematically comparing sound pressure

---

16. https://rellis.tamus.edu/facilities/energy-systems-lab/

measurements in the chamber to sound pressure measurements of the RSS, using its sound power calibration data."[17]

The Certified Product Directory provides the following typical information:

Model or Series Number: Manufacturer's product identification

Details: Specific product information like "30" (1 piece model)/Crawl Space Model" or "VER. HS+" which means Vertical High Speed or "Hor. HS+" which means Horizontal High Speed, which refers to range hoods that are either vertical or horizontal outlets and that they were tested at their high speed setting.

Static Pressure: for direct discharge fans, the static pressure rating point is 0.03 iwg because there is no ducting attached. For ducted fans the rating point is 0.1 iwg with a second rating point at 0.25 iwg being optional. Inline fans are rated at 0.20 iwg, with two additional rating points being optional.

CFM: the airflow at the rating point. Alternative airflows can be listed at alternative resistances, but the airflow at the rating point is what is listed in literature and the promotion of the product.

Sones: this is the sound level at the rating point in sones.

Watts: the power consumption of the product is an optional number, but it is the power consumption at watts at the rating point.

> The certified airflow rating is a great place to start to compare one fan to another, but the installed performance will differ from the Certified Rating point because of the resistance of the installation—the ducting and the termination fitting or hood or vent cap. Using a higher rating point like 0.25 iwg will provide a better installed performance reference, although the actual installation will probably exceed even that number.

HRV/ERV testing is commonly performed at the Bodycote Laboratories in Ontario. These devices undergo long-term temperature testing because their purpose is to provide ventilation while saving heat. The air temperatures on the incoming air stream must be brought down below freezing so that moisture that collects in the system will freeze the way it would in an actual installation. (See Appendix G for a complete description of HRV/ERV testing.)

---

17. HVI 915, Loudness Testing and Rating

The result of all this testing is the entry in the HVI Certified Directory, which provides an abundance of information on the performance of the product. The "efficiency" of the system, its "performance", is the number that most evaluation systems are looking for. The HVI directory provides "Sensible Recovery Efficiency", "Apparent Sensible Effectiveness", and "Total Recovery Efficiency". It provides different numbers for heating at different airflows and other numbers for cooling.

THESE ARE the definitions in the HVI Directory:

Sensible Recovery Efficiency (SRE): The net sensible energy recovered by the supply airstream as adjusted by electric consumption, case heat loss or heat gain, air leakage, airflow mass imbalance between the two airstreams and the energy used for defrost (when running the Very Low Temperature Test), as a percent of the potential sensible energy that could be recovered plus the exhaust fan energy. This value is used to predict and compare Heating Season Performance of the HRV/ERV unit.

Adjusted Sensible Recovery Efficiency (ASRE): The net sensible energy recovered by the supply airstream as adjusted by case heat loss or heat gain, air leakage, airflow mass imbalance between the two airstreams and the energy used for defrost (when running the Very Low Temperature Test), as a percent of the potential sensible energy that could be recovered. This value should be used for energy modeling when wattage for air movement is separately accounted for in the energy model.

Total Recovery Efficiency (TRE): The net total energy (sensible plus latent, also called enthalpy) recovered by the supply airstream adjusted by electric consumption, case heat loss or heat gain, air leakage and airflow mass imbalance between the two airstreams, as a percent of the potential total energy that could be recovered plus the exhaust fan energy. This value is used to predict and compare Cooling Season Performance for the HRV/ERV unit.

Adjusted Total Recovery Efficiency (ATRE): The net total energy (sensible plus latent, also called enthalpy) recovered by the supply airstream adjusted by case heat loss or heat gain, air leakage and airflow mass imbalance between the two airstreams, as a percent of the potential total energy that could be recovered. This value is used to predict and compare Cooling Season Performance for the HRV/ERV unit. This value should be used for energy modeling when wattage for air movement is separately accounted for in the energy model.

Since the motor or motors are in the same housing as the exchanger element, the heat generated from the work they are doing is added to the air streams. The efficiency calculation should include that information, so the SRE is the number to use. The number listed in marketing information is usually the ASRE, usually at the lowest operating speed and usually at 0° C or 32° F. Those specifications should be listed beside the efficiency percentages. It would be advisable to refer to the complete HVI directory for all the information prior to selecting an HRV or ERV. Talk to HVI or the product manufacturer for specific information if you have questions.

Chapter 10

System Troubleshooting, Service, and Maintenance

My system isn't moving any air

The first question to ask is: how do you know? What method have you used to measure it? The second question is: did this happen suddenly or has it always been this way, not moving any air? The third question is: is the air mover (fan or HRV/ERV) running at all? If it is a simple system—a bath fan on a light switch, for example, it will be much simpler to determine why it isn't working or why it isn't moving any air.

Sometimes the amount of air that is moving is difficult to measure because it is so low. The tissue or smoke methods described in Chapter 9 can give you a sense of subtle airflow. But the fact is that if the ventilation system is meant to move 90 cubic feet of air per minute and instead it is moving less than 20, there is definitely a problem that needs to be addressed. Knowing whether it is a new symptom or something that has been going on for a long time will give you a good place to start—whether a critter has recently moved into the ductwork or if the initial installation was defective.

Understanding the system is always the place to start. What sort of ventilation system is it? What are the component parts—for a fan: ducting, hood, or control, for an HRV/ERV: ducting, grilles, exterior inlet and outlet hoods, and controls? Understanding how the system is supposed to work will provide insight into why it is not working.

If there is no airflow or only occasional airflow, check to see if the air mover is running. Air pressures or wind blowing on the house could cause occasional, subtle airflow, but if there seems to be no steady airflow and no sound, chances are that the air mover isn't running. Fans are remarkably quiet these days, so sometimes it is difficult to tell.

It could be that the device is turned off. It could be that it is supposed to be off. Controls for ventilation systems are not always in obvious places, and they can be programmed to turn the system on and off throughout the day. They are occasionally buried in closets or installed in an electrical box up near the ceiling, places where they have been hidden to prevent people from interfering with a designed ventilation strategy. Timers, for example, are generally solid mechanical devices, but they do fail eventually. Microprocessor-based controls sometimes have battery backups to preserve their programming during a power failure. Although if the battery dies, they will be operating in their default mode—whatever the designer decided was the program that should take over when all else failed. Dehumidistats are misunderstood devices and can be set to work backwards - on humidity fall instead of humidity rise. If it is a linear, wall mounted humidity control (not an electronic humidity control that is built into the fan), rotate the setting counter-clockwise to a very low setting like 40% RH (not all the way to off). If it is winter, it still may be too dry for the control to activate the fan. Try breathing into it and see if that gets it running.

> Step back for a moment here and think about how you want your ventilation system to run. The original designer or installer may have had a completely different vision of how it should be working. Things might have changed. Teenagers can take longer showers than infants. You might be doing more cooking. So even if the system is running the way it was originally designed to run, it still might not be working the way you think it should and maybe that's why you're troubleshooting it. Perhaps humidity control does not suit your lifestyle no matter what you set it at.

If the control is a wall switch that controls both the fan and the light, and the light works, then the switch hasn't failed. A wire might have come loose or the fan might have failed. (Some controls switch on both the light and the fan simultaneously but delay the off cycle of the fan.)

WARNING: Disconnect power to the system before attempting to service it. Electrical shocks can damage to your health!

The covers of bath fans can be removed for cleaning and that will also provide a means to visually determine if the wheel inside is spinning. Most bath fan covers are attached by 'V' shaped spring clips on either side of the grille. If there are no obvious screws, gently but firmly pull the grille down, away from the fan. As you are pulling the clips will become obvious. When the grille stops moving, it has reached the little loops on the ends of the spring clip wires. Compressing the ends of the 'V' into each other will free the clips from the fan and allow you to remove the cover completely.

Is the fan wheel spinning? If it isn't and whatever is controlling it says it should be, the fan is probably broken and needs to be replaced.

The covers to HRV/ERVs are designed to be removed to service the system, to clean the filters and the core particularly. When you are up close and personal with an HRV/ERV, it is not a subtle device. The fans are designed to aggressively move a considerable volume of air through a considerable amount of ductwork, so if you remove the cover, the fans will stop for your safety. That's what they are designed to do. But before you remove the cover, if the fans are supposed to be running, you should be able to hear them. If you can, dig out the installation and service manual that came with the device. If you can't, most of the manufacturers have their product manuals on-line. And if you have trouble there, contact the manufacturer or the Home Ventilating Institute (HVI), and they will assist you in getting the documentation that you need.

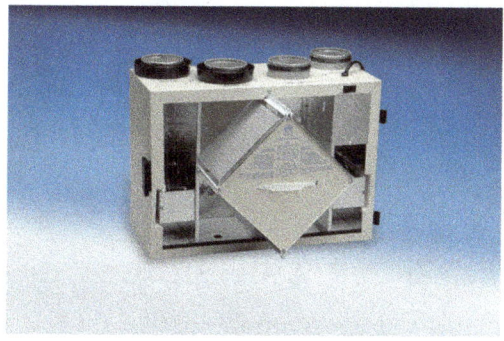

Figure 10.1 HRV Open for Service (Fantech)

But while you have the cover off the HRV/ERV, make sure that the filters and core are clean and there isn't a pile of insects or other nasty things inside there that shouldn't be. It isn't likely that you will have so much stuff in there that all the flow will be blocked, but crud will certainly reduce the air flow, and remember, what goes through this device is the good, clean, fresh air that you and your family are breathing, air that is supposed to keep you healthy.

If the air mover (fans, controls, HRV, or ERV) is working and there is still little or no airflow, the problem lies in the ducting. Does the ducting run all the way to the outside of the house and if so, is the exterior vent or termination fitting blocked? Both the fan and the exterior vent are likely to have backdraft dampers, either or both of which could be damaged and jammed shut. Sometimes in the construction process, insulators will foam the inside of ventilation ducts, so even in a new installation there might not be any air moving through a beautiful new bath fan!

If the hood isn't damaged or blocked, check the ducting. Someone may have stepped on it or dropped a trunk on it in the attic or it may be full of water or something else. If the ducting is crushed or damaged or if it is uninsulated ducting running through a cold attic, it should be replaced with a smoother, better insulated, better supported duct.

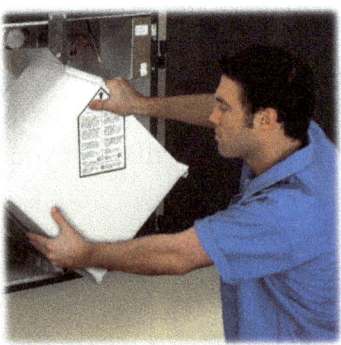

Figure 10.2 Servicing an HRV Core (Venmar)

My system is too noisy/too quiet

If the bath fan is too noisy, at least you know that's it running! If it's too quiet, maybe it isn't running, or maybe it was designed to be really, really quiet. New fans that are rated at less than 0.3 sones and can be so quiet that you might not know that they are running. Noise is not equivalent to airflow. Fans can be remarkably noisy and not be moving any air at all, or remarkably quiet and be moving a lot of air.

> It should be noted that any noise is more noticeable in a tight house. If the ventilation system operates with automatic controls, it just emphasizes the importance of having the homeowner understand what it is, what it is for, and how it works. If they are sitting in the living room and the ventilation system suddenly shifts from an unnoticeable background level to high speed because some pollutant has been sensed, the homeowner may think that the system is defective and seek to defeat it altogether.

If a fan is unacceptably noisy, it may just need to be replaced because that's the way it was made. Removing the grille (REMEMBER the warning about electrical power) should give you access to the product's model number. You can look up that model through the HVI Certified Product listing and find the sone rating or contact the manufacturer if it is no longer listed. If the fan is rated over 1.5 sones, then it will be noisy no matter what other adjustments you might make.

Fans with DC motors compensate for resistance in the airflow path. If a quiet fan has been installed and it is not quiet, there is something wrong with the installation. Check the backdraft damper in the fan to make sure that it is opening. Check the ductwork for a free flowing path to the outside. A fan rated at 0.3 sones or less should be absolutely silent unless there is an installation problem.

If a fan is unacceptably quiet (and it is running), you might need to replace it with one with a higher sone rating. Sometimes a little fan noise in a bathroom or powder room is a good thing.

Noise level may vary as pressures on the house change, making the fan's job easier or harder, pushing on the exterior backdraft damper, for example. Giving the fan the easiest path from the inside to the outside of the house will provide the best performance and the quietest operation.

Exterior dampers can flap or bang in the changing pressures and breezes on the house. Removing the damper will certainly cure that problem, but the system is then relying on the primary damper in the bathroom fan (if there is one). Inserting a spring-loaded backdraft damper in the line will provide a better seal, but be sure that the fan can overcome the back-pressure that the damper creates. A motorized damper in the line can cure the problem, but it will need to be controlled by the same control that controls the fan or by a pressure switch, sensing an increase in pressure in the duct and automatically activating the fan.

Fans can also produce motor hum that is transferred to the structure of the building. Motor hum is not part of the certification testing because it depends on how the installer installs the fan, which is not something the laboratory can verify. It is important that the installation steps described by the manufacturer be followed. Some bath fans, for example, require installing the housing, connecting the ducting, and making the electrical connections before inserting the working fan into the ceiling. That can make a difference.

If the sound level is critically important, isolating the fan from the structure is important. (Note that for the long-term satisfactory operation of the fan, it is important that it be securely mounted.) There are a variety of sources for sound isolation hardware, with extremely descriptive web sites.

Remotely mounted exhaust or supply fans are very quiet because they are mounted remotely from the space they are ventilating. Sometimes, however, they are controlled by speed controls. It should be noted that not all fans should be controlled with solid-state speed controls. If the motor has been tested for use with a solid-state speed control, it should tell you that either on the motor itself or in the installation manual. These controls provide only part of the AC electrical impulse to the motor, "chopping" the signal, turning the motor on and off rapidly. This process can be hard on the motor and also create motor hum. Sometimes the hum can be removed by adjusting the control to a slightly higher or lower speed. Sometimes these controls can also create interference with radio or television signals if they do not have adequate electronic filtration. There are DC fan products that have speed control built into them. Be sure they are wired properly in order to function as they were designed.

Because HRV/ERVs have so many components, they are more complex in resolving sound problems. If the fans are running correctly and not making noises that would indicate that the fans themselves are damaged, then noise problems are likely to be transferred to the living space through the grilles. The problems could be with restricted flow paths through the ducting, as described above for bath fans. The noise can be at the grille itself. If the velocity of the air being "thrown" out of the grille is high, it will make excessive noise. The grilles should have been matched to the system during the original installation so that the velocity of the air should not make excessive noise entering the room. If it does, chances are the system is unbalanced, that there is too much air being delivered to that room and not enough somewhere else. A balancing damper in the ducting can cure excessive airflow.

The motors in HRV/ERVs are certainly more powerful than the motors in typical bath fans so they can produce more motor hum. It is important to follow the manufacturer's installation instructions and not couple them directly to the structure of the building so that the structure itself becomes an amplifier. Some of these products come with hanging straps that will absorb motor noise or duct clamps with hanging straps that include rubber pads to absorb motor vibration.

My system is too drafty

This complaint may result from not understanding the system, it may be a poorly designed system, or the draft may result from air coming back down the ducts from the outside.

Lack of understanding should be the least of these concerns. The system should not be designed or installed in such a way that the occupants are ever uncomfortable. Air movement can be sensed as a "draft" particularly if it is unconditioned outside air blowing on people. Ventilation requires air movement, but it shouldn't be uncomfortable air movement.

In a residential installation, supply vents from positive pressure systems should be above where people sit and walk and children play and crawl. The incoming air should mix with the room air, and it shouldn't be moving at such a high velocity that people sense it as a draft. The vanes on these grilles should not be directed down into the living space. Some manufacturers have developed grilles that make use of the Coanda effect to deliver the air at the ceiling and compel the air to move across the ceiling, mixing with the room air.

"Unbalanced" exhaust-centered or supply-centered ventilation systems rely on air leaking in or leaking out around the house. Those inlets and outlets should be so small and so distributed that air moving through them can be barely sensed, if at all. If the house is too leaky, drafts will occur from both "natural ventilation" and mechanical ventilation. Those leaks should be sealed from both a comfort and an energy use point of view.

To prevent drafts from air flowing back into the house through a fan housing, most ceiling mounted bath fans include balanced backdraft dampers that allow the air to flow out but prevent the air from flowing back in. (Note that these systems rely on gravity to close. If the system has been designed for "ceiling installation", the damper is not likely to close if it is installed vertically in a wall.) Many exterior hoods include a second damper. These dampers sometimes are purposely designed to allow a small amount of leakage to flow through them even when they are closed. This small gap allows the positively pressurized air to start flowing. If the damper is completely tight all the way around its perimeter, it is possible that the damper won't open.

Spring loaded butterfly dampers can be added to the ducting to provide a better seal. They will create more back-pressure than the very light gravity damper that is usually included with the fan. These dampers can be tight enough to allow any other damper in the line can be removed, including both the exterior damper and the backdraft damper in the fan.

My system doesn't clear the moisture off the mirror

The mirror is cold. A shower creates steam in the air. The warm moist air hits the cold surface of the mirror and the moisture condenses and fogs the mirror. If the room temperature is high, the mirror temperature will be relatively warm. The warm air can hold more moisture and the mirror is much less likely to fog. Raising the room temperature is probably the most effective way to keep the mirror from fogging.

If the ventilation system's volume of air movement is high enough relative to the amount of humidity being generated, it can haul the warm moist air out of the room before it fogs the mirror. (On average, this is about 80 cfm of true airflow moving through the room.)[1] Localizing the intake vent near the mirror for a remote mounted, in-line bath fan can drag the air directly over the mirror's surface to limit the amount of fogging that will occur.

There are a variety of films that can be sprayed or wiped on the mirror to keep it from fogging. They even make a mirror for shaving in the shower. None of these are non-fogging because of airflow, however.

You could install a mirror with its own heating element![2]

---

1. Terry Brennan, https://www.camroden.com/
2. https://www.warmlyyours.com/en-US/mirror-defogger

Ventilation system maintenance

Ventilation systems run for a long time with little conscious interaction with the occupant of the home. Because of that lack of interactivity, maintaining the system is not likely to occur until there are problems. The old English system of putting a shilling in the electric meter to get heat or hot water was probably the most direct feedback system. When the shower water started getting cold, you knew that your shilling had run out!

Component failures in HRV/ERVs are likely to begin when the system has been operating for four years. If low end bath fans are required to run continuously, their motors may fail in as little as one year.

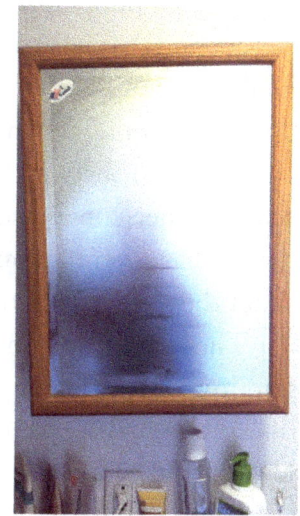

Figure 10.3 Foggy Mirror (PHR)

System issues that are most likely to be problems are not likely to be noticed. For example, if one blower in an HRV fails, and the system is connected to the air handler, air will still move around in the house, but the effectiveness of the system will be severely compromised. Energy costs will increase because the house will rely on infiltration or exfiltration for system balance. Because of the problem of out-of-sight/out-of-mind, maintenance items are over-looked.

Periodic maintenance, like balancing the airflows in an HRV or ERV, is not something that can be done by the homeowner without the proper equipment or training. It is extremely common for HRV/ERV systems to be out of balance either because they were never balanced in the first place or because the balance has not been maintained.

Homeowners rarely follow the instructions in the manuals that come with the products. Some routine maintenance issues are just as simple as changing the batteries in smoke detectors or the filter in the furnace air handler.

There is a disconnect between problems of indoor air quality (IAQ), moisture and the ventilation system. If the heat doesn't come on, the house gets cold. If moisture builds up, it is not obvious that the ventilation system isn't working.

The ventilation system is not a high priority in the minds of most homeowners when they buy an existing home, and the seller is not likely to explain the purpose or operating details of the system. The home's occupant needs to understand that it is good for their health to maintain the system.

If the homeowner is not familiar with the system and suddenly discovers that it is running when he/she thinks it shouldn't be (like when the windows are open and the weather is warm), they may shut the system off. When the cold weather comes around again, they may forget to turn it back on. Many homes have ventilation systems that have been defeated. The good news about these systems is that they generally can just be turned back on!

The operating condition of the equipment is important, but the understanding of the owner is equally important. If through lack of understanding the system has been modified (like adding an insect screen to the intake of an HRV) or the controls adjusted (like shutting off an exhaust only fan that should run continuously), the system will not function as it was designed to function. There is a lack of understanding about the purpose of the ventilation system. That it is running all the time, blowing or forcing air out of the house seems like an obvious waste of money. That lack of understanding will lead to system "failure" as surely as a burned out fan motor.

Bath fan system maintenance

There aren't a lot of maintenance issues with a bath fan that is mounted in the bathroom's ceiling. There's no filter to change and the fan motor is sealed and needs no oiling. If the fan works and moves air, clean the grille and leave the rest of it alone. (Unless the owner's manual for the particular fan in your ceiling says there are maintenance steps you should take.) If it is accessible, look at the exhaust or termination fitting on the outside of the house and make sure that there are no birds nesting in it or that the backdraft damper isn't jammed open or closed. Check out the ducting to make sure that it hasn't been crushed or been disconnected from some fitting somewhere along the way.

Remote mounted or in-line fans can collect condensation inside their housings, particularly if they are mounted horizontally. Checking that means taking the system apart, which may not be a regular maintenance task. Other than that, checking the ducting and termination fittings as described previously, is about all you need to do. If the fan has been in service for over 5 years, it probably merits taking it apart and cleaning it. A filter can be added to the grille or ducting to prolong the life of the fan.

Exhaust-centered systems should run for a long time with no maintenance or interference. Unfortunately, with products like that, they get ignored. They run quietly in the background until they are forgotten about altogether, and when they stop running, the effects may not be blatantly obvious. About the best possible maintenance that can be done is to make sure that the fan is still working.

Although this is not bath fan maintenance, supply-centered systems should have filters that need to be changed as frequently as the local environmental conditions demand—maybe every year, maybe every three months. That filter is removing the particulate pollutants in the incoming air and protecting the home's occupants.

HRV/ERV system maintenance

The maintenance information for HRV/ERVs is in Appendix H.

Chapter 11

Costs of Ventilation

We have to accept the fact that residential ventilation is not free. Unless you live in what is affectionately termed a "paradise climate" where you can leave the windows open all the time and don't have to worry about excess humidity and you have no mechanical heating or cooling concerns, you're going to have to pay something to have air moving through your house. Just leaving the windows open will entail a cost for conditioning the air. So what's it worth to be able to breathe regularly? (Of course, that's looking at the value, not the cost.)

There is a first cost for buying and installing the equipment. There is an energy cost for running the fan motors. And there is an energy cost for conditioning the air moving through the house. The life cycle cost includes all of these and adds the cost of replacing the system when it dies, removing the old equipment and taking it off to the dump or recycling facility. (It could even be extended in the other direction to include the cost of manufacture, delivery to the distribution facility, and finally to your house. It just depends on how far out you want to widen the circle.)

There are cost offsets that are virtually impossible to quantify. How much is saved for improved health for the occupants of the house with better ventilation? How much is saved for reducing the moisture effects on the structure of the house? It may be possible to quantify the savings in cooling load by reducing the temperature of the air in the attic with an attic fan (if it accomplishes that). A dehumidifier will reduce the humidity in the house, reducing the dehumidification load of the air conditioning, but it will also increase the temperature in the house, increasing the load of the air conditioning, and it will have an electrical cost.

Those are local costs. There are also global costs, carbon costs. In those terms, the most efficient, most effective, longest lasting, simplest to maintain system with the least manufacturing and delivery cost will have the least overall cost to the planet.

The way prices for almost everything are changing, today's real numbers are not particularly meaningful here except in relative terms (particularly in terms of the cost of energy), so they are only provided as an acceptable starting point.

Since putting these numbers together in 2017, the changes have not been dramatic. A low end bath fan has double in price from $10 to $20. There are many more options for extremely quiet local exhaust fans, so it isn't hard to good fans at reasonable prices. Ducting and labor costs have increased. The prices of electricity have increased in some places and down in others. The prices for a therm of gas have increased the most.

Remember that these systems are there for your health and at about $1 per day for operating cost for any of these systems, it's very cheap.

First Cost

The mechanical ventilation systems in the house consist of a variety of components. At the heart, there is the system for the occupants, the Whole Dwelling Ventilation System, the system that should run all the time, exchanging the air throughout the house. This may be a stand-alone system or it might be integrated with the heating and cooling system. Then there are the local exhaust ventilation systems—the bathroom and kitchen fans. There might (should) also be a radon or soil gas reduction fan system that runs all the time, extracting the soil gases from under the basement slab or around the foundation of the house. There might also be a garage ventilation fan controlling the build-up of carbon monoxide in the garage. There might be a whole house comfort ventilator for warm weather cooling. And there might be an attic fan for removing the heat from the attic.

The associated costs for these systems and approaches are outlined in the tables below. The total first cost is the sum of the fan or device cost, the ducting, the hood or termination fitting on the outside of the house, the control (if it is separate), and an approximation of installation cost. (Note that these are just a few representative costs. Simpler installations would cost less; more complex would obviously cost more. There is a wide variety of all these systems with many installation variations.)[1,2]

System	Installed Cost	System
Central exhaust-centered	$535	Good quality exhaust fan with ducting and installation
Central exhaust-centered with intakes	$885	Good quality exhaust fan with ducting, (3) intake vents, and installation
Central supply-centered	$1,480	Central supply fan with distributed ducting to four rooms, control, and installation
Central supply to air-handler	$580	Ducting, control, damper, installation
HRV/ERV stand only installation	$3,120	Exchanger with fans, ducting, basic control, and installation
HRV/ERV attached to an air handler	$2,520	Exchanger with fans, ducting, basic control, and installation

Table 11.1 Whole Dwelling Systems First Costs

The whole dwelling ventilation system for the occupants doesn't have to be expensive or complicated. If you consider the house to be a simple, fairly tight box of air, using a single point, exhaust only ventilation system running continuously will change all the air in the box, diluting the polluted indoor air with fresher, outdoor air—dilution of the pollution. If the leaks into the house are evenly distributed and the house is simple enough and doors are left open, a central exhaust-only system can have a good impact on improving the air quality in the house.

The simplest approach is to use a centrally located bathroom-type fan. Very low cost, "builders' special", bath fans are not a good choice for this job. Some of these fans can cost under $20. They will be too noisy (over 3 sones) to run very long. The occupants will find a way to turn them off. Indoor Envi-

---

1. [70]HomeAdvisor reported average installed cost for bathroom installation cost of $396 based on 1,561 cost profiles, but their numbers may not reflect a high quality fan.
2. [71]these numbers are for the whole dwelling ventilation system alone. An HRV/ERV exhausting from the bathrooms may eliminate the cost of the local exhaust ventilation fans that would be necessary otherwise.

ronmental Quality (IEQ) includes the elimination of noise pollution, which becomes a more important factor in a tight house. A good quality bath fan will be more expensive, but the difference is up front, installed cost will be the difference in the cost of the two fans. The installation details will be the same —same duct and same exterior hood or termination fitting (although a better fan may include better installation with larger duct and a lower resistance exterior hood). This fan could be located in a bathroom, serving as both the whole dwelling ventilation system and a spot ventilator for the bathroom. This works particularly well if a multi-speed controller controls the fan with one setting for the continuous background ventilation and a higher setting when the bathroom is occupied. (Some products do this speed shifting automatically with motion sensors or other occupancy indicators.)

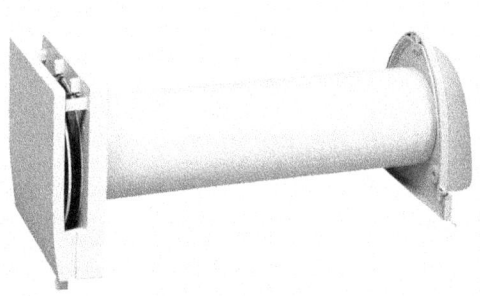

Figure 11.1 Through-Wall Fresh Air Intake (Panasonic)

An alternative to the ceiling mounted bath fan from a single bathroom is a remote mounted system that uses an in-line fan or a multi-port fan, drawing air from several points. If the system draws from a single point, its installation cost will be very similar to the ceiling mounted fan, with the cost of a grille added to the ducting, termination fitting, and control.

Some houses are tight enough to require the addition of make-up air or intake inlets. For this analysis, these are passive devices located high on the walls or "slot vents" manufactured into the windows, allowing air to flow back into the house when it is under negative pressure from the whole dwelling ventilation system. They do not provide make-up air for any other purpose.

A remote mounted, in-line fan could also be used as a supply-only system, blowing air into bedrooms, for example. It is important to add a filter box to such a system and to locate the filter in an accessible location for maintenance. The first cost of this system would be similar to the remote system described above with the addition of the filter. However, this approach works best if there are multiple distribution points, supplying air to several bedrooms, which will increase the cost of ducting, grilles and installation.

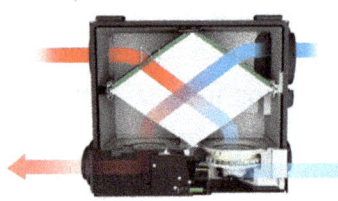

Figure 11.2 Heat Recovery Ventilator (Venmar)

A supply system added to the return side of the air handler is another inexpensive approach. There are a number of supply side devices. Some systems are primarily a duct from the outside with a flow restrictor to limit the amount of outside air that is drawn in when the air handler fan is running. Others consist of a control system, ducting, and a motorized damper. The control monitors the operation of the air handler blower and logs run-time. It compares that run-time to the programmed-in desired ventilation run-time for the house. If the blower hasn't been running long enough to satisfy the ventilation requirement, the control restarts the blower, drawing in outside air, and circulating it throughout the house. The first cost on these systems is in the $90 to $300 range. Installation is simple because it is localized to the area of the air handler and the controls are low voltage. A variation on this control is a version that is connected to both the furnace blower and a bathroom fan. Instead of activating the high-powered furnace to complete the ventilation cycle, this control will activate the energy efficient bath fan.[3]

A stand-alone HRV or ERV is fully ducted, supplying fresh air to living spaces and extracting "used" air from polluting spaces like bathrooms. Although these systems are more expensive, they can replace individual bathroom fans and their operating cost is reduced by their energy efficiency. Their first cost includes a complete ducting system that is less costly than an HVAC ducting system because the ducts are smaller.

Although it affects the effectiveness of the system, the cost of most of the ducting can be eliminated if the ERV is ducted to the air handler. Fresh, tempered air is delivered to the return side. Stale, house air can be removed from a point, further upstream, also on the return side, or better yet, extracted

---

3. https://www.aircycler.com/products/g2?variant=412050813

from the bathrooms and kitchen. Spot ventilation fans may also have to be used to achieve adequate airflow from those spaces.

Electrical costs

Operating costs can be broken down into the electrical cost of operating the equipment and the cost of conditioning the air that is being removed and replaced. The systems that run continuously, like the whole dwelling ventilation system and the radon/soil gas mitigation system, need to be electrically very efficient. Relying on a low-cost bath fan that uses 90 watts of electricity would not be a good choice for a whole dwelling ventilation system running 24/7. In Hawaii with electricity costing 43 cents per kilowatt hour (kWh) in 2023, a 90-watt fan would cost $340.59 for the year just for electrical cost. An 11.3-watt fan would cost $42.76 for the same year in the same location. At the average national electrical rate in 2024 of $0.1356 per kWh, a 90 watt fan would cost $106.91 and 11.3-watt fan would cost $13.42 per year. (The Energy Information Administration has good statistics on the cost of energy across the country for different sectors.)[4] Note that an inkjet printer/fax machine uses 5.31 watts when it's waiting—about $6.30 per year.[5,6]

---

4. https://www.eia.gov/electricity/monthly/
5. At the beginning of 2025 the national average cost of electricity in the United States was 16.94 cents per kWh. In Massachusetts it was 29.17 cents per kWh and in Louisiana it was 11.23 cents.
6. [1] A primary factor in the operating cost of the central supply system is the number of hours per day of run time or duty cycle.
   [1] The run time issue impacts the HRV/ERV system as well.

System	Wattage	Run Time (per day)	Annual Cost at $0.1356/kWh
Central exhaust-only	11.3	24	$13.42
Central exhaust-only with intakes	11.3	24	$13.42
Central supply-only	26	24	$30.88
Central supply to air-handler	400 (Air handler blower)	5.5 (average for ventilation air)	$108.89
HRV/ERV standalone installation	121	24	$143.73
HRV/ERV attached to air handler	121 + 400 (Exchanger fan + air handler blower)	5	$128.93

Table 11.2 Whole Dwelling Ventilation System Electrical Costs

A one hundred watt light bulb uses 100 watts of power. If it runs for 10 hours, it uses 1,000 watts equivalent to 1-kilowatt hour represented as 1 kWh. Electricity is sold in kWh. In 2023 one kWh in Hawaii costs $0.43. The same kWh costs $0.1035 in Idaho, with a national average of $0.1356. With the price of energy sashaying all over the place, it is difficult to predict an exact cost. Even if one-kilowatt hour is relatively cheap, accumulating a lot of them can run the price up. "A billion here, a billion there and pretty soon you're talking real money," attributed to Everett Dirksen.

Efficient bath fans operate at less than 10 watts - some as low as 6 watts. (A doorbell transformer uses 3 watts just sitting there!) Inefficient bath fans consume over a 90 watts. The electrical cost for the primary ventilation system is the power consumption of the fan in watts times the number of operating hours divided by 1000 (to convert to kWh) times the energy cost per kWh. For example, a 30 watt fan running constantly (24 x 365 = 8760) at $0.1356 per kWh:

$$(30 \times 8760)/1000 \times \$0.1356 = \$35.64 \text{ per year}$$

A 75 watt heat recovery ventilator would cost:

$$(75 \times 8760)/1000 \times \$0.1356 = \$89.09 \text{ per year}$$

If the watts aren't obvious in the specifications, multiply 120 volts times the amps. For example, if the fan is rated at .75 amps: 120 x .75 = 90 watts. This is not a perfect conversion, but it is satisfactorily close.

* * *

IF THE FURNACE fan is used for the whole dwelling ventilation system and is run continuously, it may consume as much as 400 watts or more. This may be a good approach in terms of filtration and distribution, but if all the operating cost is attributed to ventilation:

$$(400 \times 8760)/1000 \times \$0.1356 = \$475.14$$

This is just the electrical cost! Of course, a significant portion of the furnace blower's run time will be working to distribute conditioned air throughout the house, but if only 18% of the electrical cost is related to ventilation, that is $85 (at $0.1356/kWh).

The electrical cost for any of the other ventilation system can be calculated similarly. A radon mitigation fan running continuously at 19 watts would cost $22.57 per year. A garage fan running continuously at 25 watts would cost $30 per year. A whole house comfort ventilator that uses 740 watts may only run for 8 hours per day over a 3 month or 90-day period or 720 hours.

(740 watts x 720 hours)/1000 x $0.1356 = $72 for the season

All of these calculations are at the national average electrical cost of 2024. In some parts of the country, the electrical cost is going to be twice this amount. You will need to check your electric bill for the total delivered electrical cost to get an accurate number.

Conditioned Air Cost

When you blow the conditioned air out of the house, it must be replaced with unconditioned, outside, fresh air. That cost depends on the location of the house, on the amount of air moved, and on the percentage of that air that would have moved naturally into and out of the house through infiltration and exfiltration that has been mechanically displaced. The cost of conditioning the air moving naturally into and out of the house is typically 20% to 30% of the heating load. Adding a mechanical ventilation system will increase that cost slightly, perhaps 5% or 6%. So in terms of heating load, for example, if the house costs $1,000 per year to heat, 25% is from infiltration or $250. Mechanical ventilation might add $60. A 75% efficient HRV would reduce the mechanical ventilation conditioning cost for heat to $15. Per Year! That's not a lot of money to breathe good air. The cost of mechanical ventilation is small compared to the cost of conditioning unpredictable infiltration in most homes.

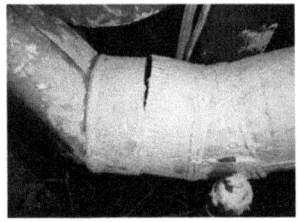

Figure 11.3 Air Leak (PHR)

	Heating/Cooling Degree Days	Exhaust or Supply-only	HRV (65% efficiency)
Boston Heating	5634	$206.55	$72.29
Boston Cooling	777	$80.92 ($0.211/kWh)	$28.32 ($0.211/kWh)
Washington Heating	4224	$109.95	$38.48
Washington Cooling	1075	$51.92 ($0.098/kWh)	$18.17 ($0.098/kWh)
Houston Heating	1396	$46.48	$18.27
Houston Cooling	2893	$162.14 ($0.114/kWh)	$62.54 ($0.114/kWh)
Phoenix Heating	1765	$53.23	$18.63
Phoenix Cooling	4355	$222.59 ($0.104/kWh)	$77.91 ($0.104/kWh)

Table 11.3 Whole Dwelling Annual Conditioned Air Costs

An exhaust-only[7] whole dwelling ventilation system is more complex to evaluate in terms of conditioned air cost. It goes back to the discussion on building

---

7. The exhaust/supply-only costs in this table are based on all 65 cfm of conditioned air. No allowance for natural infiltration/exfiltration offset. Some percentage of mechanical ventilation air will take the place of air that would otherwise naturally infiltrate and exfiltrate from the house.

pressures. An exhaust-only system will offset some of the natural infiltration that would have been moving in and out of the building even if the fan wasn't there, so not all the conditioning cost can be attributed to the fan. "Under peak [weather] conditions, the standard house will have increased driving forces and infiltration will be very high at the worst time. In tight houses with mechanical ventilation, infiltration is not driven by wind and cold but is dominated by the fan."[8] In many cases, approximately 50% of natural infiltration is offset by exhaust-only ventilation, giving it an average 50% heat recovery component, or a conditioning cost per the HRV example of $30 per year.

There are other factors like cooling cost, which would increase the conditioning cost, and reducing the runtime, which would reduce the cost. If the house is tighter, the percentage of the conditioning cost related to ventilation will increase, but the dollar amount won't change a great deal.

Other ventilation systems besides the primary system will add to the conditioning costs, but to a lesser degree. Bathroom spot ventilation systems operate for a very short period, often not much longer than when the bathroom is occupied.

A range hood exhausts air for even less time per day (often because they are too noisy). So the cost of the conditioned air they displace is very small.

A radon or soil gas mitigation system draws its air from under the slab and from outside of the house. Some basement or crawl space air may be drawn into the system depending on how it has been designed, and sometimes, that will be conditioned air. Properly designed, the amount of conditioned air drawn into the system is small enough to ignore.

A garage, spot ventilation system will have a similar impact on the cost of conditioned air. Garages are rarely conditioned spaces, so the air that is vented out will primarily leak into the garage from the outside. Some air may come from the house, but those gaps and leaks should be carefully sealed and minimized.

Whole house comfort ventilators purposely move outside air in and inside air out at a high volume. They will decrease the cooling load from a temperature standpoint because the moving air makes the occupants more comfortable at a higher temperature, but they may increase the dehumidification load depending on the local climate and use conditions.

---

8. Kelley, "Ventilation System Performance in Energy Crafted Homes", 1995

Attic exhaust fans should not be removing air from the house, but cycling outside air into the attic, through the fan, and back to the outside so they have little or no effect on conditioning loads unless the AC system is in the attic.

Motor Life/Replacement Cost

The motor is the key mechanical component in the fan. Aside from cosmetics, it is unlikely that the fan will be replaced until the motor burns out. If the fan is operating as the whole dwelling ventilation system, it is vital that it continue to run. It should be replaced as soon as it stops working; therefore, the longevity of the fan motor has to figure into the operating cost of the product.

The fan motors on inexpensive fans were never expected to run for exceptionally long periods of time in homes.[9] Until people began to understand the need for mechanical ventilation, it was expected that bath fans would be used only approximately 7 minutes per day. The motors in inexpensive fans will commonly burn out in a year or two if they are allowed to run continuously.

It is difficult for fan and motor manufacturers to predict the life expectancy of their products. There are a lot of variables involved. Much of it comes down to the type of bearings and the lubricants used. This is one of those areas where if you pay more, you get more. It costs more to make a better motor with better bearings and better lubricants.

There is a wide variety of motor types. Without taking the fan apart, it is often difficult to tell what sort of motor is spinning the blade. It is difficult to get a fan manufacturer to define the number of operating hours for their products. If all fan manufacturers defined the number of hours of motor life, we could easily compare one product with another, but they would all have to be tested to the same specifications. There are some general rules of thumb you can use to guess the longevity of the motor. Note that although programs often require or recommend fans that have been "rated for continuous operation," there is no official program to certify that feature.

Take the grille off a low-cost fan. If the part of the motor that spins is imbedded in the jaws of a 'C', you can be pretty sure that is a 'C' frame motor. The permanent split capacitor motors often have a capacitor like a small tin

---

9. In point of fact, the inexpensive fans that have been installed in filling stations, restaurants and bars run so long and are so numerous exhaust fan manufacturers never focused on fan motor life. They just work!

can strapped to their side or located somewhere else in the assembly. (Sometimes they look like a "fat domino" and are hidden in the wiring compartment.) Most of the in-line fans use motorized impellers. And if the fan uses an EC motor somewhere it will tell you because they are more expensive and very energy efficient.

Motor Type	Hours of running life
C-frame Shaded pole	20,000 to 30,000
Permanent Split Capacitor (PSC)	20,000 to 30,000
Motorized impellers	50,000 to 70,000
Electronically Commutated Motors (ECM)	80,000 to 130,000

Table 11.4 Typical Motor Hours of Running Life

There are 8,760 hours in a year. In the worst case, fans rated for 20,000 hours of life will hang in there for about two years and three months. Some fan motors are designed to run for 50,000 hours or more—well over 5 years. A fan that will be used infrequently as in a powder room doesn't need to have as long a life motor as one that will be run continuously. Furnace fans run approximately 33% of the time in their job of conditioning the air.

The following table provides a picture of expected fan lives based on the fan's use. Note that these are rough figures. The actual operating life of the fan will depend on many issues, so there will be significant variations on both sides. Motor life is obviously not the only factor, especially if we're talking a hundred years!

Application	Hours per day	Expected fan life (by fan type) hours	Years of operation
Primary Ventilation system (High quality bath fan)	24	100,000	11.4
Primary Ventilation system (ERV/HRV)	19.2 (80% run time)	70,000	10
Primary Ventilation system (ECM Motor)	24	90,000	10
Furnace Air Handler (for space conditioning only)	8	55,000	19
Furnace Air Handler (for continuous ventilation and space conditioning)	24	55,000	6.3
Radon/soil gas mitigation fan	24	64,000	7.3
Spot ventilator (powder room)	0.5	20,000	110
Range hood	0.167 (10 minutes)	20,000	A very long time

Table 11.5 Ventilation Product Life Expectancy

Insulation materials have improved to where they last indefinitely, so motor life is governed by bearing life and bearing life depends on degradation, primarily of the lubricant. Materials like steel degrade through chemical reactions like oxidation, which is accelerated by heat. Every 10°C approximately doubles the speed of the reaction. A motor designed so that the bearings are 10°C cooler will run about twice as long. Using these factors, a motor manufacturer can accelerate a life test on a motor by raising the temperature.

Ventilation Cost Summary

The total cost of operating the ventilation systems in a home is the combined cost of the equipment, the electrical cost, the conditioned air cost, and the replacement cost for all the systems. Although there are definitely costs involved, the effects of good ventilation systems on the health of the occupants and the durability of the building make those costs worthwhile. The equipment may not be as glamorous as a high-end stove in the kitchen or a spa in the bathroom and cost avoidance is never obvious, but that certainly doesn't reduce the importance. And the costs are not that high.

It takes some work to figure out the cost of the system. Unfortunately, there is no simple way of calculating the operating cost per year that could be tacked on the side of the box. Certified airflow from HVI will provide that component. Power consumption can be determined from the watts. Life expectancy of the motor can be guesstimated from the previous table (or from the manufacturer if they will provide it). The run-time can be estimated from the application. The conditioned air cost depends on the application, the airflow, the local conditions, the heat recovery efficiency, and the run-time.

You can analyze these calculations, but ventilation doesn't significantly contribute to the cost of maintaining a healthy home. It is difficult to accept the idea that if a fan is running all the time, that it isn't wasting energy, but there are many less essential components running constantly in the house that we are not even aware of. Clocks, power strips, transformers, stereo equipment, answering machines, computers, door bell transformers, all use power all the time. Background power consumption will rarely drop below 300 watts even without a ventilation system running. That is (300 x 8760)/1000 x $0.1194 = $313 per year. And if you add air conditioning and heating, water heaters, stoves, and refrigerators and freezers to that, you will get your total electrical cost. We just accept those costs as part of life. Reducing the cost of energy for the house by building it tightly allows the cost of operating a whole dwelling ventilation system twenty-four-seven-three-sixty-five to about $1 per cubic foot of air moved. A 50 cfm fan costs about $50 per year to operate continuously!

"Selling" the Ventilation System

Perhaps this needs a whole chapter for itself. Clearly, a mechanical ventilation system can only do its job if it's running. If the occupant of the house doesn't appreciate what the system is for, they won't use it. All the science in the world, all the fancy mathematical calculations in quadrature, all the efforts for good, functional installation are meaningless if the system isn't used. Codes can require it, but if the "ventilation police" don't fine the occupants, who cares? And that's the point: making people care.

HEALTH: Assuming that the air outside is of better quality than the air inside the house, the ventilation system is there to exchange the bad air inside with the good air outside. There are hundreds of studies and programs that point to good mechanical ventilation as a key component of the health of the occupants and the building itself. The difficulty is making the one-to-one connection between the mechanical ventilation system and the health of the occupants. Flick the light switch and the light goes out. Flick off the fan switch, the fan stops but the occupants don't fall over! And we are told that so many things in life are bad for us (like red wine) only to discover a couple of years later that, no, it's actually good for us. In this case, however, you can show the effect of bad air quickly with a plastic bag! And the good/bad thing has raged for hundreds of years regarding the qualities of ventilation air.

Accepting the fact that we need fresh air to breathe means that as houses get tighter to save energy, we need to breathe fresh air. Think of a scuba diver without an air tank. Think of a fireplace without a chimney. The bad air needs to go out so the good air can come in.

There are fundamental questions that come up again and again.

"You're telling me to make my house tight, and now you're telling me to make holes in it!"

"It costs a lot to run the fan all the time!"

"It's a waste of energy!"

You can provide all the logical answers to these questions, referring to the energy saved by making the house tighter, telling people doorbell transformers use 6 watts and some fans use 8 watts and you don't unplug your doorbell transformer, do you? You can wax eloquent on the impact on health that good, fresh air can provide. People don't unplug their refrigerators, they don't even shut their computers off when they are not being used - or their TVs or modems or network hubs. We allow our furnaces and air conditioners to run on automatic controls.

It's the "open window" syndrome. Isn't it dangerous to leave a window open, especially at night? It's a miasma theory of Western society: night air is poisonous - miasmaphobia! The word malaria in the original Italian meant bad air - *mal, aria*. In the 1800s, it was common to believe that the air outside somehow became poisonous at night. Even Sam Adams was lectured by Ben Franklin regarding the beneficial qualities of outside air - until he fell asleep. Social battles raged throughout the 1800s as technologies made it possible to make the house a sanctuary against outside pollutants from swamps and slums. Heating systems transformed from open fireplaces to stoves to central heating. Man's purity, sanctity, and health could all be sullied by the unknown qualities of the outside air.[10] The cyclic nature of human history has led us from wide open homes under the starry skies to sealed up houses to protect us from the night air that was only available to the upper classes through indoor plumbing, back to open windows, and finally back to hermetically sealed homes of today with the air-conditioned by mechanical systems and codes and air sealing technologies. It is reminiscent of the story of the girl who watched her mother carefully cut the ends off a ham before placing it in a pot as she was preparing for dinner. Curious, the girl asked her mother why she did that. The mother looked at her daughter as mothers do when they are not sure of the answer and admitted that she didn't have a clue, but that's what her mother had always done. Pursuing the question, the girl finally had a chance to ask her grandmother about it and the old lady replied, "Lord, child, I always used the same pot and the ham simply wouldn't fit unless I cut the ends off!"

Miasmaphobia persists - a primal fear that cannot be overcome by technology, reason, or logic.

---

10. Peter C. Baldwin, How Night Air Became Good Air, 1776-1930, Environmental History Vol 8, No. 3 (July, 2003), pp 412 - 429

Chapter 12

Ventilation Codes

The most important building code issues are those that apply locally to the building that you are working on. There is no national, universal building code that applies to every house in every neighborhood. States and local jurisdictions have adopted and adapted various national and international building, mechanical, and energy codes.

The International Code Council (ICC)[1] is "a membership association dedicated to building safety and fire prevention, and develops the codes used to construct residential and commercial buildings, including homes and schools." On their website is a map identified as "I-Code Adoptions" that allows state by state identification of what "I" codes have been adopted. For example, as of this writing Massachusetts has adopted the 2021 International Building Code (IBC), 2021 International Existing Building Code (IEBC), the 2021 International Mechanical Code (IMC) the 2021 International Residential Code (IRC), and the 2021 International Energy Conservation Code (IECC). The ninth edition of the MA State Building Code was based on the suite of 2015 I-codes. The tenth edition of the MA State Building became effective in October of 2024 and is based on the 2021 suite of I-Codes.

On the ICC webpage they have developed an "Periodic Table" of International Codes, Standards, and guidelines" that serves as a quick reference.

---

1. https://www.iccsafe.org/

The ICC bookstore sells the codebooks for states like North Carolina, California, Michigan, Virginia, Florida, Ohio, and Arkansas. Although most of the local codes are based on the ICC codes, it is important to check with local code authorities for the most pertinent codes, those that apply to the building you are working on. Some states like California, Florida, Washington, Vermont, Massachusetts, and Minnesota have specific ventilation codes or procedures.

There is an on-line service called "Up-Codes"[2] that provides updated access to building codes if you need to be kept up-to-date. And the Standard Work Specifications (SWS)[3] has basic how-to information about ventilation along with many other topics.

IMPORTANT NOTE: *The following are summaries (written in italics) and not actual Code language that applies to residential ventilation applications. There are hyperlinks to the actual code section. These summaries are not meant to be the final and comprehensive word on the codes that apply in your application at this particular moment. These summaries provide a good starting point, but the actual codes and local code officials should be consulted.*[4]

* * *

2024 INTERNATIONAL MECHANICAL Code

* * *

IMC CHAPTER 3 General Regulations
  IMC § 303.3 *Prohibited locations.*
  Fuel-fired appliances cannot be installed or draw combustion air from sleeping rooms, bathrooms, toilet rooms, storage closets, or surgical rooms. Exceptions include direct-vent appliances using outdoor air, solid fuel-fired

---

2. https://up.codes/
3. https://sws.nrel.gov/search/faceted?k=Ventilation
4. The ICC has permitted the inclusion of these code citations. The author would like to express his sincere gratitude. Please visit www.iccsafe.org for copies of the codes from their bookstore.

appliances with manufacturer-specified combustion air, and appliances in dedicated enclosures with outdoor air access and a properly sealed, self-closing door as per Chapter 7 and energy code requirements.

IMC § 304 Installation

IMC § 304.5 Hydrogen-Generating and Refueling Operations

Hydrogen-generating and refueling appliances must be installed per their listing and manufacturer's instructions, with ventilation required as specified in Section 304.5. In facilities like public and private garages, repair garages, fuel-dispensing stations, and parking garages containing such appliances, spaces connected to a private garage are treated as part of the garage if they are not part of a dwelling's living space.

IMC § 304.5.1 Natural Ventilation

Indoor spaces for hydrogen-generating or refueling operations are limited to 850 square feet and must connect to the outdoors as specified in Sections 304.5.1.1 and 304.5.1.2. Hydrogen-generating appliances cannot exceed 4 standard cubic feet per minute of hydrogen output per 250 square feet of floor area. Air openings must have a minimum dimension of 3 inches, with ducts matching the cross-sectional area of the connected openings. Ignition sources must be positioned at least 12 inches below the ceiling.

IMC § 304.5.1.1 Two Openings

Garages must have two permanent openings in the same exterior wall, one within 12 inches of the ceiling and the other within 12 inches of the floor. These openings must directly connect to the outdoors and provide a minimum free area of 1/2 square foot per 1,000 cubic feet of garage volume.

IMC § 304.5.1.2 Louvers and Grilles

The required free area for openings is based on their net free area. If the free area of louvers or grilles is known, it must be used in calculations. If unknown, wood louvers are assumed to provide 25% free area, and metal louvers or grilles 75%. Louvers and grilles must remain fixed in the open position.

IMC § 304.5.2 Mechanical Ventilation

Indoor hydrogen-generating or refueling locations must be ventilated per Section 502.16, and any ignition sources must be positioned below the mechanical ventilation outlets.

* * *

IMC Chapter 4 Ventilation

IMC § 401.1 Scope.

This chapter outlines ventilation requirements for occupied building spaces. It mandates compliance with Chapter 5 for mechanical exhaust systems, including those for clothes dryers, cooking appliances, hazardous exhaust, dust and refuse conveyors, subslab soil exhaust, smoke control, energy recovery ventilation, and other systems specified in Section 502.

IMC § 401.2 Ventilation required.

Occupied spaces must be ventilated either naturally (per Section 402) or mechanically (per Section 403). Dwelling units meeting air leakage standards from the International Energy Conservation Code or ASHRAE 90.1 require mechanical ventilation under Section 403. Mechanical ventilation is also mandatory for ambulatory care facilities and Group I-2 occupancies, as specified in Section 407.

IMC § 401.3 When required.

Ventilation is required when the room or space is occupied.

IMC § 401.4 Intake Opening location.

Air intake openings must adhere to the following rules:

1. They must be at least 10 feet away from lot lines or other buildings on the same lot.
2. Mechanical and gravity intake openings must be at least 10 feet horizontally from hazardous or noxious contaminant sources (e.g., vents, streets, parking lots), unless they are at least 25 feet vertically above such sources.
3. Openings within 10 feet of contaminant sources must be at least 3 feet below them, except when using approved intake/exhaust combination fittings.
4. In flood hazard areas, intake openings must be located at or above the required elevation for utilities specified in the International Building Code.

IMC § 401.5 Intake opening protection.

Outdoor air intake openings must be protected with corrosion-resistant screens, louvers, or grilles, sized per Table 401.5 and designed to withstand local weather conditions. In hurricane-prone areas, louvers must comply with AMCA 550. Openings in exterior walls must also meet the International Building Code requirements for exterior wall opening protectives.

TABLE 401.5 OPENING SIZES IN LOUVERS, GRILLES AND SCREENS PROTECTING OUTDOOR EXHAUST AND AIR INTAKE OPENINGS	
OUTDOOR OPENING TYPE	**MINIMUM AND MAXIMUM OPENING SIZES IN LOUVERS, GRILLES AND SCREENS MEASURED IN ANY DIRECTION**
Intake openings in residential occupancies	Not < ¼ inch and not > ½ inch
Intake openings in other than residential occupancies	> ¼ inch and not > 1 inch
For SI: 1 inch = 25.4 mm	

Table 12.1 (401.5) Opening Sizes

IMC § 401.6 *Contaminant sources.*

Stationary sources generating airborne particulates, heat, odors, fumes, vapors, smoke, or gases in harmful quantities must have an exhaust system per Chapter 5 or another method to collect and remove contaminants. The exhaust must discharge to an approved exterior location.

* * *

IMC § 402 – NATURAL VENTILATION

IMC § [B]402.1 *Natural ventilation.*

Natural ventilation in occupied spaces must use windows, doors, louvers, or other outdoor openings. These openings must have accessible controls for easy operation by occupants.

IMC § [B]402.2 *Ventilation area required*

Openings to the outdoors must be at least 4 percent of the floor area being ventilated.

IMC § [B]402.3 *Adjoining spaces*

Rooms without direct outdoor openings can be ventilated through adjoining rooms, provided the opening between them is unobstructed and at least 8% of the interior room's floor area, with a minimum of 25 square feet (2.3

m^2). Outdoor ventilation area must account for the total floor area being ventilated.

> Exception: Openings for ventilation can lead to a thermally isolated sunroom or patio cover if the openable area between them and the interior room is at least 8% of the interior room's floor area, with a minimum of 20 square feet (1.86 m^2). Outdoor ventilation requirements still apply based on the total floor area.

IMC § [B]402.4 Openings below grade

For below-grade openings providing natural ventilation, the horizontal clear space outside the opening must be at least 1.5 times the depth of the opening, measured from the average ground level to the bottom of the opening.

***

IMC § 403 MECHANICAL VENTILATION

IMC § 403.1 Ventilation system.

Mechanical ventilation must include supply and return or exhaust air systems. For Group R-2, R-3, and R-4 occupancies up to three stories, ventilation can use an exhaust system, supply system, or a combination. Supply air should approximately match return or exhaust air, and the system may create positive or negative pressure. Ventilation systems must comply with Chapter 6 design and installation requirements.[5]

IMC § 403.2 Outdoor air required.

The minimum outdoor airflow rate is determined by Section 403.3.

---

5. Author note: Residential Group R includes among others, the use of a building or structure, or a portion thereof, for sleep purposes. R-1 covers primarily transient occupancies like boarding house, hotels, motels. R-2 are more than 2 dwelling units such as apartment houses, convents, dormitories, etc. R-3 are dwelling units where the occupants are primarily permanent in nature like lodging houses, adult care facilities, foster homes, etc. R-4 includes buildings arranged for occupancy as residential care/assisted living facilities including five but not more than sixteen occupants, excluding staff.

Exception: *If a registered design professional proves that an engineered ventilation system can maintain contaminant levels equal to or lower than those achieved by the Section 403.3 rate, the minimum outdoor airflow rate may be reduced accordingly.*

IMC § 403.2.1 Recirculation of air.

Outdoor air required by Section 403.3 cannot be recirculated, but excess air may be recirculated as part of the supply air to building spaces, with the following exceptions:

1. Ventilation air cannot be recirculated from one dwelling to another or to different occupancies.
2. Supply air to swimming pools and deck areas cannot be recirculated unless dehumidified to maintain relative humidity at 60% or less, and air from these areas cannot be recirculated to other spaces if more than 10% of the supply air is recirculated.
3. When mechanical exhaust is required by Note b in Table 403.3.1.1, air recirculation from those spaces is prohibited, though recirculation within the space is allowed. All air supplied to such spaces must be exhausted.
4. When mechanical exhaust is required by Note g in Table 403.3.1.1, recirculation is prohibited if more than 10% of the supply air comes from recirculated air from those spaces. Recirculation within the space is allowed.

IMC § 403.2.2 Transfer air.

Air transferred from occupiable spaces can be used as makeup air for exhaust systems in areas like kitchens, baths, toilet rooms, elevators, and smoking lounges, unless recirculation is prohibited by Table 403.3.1.1. The amount of transfer and exhaust air must meet the flow rates specified in Section 403.3.1.1. Required outdoor airflow rates must be introduced directly into these spaces, the spaces from which air is transferred, or both.

IMC § 403.3 Outdoor airflow rate and Local Exhaust Airflow Rates

Group R-2, R-3, and R-4 occupancies up to three stories above grade must have outdoor air and local exhaust as per Section 403.3.2. All other occupied buildings must comply with outdoor air and local exhaust requirements specified in Section 403.3.1.

IMC § 403.3.1 Other Buildings Intended to Be Occupied

For occupancies other than Groups R-2, R-3 and R-4 the design of local exhaust systems and ventilation systems for outdoor air shall comply with Sections 403.3.1.1 through 403.3.1.5.

IMC § 403.3.1.1 Outdoor Airflow Rate

Ventilation systems must be designed to meet the minimum outdoor airflow rate for each occupiable space, delivering the required airflow to the breathing zone. The occupant load for the design should not be less than the estimated maximum occupant load from Table 403.3.1.1, or based on a similar occupancy classification if not listed. Ventilation must be continuous during occupancy, unless otherwise specified.

Except *for smoking lounges, ventilation rates are based on no smoking in the space. If smoking occurs elsewhere, the system must provide additional ventilation according to accepted engineering practices.*

Exception: *The occupant load does not need to follow the estimated maximum occupant load rate from Table 403.3.1.1 if statistical data supports an alternative occupant density.*

AREA TO BE EXHAUSTED	EXHAUST RATE CAPACITY
Kitchens	100 cfm intermittent or 50 cfm continuous
Bathrooms and toilet rooms	50 cfm intermittent or 25 cfm continuous

Table 403.3.1.1[6]
Minimum Ventilation Rates
Private dwellings, single and multiple

For SI: 1 cubic foot per minute = 0.0004719 m3/s, 1 ton = 908 kg,

---

6. This table has been abbreviated to consider only residential occupancies.

1 cubic foot per minute per square foot = 0.00508 m³/(s • m²),
°C = [(°F) -32]/1.8, 1 square foot = 0.0929 m².

[a] Based upon net occupiable floor area.

[b] Mechanical exhaust required and the recirculation of air from such spaces is prohibited. Recirculation of air that is contained completely within such spaces shall not be prohibited (see Section 403.2.1, Item 3).

[c] Spaces unheated or maintained below 50°F are not covered by these requirements unless the occupancy is continuous.

[f] Rates are per room unless otherwise indicated. The higher rate shall be provided where the exhaust system is designed to operated intermittently. The lower rate shall be permitted only where the exhaust system is designed to operate continuously while occupied.

[g] Mechanical exhaust is required and recirculation from such spaces is prohibited. For occupancies where there is a wheel-type energy recovery ventilation (ERV) unit in the exhaust system design, volume of air leaked from the exhaust airstream into the outdoor airstream within the ERV shall be less than 10 percent of the outdoor air volume. Recirculation of air that is contained completely within such spaces shall not be prohibited (see section 403.2.1, items 2 and 4).

IMC § 403.3.1.2 Exhaust ventilation.

Exhaust airflow rates must comply with Table 403.3.1.1. Outdoor air introduced by an exhaust system will count towards meeting the outdoor airflow requirements specified in Table 403.3.1.1.

IMC § 403.3.1.5 Balancing.

The ventilation air distribution system must include means to adjust and achieve the minimum required airflow rates as specified in Sections 403.3 and 403.3.1.2. The system must be balanced using an approved method to ensure it can supply and exhaust the required airflow rates.

IMC § 403.3.2 Group R-2, R-3, and R-4 Occupancies, three stories and less

The design of local exhaust and outdoor air ventilation systems for Group R-2, R-3, and R-4 occupancies up to three stories above grade must comply with Sections 403.3.2.1 through 403.3.2.5.

IMC § 403.3.2.1 Outdoor Air for Dwelling Units

Each dwelling unit must have an outdoor air ventilation system, which can include a mechanical exhaust system, supply system, or a combination. Local exhaust or supply systems, including outdoor air ducts connected to the return side of an air handler, are allowed. The system must provide the required outdoor airflow continuously while the building is occupied, with the minimum airflow rate determined by Equation 4-9.

$$Q_{OA} = 0.03\, A_{floor} + 7.5(N_{br} + 1) \quad (Equation\ 4\text{-}9)^7$$

where:

Q_{OA} = outdoor airflow rate, cfm
A_{floor} = floor area, ft^2
N_{br} = number of bedrooms; not to be less than one

EXCEPTION:

1. *Intermittent Operation of Ventilation System:* The outdoor air ventilation system does not need to run continuously. It can operate for at least 1 hour in every 4-hour period, as long as the average outdoor air flow rate over those 4 hours meets the requirements of Equation 4-9.
2. *Reduced Minimum Ventilation Rate:* The minimum required mechanical ventilation rate may be reduced by 30% if both of the following conditions are met:

- *Ventilation Air Distribution:* A ducted system supplies air directly to each bedroom and at least one of the following rooms:
- Living room
- Dining room
- Kitchen
- *Balanced System:* The whole-house ventilation system is balanced

---

7. Author's note: The 0.03 factor in the formula increased from 0.01 in the 2018 IMC and there are even versions of the 2021 code that list it as 0.01. The 2022 version of ASHRAE 62.2 relies on the 0.03 factor moderated by blower door testing to account for the leakiness of the house. Also note that the IRC M1505.4.3 in equation 15-1 uses the 0.01 factor.

IMC § 403.3.2.2 Outdoor Air for Other Spaces

Corridors and other common areas within the conditioned space must be supplied with outdoor air at a minimum rate of 0.06 cfm per square foot (0.0003 m³/(s • m²)) of floor area.

IMC § 403.3.2.3 Local Exhaust

Local exhaust systems must be provided in kitchens, bathrooms, and toilet rooms, with the capacity to exhaust the minimum airflow rate specified in Table 403.3.2.3.

AREA TO BE EXHAUSTED	EXHAUST RATE CAPACITY
Kitchens	100 cfm intermittent or 50 cfm continuous
Bathrooms and toilet rooms	50 cfm intermittent or 25 cfm continuous

TABLE 403.3.2.3 MINIMUM REQUIRED LOCAL EXHAUST RATES FOR GROUP R-2, R-3, AND R-4 OCCUPANCIES

For SI: 1 cubic foot per minute = 0.0004719 m³/s.

IMC § 403.3.2.4 System controls

Controls for outdoor air ventilation systems must be marked and include text or a symbol indicating the system's function.

IMC § 403.2.5 Ventilating equipment

Outdoor air and exhaust fans providing exhaust or outdoor air must be listed and labeled to provide the minimum required air flow in accordance with ANSI/AMCA 20-ANSI/ASHRAE 51.

* * *

IMC § 404 ENCLOSED PARKING GARAGES

IMC § 404.1 Enclosed parking garages.

When mechanical ventilation systems in enclosed parking garages operate intermittently, they must automatically function using carbon monoxide and nitrogen dioxide detectors compliant with UL 2075 standards and installed as recommended. The system should alternate between two modes:

1. Full-on mode with airflow at a minimum of 0.75 cfm per square foot of floor area.

2. Standby mode with airflow at a minimum of 0.05 cfm per square foot of floor area.

IMC § 405 SYSTEMS CONTROL

IMC § 405.1 General.

Mechanical ventilation systems must have controls, either manual or automatic, to ensure operation whenever the space is occupied. Air-conditioning systems supplying ventilation air must have automatic controls to maintain the required outdoor air supply rate during occupancy.

IMC § 406 VENTILATION OF UNINHABITED SPACES

IMC § 406.1 General.

Uninhabited spaces like crawl spaces and attics must have natural ventilation openings per the International Building Code or a mechanical exhaust and supply air system. Mechanical exhaust must provide at least 0.02 cfm per square foot (0.00001 m3/s • m2) and activate automatically when the relative humidity exceeds 60%.

* * *

IMC Chapter 5 Exhaust Systems

IMC § 501.1 Scope.

This chapter covers the design, construction, and installation of mechanical exhaust systems, including those for clothes dryers, cooking appliances, hazardous materials, dust and refuse conveyors, subslab soil, smoke control, energy recovery ventilation, and other systems outlined in Section 502.

IMC § 501.2 Independent system required.

Mechanical exhaust systems for environmental air must be separate from other exhaust systems. Dryer, domestic kitchen, and hazardous exhaust systems must also be independent. Type I exhaust systems must be separate unless specified in Section 506.3.5. Type II exhaust systems for food-processing operations must remain independent. Commercial kitchen exhaust systems must comply with Sections 506–509.

IMC § 501.3 Exhaust discharge.

Air removed by mechanical exhaust systems must be discharged outdoors in compliance with Section 501.2.1, avoiding public nuisances or locations where it could be reintroduced into a ventilation system. Exhaust air must not be directed into attics, crawl spaces, or walkways. Exceptions include:

1. Whole-house attic fans discharging into private attics.
2. Commercial cooking recirculating systems.
3. Domestic ductless range hoods, if installed per manufacturer instructions and ventilation requirements in Chapter 4 are met.

501.3.1 Location of exhaust outlets.

Exhaust outlets and ducts must terminate outdoors at specific minimum distances based on the type of exhaust:

1. Explosive or flammable vapors/dusts: 30 feet (9144 mm) from property lines and combustible walls in the exhaust direction, 10 feet (3048 mm) from openings into buildings, and 6 feet (1829 mm) from exterior walls/roofs.
2. Other product-conveying outlets: 10 feet (3048 mm) from property lines and building openings, 3 feet (914 mm) from walls/roofs, and 10 feet (3048 mm) above grade.
3. Environmental air exhaust: 3 feet (914 mm) from property lines, operable openings (except Group U), and 10 feet (3048 mm) from mechanical air intakes unless an approved combination fitting is used.
4. Flood hazard areas: Must meet elevation requirements in Section 1612 of the International Building Code.
5. Specific systems: Refer to designated sections for clothes dryers (504.4) and kitchen exhausts (506.3.13, 506.4, 506.5).

IMC § 501.3.2 Exhaust opening protection.

Outdoor exhaust openings must be protected by corrosion-resistant screens, louvers, or grilles with openings between ¼ inch and ½ inch in size and shielded against weather. In hurricane-prone regions, louvers must comply with AMCA Standard 550. Openings in exterior walls must meet the International Building Code requirements for wall opening protectives.

IMC § 501.4 Pressure equalization.

Mechanical exhaust systems must be sized to remove the required air and operate whenever air needs to be exhausted. For spaces other than R-3 occupancies and R-2 dwelling units, the space must maintain neutral or negative pressure. If the supply system provides more air than the exhaust system removes, additional exhaust must be provided. If the exhaust removes more air than the supply system provides, make-up air must be supplied to balance the deficit.

IMC § 501.5 Ducts

Exhaust ducting not described in this chapter must comply with Chapter 6.

* * *

IMC § 504 CLOTHES DRYER EXHAUST

IMC § 504.1 Installation.

Clothes dryers must be exhausted per the manufacturer's instructions, directing moisture and combustion products outside the building.

Exception: Condensing (ductless) dryers are exempt from this requirement if they are listed and labeled.

IMC § 504.2 Exhaust penetrations.

When a clothes dryer exhaust duct penetrates a wall or ceiling, the space around the duct must be sealed with noncombustible material, approved fire caulking, or a noncombustible dryer exhaust wall receptacle. Dryer exhaust ducts cannot penetrate or be located within fire blocking, draft stopping, or any fire-resistant assemblies, unless the duct is made of galvanized steel or aluminum as specified in Section 603.4, maintaining the required fire-resistance rating. Fire dampers or similar devices that could block exhaust flow are prohibited in dryer exhaust ducts.

IMC § 504.3 Cleanout.

Cleanout must be provided for each vertical riser.

IMC § 504.4 Exhaust installation.

Dryer exhaust ducts must terminate outside the building and be equipped with a backdraft damper. Screens are not allowed at the duct termination. Ducts should not be connected with sheet metal screws or other fasteners that block airflow, and they cannot be connected to a vent connector, vent, or chimney. Additionally, dryer exhaust ducts should not extend into or pass through ducts or plenums.

IMC § 504.4.1 Termination location.

Exhaust duct terminations must follow the dryer manufacturer's installation instructions. If the instructions do not specify a termination location, the duct must terminate at least 3 feet 914mm)from any openings into buildings, including those in ventilated soffits.

IMC § 504.4.2 Exhaust termination outlet and passageway size.

Dryer ducting must not be crushed and must provide an open area of not less than 12.5 square inches (8065mm2).

IMC § 504.5 Dryer Exhaust Power Ventilators[8].

Domestic dryer exhaust duct power ventilators must comply with UL 705 standards and be installed according to the manufacturer's instructions.

IMC § 504.6 Booster fans prohibited.

Booster fans must not be installed in dryer exhaust systems.

IMC § 504.7 Makeup air.

Exhaust systems exceeding 200 cfm (0.09 m3/s) require makeup air. For dryer installations in a closet, the closet must have a minimum 100-square-inch (0.0645 m2) opening or an alternative approved source of makeup air.

IMC §504.8 Protection Required

Protective steel shield plates, 0.062 inches (1.6 mm) thick, must be installed on framing members where nails or screws could penetrate dryer exhaust ducts. These plates are required if the duct is less than 1 1/4 inches (32 mm) from the framing surface and must extend at least 2 inches (51 mm) above sole plates and below top plates.

IMC § 504.9 Domestic clothes dryer ducts.

Clothes dryer exhaust ducts must conform to the requirements of Sections 504.9.1 through 504.9.6.

IMC § 504.9.1 Material and size.

Exhaust ducts must have a smooth interior finish and be constructed of metal a minimum 0.016 inch (0.4 mm) thick. The exhaust duct must be nominally 4 inches (102 mm) in diameter.

---

8. Note that there is a difference between Dryer Exhaust Power Ventilators or DEDPV products that are UL-705 listed and booster fans. The lint contained in dryer exhaust air is highly flammable. DEDPV products are specifically tested for gas and electric clothes dryers.

IMC § 504.9.2 Duct installation.

Exhaust ducts must be supported every 4 feet (1219 mm), secured in place, and connected so the insert end aligns with airflow direction. Fasteners inside the duct must not protrude more than 1/8 inch (3.2 mm).[9]

IMC § 504.9.3 Transition ducts.

Transition ducts connecting dryers to exhaust systems must be a single, UL 2158A-certified length, no longer than 8 feet (2438 mm), and not concealed within construction.

IMC § 504.9.4. Duct length.

Determine the maximum allowable exhaust duct length by one of the methods specified in Sections 504.9.4.1 through 504.9.4.3.

IMC § 504.9.4.1. Specified length.

The exhaust duct length must not exceed 35 feet (10,668 mm)[10] from the dryer connection to the outlet. Fittings reduce the maximum allowable length as specified in Table 504.9.4.1.

Dryer Exhaust Duct Fitting Type	Equivalent Length
4" radius mitered 45-degree elbow	2 feet 6 inches
4" radius mitered 90-degree elbow	5 feet
6" radius smooth 45-degree elbow	1 foot
6" radius smooth 90-degree elbow	1 foot 9 inches
8" radius smooth 45-degree elbow	1 foot
8" radius smooth 90-degree elbow	1 foot 7 inches
10" radius smooth 45-degree elbow	9 inches
10" radius smooth 90-degree elbow	1 foot 6 inches

Table 504.9.4.1
Dryer Exhaust Duct Fitting Equivalent Length

For SI: 1 inch=25.4 mm, 1 foot = 304.8 mm, 1 degree = 0.0175 rad.

IMC § 504.9.4.2 Manufacturer's instructions.

The exhaust duct length must follow the dryer manufacturer's instructions, which must be provided to the code official. For concealed ducts, these instruc-

---

9. Note that in IRC M1502.4.2 ducts "shall be supported at intervals not to exceed 12 feet (3658 mm)"
10. The International Residential Code specifies the maximum length allowed to be 25 feet (7620 mm) in M1502.4.4.1.

tions must be submitted before inspection. If the manufacturer doesn't provide fitting length calculations, use Table 504.9.4.1.

IMC § 504.9.4.3 *Dryer Exhaust Duct Power Ventilator Length.*

The dryer exhaust duct power ventilator manufacturers installation instructions shall determine the maximum duct length.

504.9.5 Length identification.

If the exhaust duct's equivalent length exceeds 35 feet (10 668 mm), a permanent label or tag indicating the length must be placed within 6 feet (1829 mm) of the duct connection.

504.9.6 Exhaust duct required.

If space is provided for a clothes dryer, an exhaust duct system must be installed. If no dryer is present at occupancy, the duct must be capped.

Exception: *This does not apply if a listed condensing dryer is installed.*

* * *

IMC § 505 DOMESTIC KITCHEN EXHAUST EQUIPMENT

IMC § 505.2 *Domestic cooking exhaust.*

Domestic cooking exhaust equipment must comply with the following:

1. *Fans for overhead range hoods and non-integral downdraft exhausts must meet UL 507 standards.*
2. *Overhead range hoods and downdraft exhausts with built-in fans must comply with UL 507.*
3. *Cooking appliances with integral downdraft exhausts must meet UL 858 or ANSI Z21.1 standards.*
4. *Over-the-range microwave ovens with integral exhausts must comply with UL 923.*

IMC § 505.3 *Exhaust ducts.*

Domestic cooking exhaust equipment must discharge outdoors through sheet metal ducts made of galvanized steel, stainless steel, aluminum, or copper, with smooth inner walls, airtight construction, and a backdraft damper. Installations in Group I-1 and I-2 occupancies must follow the International Building Code and Fire Code.

Exceptions:

1. In non-Group I-1 and I-2 settings, ductless range hoods that follow the manufacturer's instructions and meet ventilation requirements do not need to discharge outdoors.
2. Ducts for downdraft exhaust systems can be made of Schedule 40 PVC if installed under a concrete slab, backfilled with sand or gravel, and with specific installation conditions.

IMC § 505.4 Makeup air required.

Exhaust hood systems that exhaust over 400 cfm must have makeup air provided at a similar rate. The makeup air system must include a closure mechanism and be automatically controlled to start and operate with the exhaust system.

* * *

IMC § 512 SUBSLAB SOIL EXHAUST SYSTEMS

IMC § 512.1 General.

Subslab ducting must conform to the requirements of this section.

IMC § 512.2 Materials.

Subslab soil exhaust system ducts must either be air ducts meeting UL 181 Class 0 standards or piping materials compliant with the International Plumbing Code for sanitary drainage and vent pipes, such as cast iron, galvanized steel, brass, copper (Type DWV or heavier), or approved plastic piping.

IMC § 512.3 Grade.

Exhaust system ducts must have a minimum slope of one-eighth unit vertical in 12 units horizontal (1-percent slope) and must not be trapped.

IMC § 512.4 Termination.

Subslab soil exhaust system ducts must extend at least 6 inches (152 mm) above the roof and be located at least 10 feet (3048 mm) away from any operable openings or air intakes.

IMC § 512.5 Identification.

Permanently identify subslab soil exhaust ducts within each floor level by means of a tag, stencil or other approved marking.

* * *

IMC § 513 ENERGY RECOVERY VENTILATION SYSTEMS

IMC § 513.1 General.

Energy recovery ventilation systems must follow this section's requirements and comply with the International Energy Conservation Code when used for energy conservation. Ducted heat recovery ventilators must meet UL 1812 standards, while nonducted ones must meet the UL 1815 standard.

IMC § 514.2 Prohibited applications.

Energy recovery ventilation (ERV) systems are prohibited in hazardous exhaust, explosive or flammable dust systems, smoke control systems, Type I commercial kitchen exhausts, and clothes dryer exhausts. However, ERV equipment using coil-type heat exchangers to recover only sensible heat is exempt from these restrictions.

IMC § 513.3 Access.

The heat exchanger and other components of the system must be accessible as required for service, maintenance, repair or replacement.

IMC § 513.4 Recirculated Air

Air in energy recovery systems is not classified as recirculated if the system limits cross-leakage between air streams to less than 10% of the total airflow capacity.

* * *

IMC CHAPTER 6 Duct Systems

IMC § 601 GENERAL

IMC § 601.1 Scope.

Duct systems for air movement in HVAC and exhaust systems must comply with this chapter unless specified otherwise in Chapters 5 and 7.

Exception: Ducts discharging combustible material into a combustion chamber must meet NFPA 82 standards.

[B]IMC § 601.2 Air movement in egress elements.

Corridors cannot be used as supply, return, exhaust, relief, or ventilation air ducts, with exceptions:

1. Corridors can supply makeup air for exhaust systems in adjacent rooms (e.g., restrooms or janitor closets) if they are directly supplied with more outdoor air than the makeup air taken.
2. Corridors within dwelling units can be used for return air.

3. Corridors in tenant spaces under 1,000 square feet can also convey return air.

IMC § 601.2.1 Corridor Ceiling

The space between a corridor ceiling and the floor or roof above can be used as a return air plenum under these conditions:

1. The corridor doesn't require fire-resistance-rated construction.
2. The plenum is separated by fire-resistance-rated construction.
3. The air-handling system shuts down when smoke detectors activate.
4. The air-handling system shuts down upon sprinkler waterflow detection in fully sprinklered buildings.
5. The space is part of an approved smoke control system.

[B]IMC § 601.3 Exits.

Ventilation equipment and ductwork for exit enclosures must follow one of these options:

1. Be located outside the building and connected to the exit enclosure via ducts enclosed in shaft-rated construction.
2. If inside the exit enclosure, intake and exhaust air must come directly from and discharge to the outdoors, or use ducts enclosed in shaft-rated construction.
3. If within the building, the equipment and ductwork must be separated from the rest of the building by shaft-rated construction.

Openings in fire-rated construction are limited to those necessary for maintenance and must have self-closing fire-rated devices. Exit enclosure ventilation systems must operate independently from other building ventilation systems.

IMC § 601.4 Contamination prevention.

Exhaust ducts under positive pressure, chimneys, and vents cannot pass through ducts or plenums, with these exceptions:

1. Exhaust systems in ceiling return air plenums are allowed if the space permits 10% recirculation, and duct joints and seams meet Section 603.9.

2. Chimneys and vents can pass through plenums if they comply with one of the following:

- Listed for positive pressure and sealed per manufacturer instructions.
- Installed without fittings or joints in the above-ceiling space.
- Enclosed in a sealed conduit separating it from the ceiling space.

IMC §601.5 Return Air Openings

HVAC Return air openings must comply with all of the following:

1. Location Restrictions: Return air openings must be at least 10 feet (3048 mm) from open combustion chambers or draft hoods of other appliances in the same room.
2. Prohibited Areas: Return air cannot be taken from hazardous, unsanitary areas, refrigeration rooms, closets, bathrooms, kitchens, garages, unconditioned attics, boiler rooms, or furnace rooms.
3. Proportional Airflow: Return air volume must not exceed the supply air delivered to the same space.
4. Sizing Standards: Openings must follow manufacturer instructions, ACCA Manual D, or professional designs.
5. Single Dwelling Use: Air from one dwelling unit cannot be discharged into another unit.
6. Crawl Spaces: Direct connections to forced air furnaces are not allowed; transfer openings in crawl space enclosures are acceptable.
7. Closet Specifications: Return air from closets must serve only the closet, and small closets (<30 sq. ft. (2.8 m2)) need undercut doors, louvered doors, or air transfer grilles with specific free area dimensions.
8. Swimming Pool Areas: Return air cannot be taken from pool enclosures unless the air is dehumidified or served by a dedicated HVAC system.

Exceptions:
•Kitchens may have return air openings if located at least 10 feet (3048

mm) from cooking appliances (or 5 feet if the appliance is electric and part of a combined kitchen-living space).

* * *

IMC § 602 PLENUMS

IMC § 602.1 General.

Supply, return, exhaust, relief, and ventilation air plenums must comply with specified requirements. Fuel-fired appliances are not allowed to be installed within a plenum.

IMC § 602.1.1 Locations limited.

Plenums are permitted only in uninhabited crawl spaces, attics, spaces above ceilings or below floors, mechanical equipment rooms, and specific framing cavities as outlined in Section 602.2.

IMC § 602.1.2 Limited to a fire area.

Plenums must be confined to a single fire area, with air systems ducted directly from the fire area boundary to the air-handling equipment.

IMC § 602.1.3 Fuel-fired appliances.

Plenums must not contain fuel-fired appliances.

IMC § 602.2 Constructions of plenums.

Materials used for plenum enclosures exposed to airflow must meet Section 703.5 of the International Building Code or have a flame spread index ≤25 and a smoke-developed index ≤50 (per ASTM E 84 or UL 723). Gypsum boards can only be used in plenums where air temperatures stay below 125°F (52° C), surfaces remain above the dew-point temperature, and evaporative coolers are not used in the system.

IMC § 602.2.1 Stud Cavity and Joist Space Plenums[11]

Stud wall cavities and spaces between floor joists used as air plenums must meet these conditions:

1. *They cannot be used for supply air.*
2. *They cannot be part of a fire-resistance-rated assembly.*
3. *They should not convey air between floors.*
4. *They must comply with floor penetration protection requirements of the International Building Code.*

---

11. See IECC R403.3.2 "Building framing cavities shall not be used as ductwork or plenums."

5. They must be fireblocked to isolate them from adjacent concealed spaces.
6. Outside wall cavities in the building envelope cannot be used as air plenums.

IMC § 602.3 Materials within plenums.

Materials inside plenums must be noncombustible or comply with Sections 602.3.1–602.3.10, with exceptions:

1. Materials exposed in plenums of one- and two-family homes.
2. Combustible materials fully enclosed in:

- Noncombustible raceways or enclosures,
- Approved gypsum board assemblies, or
- Materials listed for plenum use.

3. Materials in Group H, Division 5 fabrication areas and related air circulation paths.

IMC § 602.3.1 Ducts, connectors, duct coverings, linings and tape.
Rigid and flexible ducts, connectors, coverings, linings, tape, and connectors must comply with the requirements of Sections 603 and 604.

IMC § 602.3.2 Smoke detectors.
Use smoke detectors that are listed and labeled.

* * *

IMC § 603 Duct Construction and installation[12]

IMC § 603.9 Joints, seams and connections.

Duct joints, seams, and connections must follow SMACNA and NAIMA standards, using approved fastening and sealing methods like welds, gaskets, mastics, tapes, or liquid sealants. Fibrous glass ductwork sealing materials must meet UL 181A standards, while metallic and flexible ducts require UL 181B-

---

12. There are numerous subsections at the beginning of Section 603 that apply to the design and installation of heating and air conditioning ducting. Those sections are not included here although they must be considered particularly if the ventilation system is combined with the conditioned air system.

compliant materials. Duct connections to air system equipment must be sealed and mechanically fastened. Closure systems must be installed per manufacturer instructions.

Exception: Ducts with static pressure under 2 inches of water column and certain welded or locking joints outside conditioned spaces do not require additional closure systems.

* * *

IMC § 605 AIR FILTERS

IMC § 605.1 General.

Central heating and air-conditioning systems must have approved air filters that filter all return, outdoor, and makeup air before it reaches any heat exchanger or coil. Liquid adhesive coatings on filters must have a flash point of at least 325°F (163°C).

IMC § 605.2 Approval.

Media and electrostatic air filters must be listed and labeled, with media filters complying with UL 900, HEPA filters with UL 586, and electrostatic filters with UL 867. Filters used in dwelling units do not require listing or labeling but must be suitable for their intended application.

IMC § 605.3 Airflow over the filter.

Air must be allowed to flow evenly across the entire filter.

* * *

2024 International Energy Conservation Code

2024 International Energy Conservation Code

IECC § 403.3 Duct Systems.[13]

Install ducts in accordance with Section R403.3.1 through R403.3.9

Exception: Ventilation ductwork not integrated with duct systems serving heating or cooling systems.

---

13. Although it is not required by code, it is good practice that ventilation ductwork connected to the heating and cooling distribution system be considered as part of that system and comply with the installation requirements of that system.

IECC § 403.6 Mechanical ventilation.

Buildings and dwelling units that meet Section R402.5.1.1 must have ventilation systems that comply with Section M1505 of the International Residential Code, the International Mechanical Code, or other approved methods. Outdoor air intakes and exhausts must include automatic or gravity dampers that close when the ventilation system is off.

IECC § R403.6.1 Heat or energy recovery ventilation

In Climate Zones 6, 7, and 8, dwelling units must have a balanced heat recovery or energy recovery ventilation system with a sensible recovery efficiency (SRE) of at least 65% at 32°F (0°C) and at or above the design airflow. The SRE must be based on listed values or interpolated from them.

IECC § R403.6.2 Fan efficacy for whole-house mechanical ventilation systems and outdoor air ventilation systems.

Fans used for whole-dwelling mechanical ventilation must meet the efficacy requirements in Table R403.6.2 and be tested according to its referenced procedure. Airflow and fan efficacy must be listed or derived from reported input power and airflow values. Fully ducted HRV, ERV, balanced systems, and in-line fans must be tested at a static pressure of at least 0.2 inches water gauge, while ducted range hoods, bathroom, and utility fans must be tested at 0.1 inches water gauge.

System Type	Air Flow Minimum (CFM)	Minimum Efficacy (CFM/WATT)	Test Procedure
HRV or ERV	Any	1.2^a	CAN/CSA C439
Balanced ventilation system without heat or energy recovery	Any	1.2^a	
Range hood	Any	2.8	ANSI/AMCA 210 – ANSI/ASHRAE 51
In-line fan supply or exhaust fan	Any	3.8	
Other exhaust fan	< 90	2.8	
	≥ 90 and < 200	3.5	
	≥ 200	4.0	
Air-handling unit that is integrated to tested and listed HVAC equipment	Any	1.2	Outdoor airflow as specified. Air-handing unit fan power determined in accordance with the applicable US Department of Energy Code of Federal Regulation DOE 10 CFR 430 or other approved test method

TABLE R403.6.2
FAN EFFICACY FOR WHOLE-HOUSE MECHANICAL VENTILATION SYSTEMS AND OUTDOOR AIR VENTILATION SYSTEMS[a]

For SI: 1 cfm = 28.3 L/min.

[a]For balanced ventilation systems, HRVs and ERVs, determine the efficacy as the outdoor airflow divided by the total fan power.

IECC § R403.6.3 Testing

Mechanical ventilation systems must be tested and verified to meet the minimum flow rates of Section R403.6 per ANSI/RESNET/ICC 380, with testing by an approved third party if required. A written, signed report must be submitted to the code official.

Exceptions:

1. Ducted kitchen range hoods (6-inch diameter, ≤ 10 feet length, ≤ two 90-degree elbows) do not require testing.
2. Systems with integrated diagnostic tools that measure and display airflow rates do not need third-party testing.
3. Testing is not required if performed per Section R403.6.4.

IECC § R403.6.4 Unit sampling.

For buildings with eight or more dwelling or sleeping units, mechanical ventilation systems must be tested in the greater of seven units or 20% of the total units, including units on the top, middle, and ground floors, as well as the largest unit. If the building has fewer than eight units, all units must be tested. Systems that fail to meet the minimum ventilation flow rate must be corrected and retested. Additionally, for each failed unit, three more systems, including the corrected one, must be tested.

IECC § R403.6.5 Intermittent exhaust control for bathrooms and toilet rooms.

For bathrooms or toilet rooms with exhaust systems designed for intermittent operation, the controls must include one or more of the following:

1. *Timer control: Automatically turns off fans with at least one delay setpoint of 30 minutes or less.*

2. *Occupant sensor: Turns off fans after detecting the space is vacant, with at least one delay setpoint of 30 minutes or less.*
3. *Humidity control: Turns off fans when humidity, adjustable between 50% and 80%, reaches the setpoint.*
4. *Contaminant control: Turns off fans based on particle or gas concentration setpoints.*

A manual off function cannot replace the required minimum setpoints.

Exception: *Systems that are part of an outdoor air or whole-house mechanical ventilation system.*

Building Component	Standard Reference Design	Proposed Design
Air leakage rate	For detached one-family dwellings, the air leakage rate at a pressure of 0.2 inch water gauge (50 Pa) shall be as follows: Climate Zones 0 through 2: 4.0 air changes per hour. Climate Zones 3, 4, and 5: 3.0 air changes per hour. Climate Zone 6 through 8: 2.5 air changes per hour. For detached one-family dwellings that are 1,500 ft^2 or smaller and attached dwelling units or sleeping units, the air leakage rate at a pressure of 0.2 inch water gauge (50 Pa) shall be 0.27 cfm/ft^2 of the testing unit enclosure area.	The measured air leakage rate.[a]
Mechanical ventilation rate	The mechanical ventilation rate shall be in addition to the air leakage rate and shall be the same as the proposed design but not greater than $B \times M$ where $B = 0.01 \times CFA + 7.5 \times (N_{br} + 1)$, cfm $M = 1.0$ where the measure air leakage rate is $\geq$ 3.0 air changes per hour at 50 Pascals, and otherwise, M = minimum $(1.7 Q/B)$. Q = the proposed mechanical ventilation rate CFM. CFA = conditioned floor area, ft2. N_{br} = number of bedrooms.	The measured mechanical ventilation rate[b] (Q) shall be in addition to the measured air leakage rate.
Mechanical ventilation fan energy	The mechanical ventilation system type shall be the same as in the proposed design... Heat recovery or energy recovery shall be modeled for mechanical ventilation where required by Section R403.6.1. Heat recovery or energy recovery shall not be modeled for mechanical ventilation where not required by Section R403.6.1. Where mechanical ventilation is not specified in the proposed design: None Where mechanical ventilation is specified in the proposed design, the annual vent fan energy use, in units of kWh/yr, shall equal $(8.76 \times B \times M)e_f$ where: B and M are determined in accordance with the air exchange mechanical ventilation rate row of this table. e_f = the minimum fan efficacy, as specified in Table R403.6.2, corresponding to the system type at a flow rate of $B \times M$.	As proposed

For SI: 1 square foot = 0.93 m^2, 1 British thermal unit = 1055 J, 1 pound per square foot = 4.88 kg/m^2, 1 gallon (US) = 3.785 L, °C = (°F-32)/1.8, 1 degree = 0.79 rad, 1 cubic foot per minute = 28.317 L/min

[a] Hourly calculations as specified in the ASHRAE *Handbook of Fundamentals*, or the equivalent shall be used to determine the energy loads resulting from infiltration.

[b] The combined air exchange rate for infiltration and mechanical ventilation shall be determined in accordance with Equation 43 of 2001 ASHRAE *Handbook of Fundamentals*, page 26.24 and the "Whole-house Ventilation" provisions of 2001 ASHRAE *Handbook of Fundamentals*, page 26.19 for intermittent mechanical ventilation.

TABLE R405.5.2(1)
SPECIFICATIONS FOR THE STANDARD REFERENCE AND PROPOSED DESIGNS

a. Hourly calculations as specified in the ASHRAE *Handbook of Fundamentals*, or the equivalent shall be used to determine the energy loads resulting from infiltration.

b. The combined air exchange rate for infiltration and mechanical ventilation shall be determined in accordance with Equation 43 of 2001 ASHRAE *Handbook of Fundamentals*, page 26.24 and the "Whole-house Ventilation" provisions of 2001 ASHRAE *Handbook of Fundamentals*, page 26.19 for intermittent mechanical ventilation.

* * *

2024 International Building Code

2024 International Building Code

IBC § 1202 VENTILATION[14]

IBC §1202.1 General.

Buildings must have either natural ventilation per Section 1202.5 or mechanical ventilation per the International Mechanical Code (IMC). Dwelling units meeting air leakage requirements of the International Energy Conservation Code or ASHRAE 90.1 must use mechanical ventilation as specified in IMC Section 403.

IBC §1202.2 Roof ventilation.

Roof assemblies must be ventilated in accordance with this section or comply with Section 1202.3.

IBC § 1202.2.1 Ventilated attics and rafter spaces.

Enclosed attics and rafter spaces with ceilings applied directly to roof framing must have cross ventilation with openings protected from rain and snow. Air movement must not be obstructed, and at least 1 inch of airspace is required between insulation and roof sheathing. The net free ventilating area must be at least 1/150 of the ventilated space area, with installation following manufacturer instructions.

. . .

---

14. https://codes.iccsafe.org/content/IBC2024P1/chapter-12-interior-environment#IBC2024P1_Ch12_Sec1202

EXCEPTION: *Ventilation area may be reduced to 1/300 if:*

1. *In Climate Zones 6, 7, and 8, a Class I or II vapor retarder is installed on the warm side of the ceiling.*
2. *40–50% of ventilation is in the upper attic, within 3 feet of the ridge, with the remainder at eave or cornice vents. Exceptions are allowed where framing prevents ideal upper vent placement.*

IBC § 1202.2.2 Openings into attic.

Exterior openings into attic spaces of occupied buildings must be protected to prevent entry by animals like birds, rodents, and snakes. Ventilation openings between 1/16 inch (1.6 mm) and 1/4 inch (6.4 mm) are allowed. Larger openings must be covered with corrosion-resistant screening or similar material with openings within the 1/16 inch to 1/4 inch range. Combustion air drawn from attics must comply with Chapter 7 of the International Mechanical Code.

IBC § 1202.3 Unvented Attic and Unvented Enclosed Rafter Assemblies

Unvented attics and enclosed roof framing assemblies are allowed if the following conditions are met:

1. *The attic space is fully within the building's thermal envelope.*
2. *No Class I vapor retarders are installed on the ceiling side of the assembly.*
3. *For wood shingles or shakes, a 1/4-inch vented airspace must separate them from the roofing underlayment.*
4. *In Climate Zones 5–8, air-impermeable insulation must act as or be covered by a Class II vapor retarder.*
5. *Insulation must follow these guidelines based on air permeability:*

- *5.1.1: Air-impermeable insulation must directly contact the underside of the roof sheathing.*
- *5.1.2: Air-permeable insulation must be paired with rigid insulation above the roof sheathing for condensation control (per Table 1202.3).*
- *5.1.3: Combined insulation types require air-impermeable insulation directly under the sheathing and air-permeable insulation beneath it.*

- 5.1.4: *Alternatively, rigid insulation above the sheathing must keep the underside temperature above 45°F (7°C), assuming an interior temperature of 68°F (20°C).*

Exceptions:

1. *Special-use enclosures like pools, hospitals, or art galleries are exempt.*
2. *Enclosures in Climate Zones 5–8 with humidity levels above 35% in the coldest months are exempt.*

CLIMATE ZONE	MINIMUM R-VALUE OF AIR-IMPERMEABLE INSULATION[a]
2B and 3B tile roof only	0 (none required)
1, 2A, 2B, 3A, 3B, 3C	10%
4C	20%
4A, 4B	30%
5	40%
6	50%
7	60%
8	70%

TABLE 1202.3 INSULATION FOR CONDENSATION CONTROL

[a.] Contributes to, but does not supersede, thermal resistance requirements for attic and roof assemblies in Section C402.2.1 of the *International Energy Conservation Code*.

IBC § 1202.4 *Under-floor ventilation.*

The space between the bottom of the floor joists and the earth under any building except spaces occupied by basements or cellars shall be provided with ventilation in accordance with Section 1202.4.1, 1202.4.2 or 1202.4.3.

IBC § 1202.4.1 *Ventilation openings.*

Ventilation openings through foundation walls must be provided to allow cross ventilation of the under-floor space. The net area of these openings must meet the requirements in Section 1202.4.1.1 or 1202.4.1.2. The openings must be covered with materials that have a maximum dimension of 1/4 inch (6.4 mm), such as:

1. *Perforated sheet metal (at least 0.070 inch (1.8mm) thick)*
2. *Expanded sheet metal (at least 0.047 inch (1.2mm) thick)*
3. *Cast-iron grilles or gratings*

Ventilation Codes 221

4. Extruded load-bearing vents
5. Hardware cloth (0.035-inch (0.89mm) wire or thicker)
6. Corrosion-resistant wire mesh (maximum 1/8-inch (3.2 mm) openings)
7. Operable louvres (if ventilation meets Section 1202.4.1.2 requirements)

IBC § 1202.4.1.1 *Ventilation area for crawl spaces with open earth floors.*

Ventilation openings for crawl spaces with uncovered earth floors must have openings that are not less than 1 square foot for each 150 square feet (0.67 m2 for each 100 m2) of crawl space area.

IBC § 1202.4.1.2 *Ventilation area for crawl spaces with covered floors.*

Ventilation openings for crawl spaces with the ground surface covered with a Class I vapor retarder must not be less than 1 square foot for each 1,500 square feet (0.67 m2 for each 1000 m2) of crawl space area.

IBC § 1202.4.2 *Ventilation in cold climate.*

In extremely cold climates, if ventilation openings would result in significant energy loss, ventilation openings must be provided to the interior of the structure instead.

IBC § 1202.4.3 *Mechanical ventilation.*

Mechanical ventilation must be provided to crawl spaces with a Class I vapor retarder on the ground surface, following the requirements in Section 1202.4.3.1 or 1202.4.3.2.

IBC § 1202.4.3.1 *Continuous mechanical ventilation.*

Continuously operated mechanical ventilation must be provided at a rate of 1.0 cubic foot per minute (cfm) (1.02 L/s for each 10 m2) for every 50 square feet of crawl space ground area, and the ground surface must be covered with a Class I vapor retarder.

IBC § 1202.4.3.2 *Conditioned space.*

The crawl space must be conditioned according to the International Mechanical Code, and its walls must be insulated according to the International Energy Conservation Code.

IBC § 1202.4.4 *Flood hazard areas.*

For buildings in flood hazard areas, under-floor ventilation openings are considered to meet the flood opening requirements of ASCE 24 if they are designed and installed in accordance with ASCE 24.

* * *

IBC § 1202.5 *Natural ventilation.*

Natural ventilation of an occupied space must be through windows, doors, louvers, or other openings to the outdoors. The operating mechanisms for these openings must be easily accessible, allowing building occupants to control them easily.

IBC § 1202.5.1 *Ventilation area required.*

The minimum openable area to the outdoors must be 4% of the floor area being ventilated.

IBC § 1202.5.1.1 *Adjoining spaces.*

When rooms or spaces without direct outdoor openings are ventilated through an adjoining room, the opening to the adjoining room must be unobstructed and at least 8% of the floor area of the interior room, but no less than 25 square feet (2,3 m^2). The openable area to the outdoors is based on the total floor area being ventilated.

EXCEPTION: Exterior openings for ventilation may lead into a sunroom with thermal isolation or a patio cover, provided the openable area between the sunroom or patio cover and the interior room is at least 8% of the interior room's floor area, but no less than 20 square feet (1.86m^2). The openable area to the outdoors is still based on the total floor area being ventilated.

IBC § 1202.5.1.2 *Openings Below Grade*

When openings below grade provide required natural ventilation, the outside horizontal clear space, measured perpendicular to the opening, must be one and a half times the depth of the opening. The depth is measured from the average ground level to the bottom of the opening.

IBC § 1202.5.2 *Contaminants Exhausted*

Contaminant sources in naturally ventilated spaces must be removed in accordance with the International Mechanical Code and the International Fire Code.

IBC § 1202.5.2.1 *Bathrooms*

Rooms with bathtubs, showers, spas, or similar bathing fixtures must be mechanically ventilated in accordance with the International Mechanical Code.

IBC § 1202.5.3 *Openings on yards or courts.*

If natural ventilation is provided through openings onto yards or courts, those yards or courts must comply with Section 1205.

IBC § 1202.6 *Other ventilation and exhaust systems.*

Ventilation and exhaust systems for occupancies with flammable hazards or other contaminant sources must be provided as required by both the International Mechanical Code and the International Fire Code.

* * *

2024 International Residential Code

IRC § R408 UNDER-FLOOR SPACE

IRC § R408.1 *Ventilation.*

The under-floor space between the bottom of the floor joists and the earth under any building (except space occupied by a basement) shall comply with Section R408.2 or R408.3.

IRC § R408.2 *Openings for under-floor ventilation.*

Ventilation Openings:

- *Openings must total at least 1 square foot (0.0929 m2) per 150 square feet (14 m2) of under-floor space.*
- *At least one opening must be within 3 feet (915 mm) of each building corner.*
- *Openings must be covered with specific materials, including perforated/expanded metal plates, cast-iron grates, brick vents, hardware cloth, or corrosion-resistant wire mesh, with openings not exceeding ¼ inch (6.4 mm).*

Exceptions:

- *Ventilation can be reduced to 1/1,500 of the under-floor area if the ground has an approved Class 1 vapor retarder.*
- *If a vapor retarder is used, openings near corners are not required, provided cross ventilation is avoided.*

IRC § R408.3 *Unvented crawl space.*

Vapor Retarder:

- *Exposed earth must be covered with a Class 1 vapor retarder.*
- *Joints must overlap 6 inches (152 mm) and be sealed or taped.*
- *Edges must extend 6 inches (152 mm) up the stem wall, attached and sealed.*

Ventilation or Conditioning Options (one must be provided):

- *Mechanical Exhaust: Continuous ventilation at 1 CFM per 50 ft² with an air pathway and insulated perimeter walls.*
- *Conditioned Air Supply: Air delivered at 1 CFM (0.47 L/s) per 50 ft² (4.7 m2) with a return pathway and insulated perimeter walls.*
- *Plenum: Compliance with Section M1601.5 if the space is used as a plenum.*
- *Dehumidification: Sized per the manufacturer's specifications.*

IRC § R806 Roof Ventilation[15]

IRC § R806.1 Ventilation required.

Enclosed attics and rafter spaces require cross ventilation through protected openings to prevent rain or snow entry. Key requirements include:

- Opening Size:

  - *Minimum 1/16 inch (1.6 mm) and maximum ¼ inch (6.4 mm).*
  - *Larger openings must have corrosion-resistant screening or similar material with openings between 1/16 inch (1.6 mm) and ¼ inch (6.4 mm).*

- *Protection: Openings must prevent entry of birds, rodents, snakes, and similar creatures.*

  - *Placement: Openings must connect directly to outside air.*
  - *Openings in roof framing must comply with Section R802.7.*

IRC § R806.2 Minimum vent area.

---

15. See IRC § R806.4 for a description of "Unvented Attic Assembly" requirements.

The minimum net free ventilating area for vented spaces is 1/150 of the space area.

Exception: The area can be reduced to 1/300 if:

1. In Climate Zones 6, 7, and 8, a Class I or II vapor retarder is installed on the warm side of the ceiling.
2. 40% to 50% of the ventilation is located in the upper portion of the attic (within 3 feet below the ridge), with the rest in the lower third of the space.

- If framing conflicts, upper vents can be placed more than 3 feet (914 mm) below the ridge.

IRC § R806.3 Vent and Insulation Clearance

When eave or cornice vents are installed, insulation must not block airflow. A minimum 1-inch (25 mm)

space must be maintained between the insulation and the roof sheathing at the vent location.

IRC § R806.4 Installation and Weather Protection

Ventilators must be installed following the manufacturer's instructions. For roof systems, installation must comply with Section R903, and for wall systems, it must comply with Section R703.1.

IRC § R806.5 Unvented Attic and Unvented Enclosed Rafter Assemblies

Unvented attics and enclosed roof framing assemblies are allowed if the following conditions are met:

1. The attic space is entirely within the building thermal envelope.
2. No Class I vapor retarders are on the ceiling side of the attic or roof assembly.
3. For wood shingles/shakes, a ¼-inch vented airspace is required above the structural sheathing.
4. In Climate Zones 5–8, air-impermeable insulation must act as a Class II vapor retarder or have a vapor retarder coating in direct contact with it.
5. Insulation must meet specific requirements:

- *Air-impermeable insulation must contact the roof sheathing directly.*
- *If air-permeable insulation is used, rigid insulation must be placed above the sheathing to prevent condensation (per Table R806.5).*
- *For combined insulation, air-impermeable insulation must contact the roof sheathing, with air-permeable insulation below it.*
- *Alternatively, sufficient rigid insulation above the sheathing can maintain temperatures to prevent condensation.*

6. *Preformed insulation boards must be sealed at the edges to create a continuous air-impermeable layer.*

CLIMATE ZONE	MINIMUM RIGID BOARD ON AIR-IMPERMEABLE INSULATION R-VALUE[a, b]
2B and 3B tile roof only	0 (none required)
1, 2A, 2B, 3A, 3B, 3C	R-5
4C	R-10
4A, 4B	R-15
5	R-20
6	R-25
7	R-30
8	R-35

TABLE R806.5 INSULATION FOR CONDENSATION CONTROL

[a] Contributes to but does not supersede the requirements in Section N1102.

[b] Alternatively, sufficient continuous insulation shall be installed directly above the structural roof sheathing to maintain the monthly average temperature of the underside of the structural roof sheathing above 45°F (7°C). For calculation purposes, an interior air temperature of 68°F (20°C) is assumed and the exterior air temperature is assumed to be the monthly average outside air temperature of the three coldest months.

* * *

IRC § M1501 Exhaust systems

IRC § M1501.1 *Outdoor discharge.*

Air from mechanical exhaust systems must be discharged outdoors and not into attics, soffits, ridge vents, or crawl spaces.

Exception: *Whole-house ventilation attic fans are allowed to discharge into private attic spaces.*

* * *

IRC § M1502 CLOTHES DRYER EXHAUST

IRC § M1502.1 *General.*

Exhaust clothes dryers according to the manufacturer's instructions.

IRC § M1502.2 *Independent exhaust systems.*

Dryer exhaust systems must be separate from other systems and vent moisture directly outdoors.

EXCEPTION: *This does not apply to condensing (ductless) clothes dryers that are listed and labeled.*

IRC § M1502.3 *Duct termination.*

Dryer exhaust ducts must terminate outside the building and follow the manufacturer's installation instructions. If no location is specified, the duct must terminate at least 3 feet (914 mm) away from any building openings. Terminations must have a backdraft damper, and screens are not allowed at the duct termination.

IRC § M1502.3.1 *Exhaust termination outlet and passageway size.*

Dryer exhaust duct terminals must maintain their full size and provide an open area of at least 12.5 square inches (8065 mm^2).

IRC § M1502.4 *Dryer Exhaust ducts.*

Dryer exhaust ducts must conform to the requirements of Sections M1502.4.1 through M1502.4.8.[16]

IRC § M1502.4.1 *Material and Size*

Exhaust ducts must have a smooth interior finish, be made of metal with a

---

16. The provisions of this section are the same or very similar to the provisions in the International Mechanical Code cited above in section 504. One significant difference is in the length of ducting allowed – 25 feet in the Residential Code and 35 feet in the Mechanical Code.

minimum thickness of 0.0157 inches (0.3950 mm) (28 gauge), and have a nominal diameter of 4 inches (102 mm).

IRC § M1502.4.2 Duct Installation

Exhaust ducts must be:

- Supported every 12 feet (3658 mm) or less and secured in place.
- Inserted with the end extending into the adjoining duct or fitting in the direction of airflow.
- Sealed per Section M1601.4.1 and mechanically fastened.
- Free from screws or fasteners protruding more than 1/8 inch (3.2 mm) into the duct interior.
- Installed in wall or ceiling cavities large enough to prevent duct deformation.

IRC § M1502.4.3 Transition Duct

Transition ducts connecting the dryer to the exhaust system must:

- Be a single length, listed, and labeled per UL 2158A.
- Not exceed 8 feet (2438 mm) in length.
- Remain unconcealed within construction.

IRC § M1502.4.4 Dryer Exhaust Duct Power Ventilators

Domestic dryer exhaust duct power ventilators must comply with UL 705 and be installed following the manufacturer's instructions.

IRC § M1502.4.5 Booster fans prohibited.

Domestic booster fans must not be installed in dryer exhaust systems.

IRC § M1502.4.6 Duct Length.

The maximum allowable exhaust duct length must be determined by one of the methods specified in Sections M1502.4.6.1 through M1502.4.6.3.

IRC § M1502.4.6.1 Specified Length.

The maximum length of a dryer exhaust duct is 35 feet (10,668 mm) from the connection to the transition duct to the outlet terminal. This length is reduced based on fittings, as specified in Table M1502.4.6.1. The transition duct length is not included in this maximum measurement.

DRYER EXHAUST DUCT FITTING TYPE	EQUIVALENT LENGTH
4 inch radius mitered 45 degree elbow	2 feet 6 inches
4 inch radius mitered 90 degree elbow	5 feet
6 inch radius smooth 45 degree elbow	1 foot
6 inch radius smooth 90 degree elbow	1 foot 9 inches
8 inch radius smooth 45 degree elbow	1 foot
8 inch radius smooth 90 degree elbow	1 foot 7 inches
10 inch radius smooth 45 degree elbow	9 inches
10 inch radius smooth 90 degree elbow	1 foot 6 inches

TABLE M1502.4.6.1 DRYER EXHAUST DUCT FITTING EQUIVALENT LENGTH

For SI: 1 inch = 25.4 mm, 1 foot = 304.8 mm, 1 degree = 0.0175 rad.

IRC § M1502.4.6.2 *Manufacturer's Instructions.*

The size and maximum length of the exhaust duct must follow the dryer manufacturer's installation instructions. A copy of these instructions must be provided to the code official during the concealment inspection. If the manufacturer does not provide fitting length calculations, use Table M1502.4.6.1.

IRC § M1502.4.6.3 *Dryer Exhaust Duct Power Ventilator*

The maximum length of the exhaust duct must comply with the manufacturer's instructions for the dryer exhaust duct power ventilator.

IRC § M1502.4.7 *Length Identification*

If the exhaust duct equivalent length exceeds 35 feet (10,668 mm), the equivalent length must be marked on a permanent label or tag. This label must be placed within 6 feet (1829 mm) of the exhaust duct connection.

IRC § M1502.4.8 *Exhaust Duct Required.*

An exhaust duct system must be installed where a clothes dryer space is provided. If the dryer is not installed at occupancy, the exhaust duct must be capped or plugged and marked as "future use."

Exception: *This does not apply if a listed condensing clothes dryer is installed before occupancy.*

IRC § M1502.5 *Protection required.*

Protective shield plates must be installed where nails or screws might penetrate the dryer exhaust duct. These plates should be placed on the finished face of framing members when there is less than 1 ¼ inches between the duct and the framing. The plates must be made of steel, at least 0.062 inches (1.6 mm) thick, and extend 2 inches (51 mm) above the sole plate and below the top plate.

IRC § M1502.6 *Makeup air.*

Makeup air must be provided for installations exhausting more than 200 cubic feet per minute (0.09 m3/s).

IRC § M1502.6.1 *Closet installation.*

If a closet is designed for a clothes dryer, makeup air must be provided according to the dryer manufacturer's instructions. If no instructions are provided, the closet must have one or more permanent openings totaling at least 100 square inches (645 mm²), or makeup air must be provided by other approved methods.

* * *

IRC § M1503 Domestic Cooking Exhaust Equipment

IRC § M1503.1 *General.*

Domestic cooking equipment must comply with the requirements of this section.

IRC § M1503.2 *Domestic cooking exhaust.*

Domestic cooking exhaust equipment must meet one of the following requirements:

1. *Fans for overhead range hoods and downdraft exhaust systems (not integral with the appliance) must be listed and labeled according to UL 507.*
2. *Overhead range hoods and downdraft exhaust systems with integral fans must comply with UL 507.*
3. *Domestic cooking appliances with integral downdraft exhaust must be listed and labeled per ANSI Z21.1 or UL 858.*

4. Microwave ovens with integral exhaust for installation above the cooking surface must be listed and labeled according to UL 923.

IRC § M1503.2.1 Open-top broiler exhaust

Domestic open-top broiler units must have a metal exhaust hood with a minimum thickness of 0.0157 inches (0.3950 mm) (28 gauge). The hood should be installed with at least ¼ inch (6.4 mm) clearance from combustible materials or cabinets, and 24 inches (610 mm) clearance from the cooking surface to combustible materials or cabinets. The hood must cover the entire broiler unit and be at least as wide as the unit.

EXCEPTION: Broiler units with an integral exhaust system that are listed and labeled for use without an exhaust hood do not require one.

IRC § M1503.3 Exhaust discharge.

Domestic cooking exhaust equipment must discharge to the outdoors through a duct with a smooth interior, airtight construction, a backdraft damper, and be independent of other exhaust systems. The duct should not terminate in an attic, crawl space, or any indoor areas.

EXCEPTION: Ductless range hoods, when installed according to the manufacturer's instructions and with proper ventilation, are not required to discharge to the outdoors.

IRC § M1503.4 Duct Material

Ducts for domestic cooking exhaust equipment must be made of galvanized steel, stainless steel, or copper.

EXCEPTION: Ducts for kitchen appliances with down-draft exhaust systems may be made of schedule 40 PVC if all the following conditions are met:

1. The duct is installed under a concrete slab on grade.
2. The trench for the duct is filled with sand or gravel.
3. The PVC duct is no more than 1 inch (25 mm) above the indoor concrete floor.

4. The PVC duct is no more than 1 inch (25 mm) above grade outside.
5. The PVC ducts are solvent cemented.

IRC § M1503.5 Kitchen Exhaust Rates

For domestic kitchen appliances with ducted range hoods or down-draft exhaust systems, the exhaust rate must meet or exceed the airflow requirements specified in Table M1505.5 at one or more speed settings.

IRC § M1503.6 Makeup Air Required

If a dwelling unit has one or more gas, liquid, or solid fuel-burning appliances (that are not direct-vent or using a mechanical draft system) within its air barrier, any exhaust system capable of exhausting more than 400 cubic feet per minute (0.19 m^3/s) must have makeup air supplied at a rate roughly equal to the exhaust rate. The makeup air system must include at least one outdoor air duct and damper as per Section M1503.6.2.

EXCEPTION: Makeup air is not required for exhaust systems used solely for space cooling when operated only when windows or air inlets are open.

IRC § M1503.6.1 Location

Kitchen exhaust makeup air ducted from the outdoors must be discharged into the same room as the exhaust system or into rooms or ducts that are connected by permanent openings. These openings must have a net cross-sectional area at least as large as the required area of the makeup air supply openings.

IRC § M1503.6.2 Makeup air dampers.

When makeup air dampers are required (per Section M1503.6), they must comply with the following:

1. Dampers must be either gravity dampers or electrically operated dampers that automatically open when the exhaust system is running.

2. Dampers must be accessible for inspection, service, repair, and replacement without removing permanent structures or unrelated ducts.
3. Gravity or barometric dampers are not allowed in passive systems unless they are rated to deliver the required airflow at a pressure differential of 0.01 in. w.c. (3 Pa) or less.

* * *

IRC § M1504 Exhaust Ducts and Exhaust Openings
  IRC § M1504.1 Duct Construction
Exhaust ducting not specified in this chapter it must comply with Chapter 16.
  IRC § M1504.2 Duct Length
The length of exhaust and supply ducts for ventilating equipment must follow the limits in Table M1504.2.

EXCEPTION: Duct length is unlimited if:

1. The system complies with the manufacturer's design criteria, or
2. The installed airflow rate is verified using a flow hood, flow grid, or another approved airflow measurement device.

Duct Type	Flex Duct								Smooth Wall Duct							
CFM @ 0.25 in. w.c.	50	80	100	125	150	200	250	300	50	80	100	125	150	200	250	300
Diameter (inches)	Maximum Length (feet)[c,d,e]															
3	X	X	X	X	X	X	X	X	5	X	X	X	X	X	X	X
4	56	4	X	X	X	X	X	X	114	31	10	X	X	X	X	X
5	NL	81	42	16	2	X	X	X	NL	152	91	51	28	4	X	X
6	NL	NL	158	91	55	18	1	X	NL	NL	NL	168	112	53	25	9
7	NL	NL	NL	NL	161	78	40	19	NL	NL	NL	NL	NL	NL	88	54
8 +	NL	NL	NL	NL	NL	189	111	69	NL	NL	NL	NL	NL	NL	198	133

TABLE M1504.2 DUCT LENGTH

For SI: 1 foot = 304.8 mm.

a. Fan airflow rating shall be in accordance with ANSI/AMCA 210-ANSI/ASHRAE 51.

b. For noncircular ducts, calculate the diameter as four times the cross-sectional area divided by the perimeter.

c. This table assumes that elbows are not used. Fifteen feet of allowable duct length shall be deducted for each elbow installed in the duct run.

d. NL = no limit on duct length of this size.

e. X = not allowed. Any length of duct of this size with assumed turns and fittings will exceed the rated pressure drop.

IRC § M1504.3 Exhaust Openings

Air exhaust openings must comply with the following clearance requirements:

1. 3 feet (914 mm) minimum from property lines.
2. 3 feet (914 mm) minimum from gravity air intakes, windows, and doors, unless the exhaust is 1 foot (305 mm) above them.
3. 10 feet (3048 mm) minimum from mechanical air intakes, except when:

- The exhaust is 3 feet (914 mm) above the intake.
- It uses a factory-built combination fitting installed per the manufacturer's instructions, and the exhaust air is from a living space.

4. Must also comply with Sections R303.5.2 and R303.6.

* * *

IRC § M1505 MECHANICAL VENTILATION

IRC § M1505.1 General.

Local exhaust or whole-house mechanical ventilation shall be designed in accordance with this section.

IRC § M1505.2 Recirculation of air.

Bathroom, toilet room, and kitchen exhaust air must be discharged directly to the outdoors and cannot be recirculated within a residence, discharged to another dwelling, or vented into attics, crawl spaces, or interior building areas. However, ductless range hoods are allowed if installed per Section M1503.3 exceptions.

IRC § M1505.3 Exhaust equipment.

Exhaust fans and whole-house mechanical ventilation fans must be listed and labeled to meet the minimum required airflow standards as per ANSI/AMCA 210-ANSI/ASHRAE 51 or HVI 916.

IRC § M1505.4 Whole-house mechanical ventilation system.

Whole-house mechanical ventilation systems must be designed in accordance with Sections M1505.4.1 through M1505.5.

IRC § M1505.4.1 System Design

A whole-house ventilation system may include supply or exhaust fans, or both, along with related ducts and controls. Local exhaust or supply fans can be part of the system, and outdoor air ducts connected to the return side of an air handler qualify as supply ventilation.

IRC § M1505.4.2 System Controls

Whole-house mechanical ventilation systems must have controls that allow manual override and include labels or symbols indicating their function.

IRC § M1505.4.3 Mechanical Ventilation rate.[17]

Whole-house mechanical ventilation systems must supply outdoor air continuously at rates specified in Table M1505.4.3(1) or calculated using Equation 15-1.

Ventilation rate in cfm = (0.01 x total square foot area of house) + (7.5 x (number of bedrooms + 1))

Equation 15-1

Exceptions allow adjustments to whole-house mechanical ventilation rates under two conditions:

1. *Ventilation Rate Credit:* The rate can be reduced by 30% if the system delivers air directly to each bedroom and at least one of the following: living room, dining room, or kitchen, and if the system is balanced.

---

17. See footnote for the IMC 403.3.2.1 regarding the square footage factor of 0.01 or 0.03.

2. *Intermittent Operation: The system may operate intermittently if it runs for at least 25% of each 4-hour period, with the ventilation rate adjusted by a factor from Table M1505.4.3(2).*

DWELLING UNIT FLOOR AREA (square feet)	NUMBER OF BEDROOMS				
	0 – 1	2 – 3	4 – 5	6 – 7	> 7
	Airflow in CFM				
< 1,500	30	45	60	75	90
1,501 – 3,000	45	60	75	90	105
3,001 – 4,500	60	75	90	105	120
4,501 – 6,000	75	90	105	120	135
6,001 – 7,500	90	105	120	135	150
> 7,500	105	120	135	150	165

TABLE M1505.4.3(1) CONTINUOUS WHOLE-HOUSE MECHANICAL VENTILATION SYSTEM AIRFLOW RATE REQUIREMENTS

For SI: 1 square foot = 0.0929 m², 1 cubic foot per minute = 0.0004719 m³/s.

RUN-TIME PERCENTAGE IN EACH 4-HOUR SEGMENT	25%	33%	50%	66%	75%	100%
Factor[a]	4	3	2	1.5	1.3	1.0

TABLE M1505.4.3(2) INTERMITTENT WHOLE-HOUSE MECHANICAL VENTILATION RATE FACTORS[a, b]

a. For ventilation system run-time values between those given, the factors are permitted to be determined by interpolation.
b. Extrapolation beyond the table is prohibited.

IRC § M1507.4 *Local Exhaust Rates*

Local exhaust systems must meet the minimum airflow rates specified in Table M1505.5 at one or more speed settings. Bathroom or toilet exhaust fans must provide airflow at or above these rates, tested at a static pressure of 0.25 inch wc, as per Section M1505.3.

AREA TO BE EXHAUSTED	EXHAUST RATES
Kitchens	100 cfm intermittent or 25 cfm continuous
Bathrooms-Toilet Rooms	Mechanical exhaust capacity of 50 cfm intermittent or 20 cfm continuous

TABLE M1505.5 MINIMUM REQUIRED LOCAL EXHAUST RATES FOR ONE- AND TWO-FAMILY DWELLINGS

* * *

2024 International Property Maintenance Code

IPMC § 403.1 Habitable spaces.

Every habitable space must have at least one openable window, with the openable area being at least 45% of the minimum required glazed area in Section 402.1.

EXCEPTION: *If a room lacks openings to the outdoors and is ventilated through an adjoining room, the opening to the adjoining room must be at least 8% of the interior room's floor area, or 25 square feet (2.33 m2) minimum. Ventilation openings to the outdoors are based on the total floor area being ventilated.*

IPMC §403.2 Bathrooms and toilet rooms.

Every bathroom and toilet room must meet the ventilation requirements for habitable spaces, as outlined in Section 403.1. However, a window is not required if the space is equipped with a mechanical ventilation system. The air exhausted by the system must be discharged outdoors and not recirculated.

IPMC §403.5 Clothes dryer exhaust.

Clothes dryer exhaust systems must be separate from all other systems and vented outside the building according to the manufacturer's instructions. However, listed and labeled condensing (ductless) clothes dryers are exempt from this requirement.

* * *

State Ventilation Codes

Some states have individual, specific ventilation codes often integrated with their energy efficiency programs. This is by no means a complete list and because these codes are changing regularly, what is listed here may not be the most up-to-date standard. It is important to check with local code officials.

California

California has some complex ventilation codes[18] mainly built on the ASHRAE 62.2-2010 Standard. Some of the ventilation requirements and energy efficiency are described in Title 24, Part 6 of the California Code of Regulations[19].

Starting on January 1, 2010 all new homes (and existing homes with additions over 1000 square feet) were required to be equipped with mechanical whole house ventilation. But there are a bunch of other refinements in the 2016 California Mechanical Code[20] and in the California 2016 Building Energy Efficiency Standard.

From the Energy Efficiency Standard:

(o) *Ventilation for Indoor Air Quality.*

All dwelling units shall meet the requirements of ASHRAE, Ventilation and Acceptable Indoor Air Quality in Low-Rise Residential Buildings. Window operation is not a permissible method of providing the Whole-Building Ventilation airflow required in Section 4 of ASHRAE Standard 62.2. Continuous operation of central forced air system air handlers used in central fan integrated ventilation systems is not a permissible method of providing the whole-building ventilation airflow required in Section 4 of ASHRAE Standard 62.2. Additionally, all dwelling units shall meet the following requirements:

1. Field Verification and Diagnostic Testing.

A. Airflow Performance.

---

18. https://energycodeace.com/
19. http://www.title24express.com/what-is-title-24/title-24-continuous-ventilation/
20. http://www.iapmo.org/Pages/2016CaliforniaMechanicalCode.aspx

The Whole-Building Ventilation airflow required by Section 4 of ASHRAE Standard 62.2 shall be confirmed through field verification and diagnostic testing in accordance with the applicable procedures specified in Reference Residential Appendix RA3.7.

California has an extensive description of ventilation testing procedures as part of the 2016 Building and Appliance Efficiency Regulations. These even include in section RA3.7.3 instructions for the manufacturers of diagnostic equipment!

CALIFORNIA VENTILATION and Indoor Air Quality

§ 150.0(o)1: Requirements for Ventilation and Indoor Air Quality. All dwelling units must meet the requirements of ASHRAE Standard 62.2,Ventilation and Acceptable Indoor Air Quality in Residential Buildings subject to the amendments specified in § 150.0(o)1. [Exceptions may apply]

§ 150.0(o)1B: Central Fan Integrated (CFI) Ventilation Systems. Continuous operation of CFI air handlers is not allowed to provide the whole-dwelling unit ventilation airflow required per §150.0(o)1C. A motorized damper(s) must be installed on the ventilation duct(s) that prevents all airflow through the space conditioning duct system when the damper(s) is closed and controlled per §150.0(o)1Biii&iv. CFI ventilation systems must have controls that track outdoor air ventilation run time, and either open or close the motorized damper(s) for compliance with §150.0(o)1C.

§ 150.0(o)1C: Whole-Dwelling Unit Mechanical Ventilation for Single-Family Detached and townhouses. Single-family detached dwelling units, and attached dwelling units not sharing ceilings or floors with other dwelling units, occupiable spaces, public garages, or commercial spaces must have mechanical ventilation airflow specified in § 150.0(o)1Ci-iii.

§ 150.0(o)1G: Local Mechanical Exhaust. Kitchens and bathrooms must have local mechanical exhaust; nonenclosed kitchens must have demand-controlled exhaust system meeting requirements of §150.0(o)1Giii,enclosed kitchens and bathrooms can use demand-controlled or continuous exhaust meeting §150.0(o)1Giii-iv. Airflow must be measured by the installer per §150.0(o)1Gv, and rated for sound per §150.0(o)1Gvi. [Exceptions may apply]

§ 150.0(o)1H&I: Airflow Measurement and Sound Ratings of Whole-Dwelling Unit Ventilation Systems. The airflow required per § 150.0(o)1C must be measured by using a flow hood, flow grid, or other airflow measuring device at the fan's inlet or outlet terminals/grilles per Reference Residential Appendix RA3.7. Whole-Dwelling unit ventilation systems must be rated for sound per ASHRAE 62.2 §7.2 at no less than the minimum airflow rate required by §150.0(o)1C.

§ 150.0(o)2: Field Verification and Diagnostic Testing. Whole-Dwelling Unit ventilation airflow, vented range hood airflow and sound rating, and HRV and ERV fan efficacy must be verified in accordance with Reference Residential Appendix RA3.7. Vented range hoods must be verified per Reference Residential Appendix RA3.7.4.3 to confirm if it is rated by HVI or AHAM to comply with the airflow rates and sound requirements per §150.0(o)1G

California Reference Appendix

RA3.7 Field Verification and Diagnostic Testing of Mechanical Ventilation Systems

RA3.7.1 Purpose and Scope

RA3.7 contains procedures for measuring the airflow in mechanical ventilation systems to confirm compliance with the requirements of ASHRAE 62.2.

RA3.7 is applicable to mechanical ventilation systems in low-rise residential buildings.

RA3.7 provides required procedures for installers, HERS raters and others who are required to perform field verification of mechanical ventilation systems for compliance with Part 6.

Diagnostic	Description	Procedure
Whole-Building Mechanical Ventilation Airflow – Continuous Operation	Verify that whole-building ventilation system complies with the airflow rate required by ASHRAE Standard 62.2.	RA7.4.1 Continuous Operation
Whole-Building Mechanical Ventilation Airflow – Intermittent Operation	Verify that whole-building ventilation system complies with the airflow rate required by ASHRAE Standard 62.2.	RA7.4.2. Intermittent Operation

Table RA3.7-1 – Summary of Verification and Diagnostic procedures

RA3.7.2 Instrumentation Specifications

The instrumentation for the air distribution diagnostic measurements shall conform to the following specifications:

RA3.7.2.1 Pressure Measurements

All pressure measurements shall be measured with measurement systems (i.e., sensor plus data acquisition system) having an accuracy equal to or better than ± 1% of pressure reading or ± 0.2 Pa (0.0008 inches water) (whichever is greater). All pressure measurements within the duct system shall be made with static pressure probes such as Dwyer A303 or equivalent.

RA3.7.2.2 Airflow Rate Measurements

All measurements of ventilation fan airflow rate shall be made with an airflow rate measurement apparatus (i.e., sensor plus data acquisition system) having an accuracy equal to or better than ± 10% of reading. The apparatus shall have an accuracy specification that is applicable to the airflow rates that must be verified utilizing the procedures in Section RA3.7.4.

RA3.7.2.3 Calibration

All instrumentation used for mechanical ventilation system airflow rate diagnostic measurements shall be calibrated according to the manufacturer's calibration procedure to ensure the airflow measurement apparatus conforms to the accuracy requirement specified in Section RA3.7.2.2.

RA3.7.3 Diagnostic Apparatus for Measurement of Ventilation System Airflow

Ventilation system airflow rate shall be measured using one of the apparatuses listed in Section RA3.7.3. The apparatus shall produce airflow rate measurements that conform to the accuracy requirements specified in Section RA3.7.2 for measurements of residential mechanical ventilation system airflow at system grilles or registers for single or multiple branch ventilation duct systems.

The airflow rate measurement apparatus manufacturers shall publish in their product documentation, specifications for how their airflow measurement apparatuses are to be used for accurately measuring residential mechanical ventilation system airflow at system grilles or registers of single or multiple branch ventilation systems.

The airflow measurement apparatus manufacturers shall certify to the Energy Commission that use of the apparatus in accordance with the specifications given in the manufacturer's product documentation will produce measurement results that are within the accuracy required by Section RA3.7.2.2.

For the airflow measurement apparatuses that are certified to the Commission as meeting the accuracy required by Section RA3.7.2.2, the following information will be posted on the Energy Commission website, making the information available to all people involved in the airflow verification compliance process:

- (a) The product manufacturers' model numbers for the airflow measurement apparatuses.
- (b) The product manufacturers' product documentation that gives the specifications for use of the airflow measurement apparatuses to accurately measure residential mechanical ventilation system airflow at system grilles or registers of single or multiple branch ventilation systems.

A manufacturer's certification to the Commission of the accuracy of the airflow measurement apparatus, and submittal to the Commission of the product documentation that specifies the proper use of the airflow measurement apparatus to produce accurate airflow rate measurements shall be prerequisites for allowing the manufacturer's airflow measurement apparatus to be used for conducting the system airflow verification procedures in Section RA3.7 for demonstrating compliance with Part 6.

RA3.7.3.1 Residential Mechanical Exhaust Airflow Measurement Device

A flowmeter that meets the applicable instrument accuracy specifications in RA3.7.2 shall be used to measure the mechanical exhaust airflow.

RA3.7.3.2 Powered Flow Capture Hood Airflow Measurement Device

A powered and pressure balanced flow capture hood (subsequently referred to as a Powered Flow Hood) that has the capability to balance the flow capture static pressure difference between the room and the flow capture hood enclosure to 0.0 ± 0.2 Pa (0.0008 inches water) and meets the applicable instrumentation specifications in Section RA3.7.2 may be used to verify the ventilation airflow rate if the powered flow hood has a flow capture area at least as large as the ventilation system register/grille in all dimensions. The fan adjustment needed to balance the flow capture static pressure difference between the room and the flow capture hood enclosure to 0.0 ± 0.2 Pa (0.0008 inches water) shall be provided by either an automatic control or a manual control operated in accordance with the apparatus manufacturer's instructions specified in the manufacturer's product documentation.

RA3.7.3.3 Traditional Flow Capture Hood

A traditional flow capture hood meeting the applicable instrumentation specifications in Section RA3.7.2 may be used to verify the ventilation system airflow rate if the non-powered flow hood has a capture area at least as large as the ventilation system register/grille in all dimensions.

RA3.7.4 Procedures

This section describes the procedures used to verify Mechanical ventilation system airflow.

RA3.7.4.1 Whole-Building Mechanical Ventilation Airflow Rate Measurement - Continuous Operation

RA3.7.4.1.1 Exhaust Ventilation Systems

A flow measuring device that meets the applicable instrumentation requirements of Section RA3.7.2 shall be used. If the measured airflow is equal to or greater than the value for whole-building ventilation airflow rate required by Section 4 of ASHRAE, the mechanical ventilation system complies with the requirement for whole-building mechanical ventilation airflow. If the measured airflow is less than the required whole-building ventilation airflow rate, the mechanical ventilation system does not comply, and corrective action shall be taken.

RA3.7.4.1.2 Supply Ventilation Systems

The Executive Director may approve supply mechanical ventilation systems, devices, or controls for use for compliance with the HERS Rater field verification and diagnostic testing requirement for whole-building mechanical ventilation airflow, subject to a manufacturer providing sufficient evidence to the Executive Director that the installed mechanical ventilation systems, devices, or controls will provide at least the minimum whole-building ventilation airflow required by ASHRAE, and subject to consideration of the manufacturer's proposed field verification and diagnostic test protocol for these ventilation system(s).

Approved systems, devices, or controls, and field verification and diagnostic test protocols for Supply Ventilation Systems shall be listed in directories published by the Energy Commission.

RA3.7.4.2 Whole-Building Mechanical Ventilation Airflow Rate Measurement – Intermittent Operation

The Executive Director may approve intermittent mechanical ventilation systems, devices, or controls for use for compliance with the HERS Rater field verification and diagnostic testing requirement whole-building mechanical ventilation airflow, subject to a manufacturer providing sufficient evidence to the Executive Director that the installed mechanical ventilation systems, devices, or controls will provide at least the minimum whole-building ventilation airflow required by ASHRAE, and subject to consideration of the manufacturer's proposed field verification and diagnostic test protocol for the ventilation system(s).

Approved systems, devices, or controls, and field verification and diagnostic test protocols for intermittent mechanical ventilation systems shall be listed in directories published by the Energy Commission.

Energy Code Ace insights to the California Code[21]

The 2022 Energy Code incorporated updated versions of Standard 62.2 and extended its requirements to multifamily buildings. (Note that the language on the Energy Code Ace site is commentary and not the actual code language. The site does include links to the code.)

The California Code language can be found in Subchapter 7 Section 150.0 of the 2022 California Code of Regulations. The mandatory features are in Section 150.0(o)[22].

MULTIFAMILY

11.4.2.3 Differences between Energy Code and ASHRAE Standard 62.2

The Energy Code mandatory requirements include the adopted 2019 ASHRAE Standard 62.2 with amendments. The key differences in the Energy Code compared to the 2019 ASHRAE Standard 62.2 include the following:

- While ASHRAE Standard 62.2 requires compartmentalization but does not require balanced ventilation, the Energy Code provide two options for compliance with dwelling unit ventilation: 1) installation of a balanced ventilation system or 2) installation of an exhaust or supply-only system accompanied

---

21. https://energycodeace.com/
22. https://energycodeace.com/content/section-1500-mandatory-features-and-devices-single-family-r#ra-chunk--135347

by compartmentalization: sealing to a leakage rate of not more than 0.3 CFM50 per square feet of dwelling unit enclosure surface area.
- The Energy Code require MERV 13 filtration for all recirculated air and outdoor air, including outdoor air provided by supply air ventilation systems or the supply side of balanced ventilation systems, while ASHRAE Standard 62.2 requires MERV 6 filtration for HVAC systems with at least 10 ft. of ductwork. The additional filtration requirements in the Energy Code are important for reducing particulate matter which can pose a health to residents.
- Both standards require kitchen exhaust systems vented to the outdoors and allow three systems for kitchen exhaust systems in multifamily dwelling units: 1) demand-controlled range hood, 2) downdraft exhaust or 3) continuous kitchen exhaust for enclosed kitchens only.
   - For demand-controlled range hoods, the Energy Code require that they either meet a minimum airflow or capture efficiency that depends on the type and dwelling unit floor area as shown in Table 11-22. There are no capture efficiency requirements in ASHRAE Standard 62.2. Additionally, the required minimum hood airflows are higher in the Energy Code, as shown in Table 11-22, than the requirement in ASHRAE Standard 62.2, which is 100 CFM for all demand-controlled range hoods.

Dwelling unit floor area (sq. ft)	Hood over electric range	Hood over gas range
≤ 750	65% CE or 160 CFM	85% CE or 280 CFM
750 – 1,000	55% CE or 130 CFM	85% CE or 280 CFM
> 1,000 – 1,500	50% CE or 110 CFM	80% CE or 250 CFM
>1,500	50% CE or 110 CFM	70% CE or 180 CFM

Table 11-22: Minimum Capture Efficiency (CE)[23] or Airflow (CFM) for Demand-Controlled Range Hoods

---

23. Range hood capture efficiency defines the effectiveness of a range hood to capture cooking effluents. This work has been done at the Lawrence Berkely Laboratories developing a standardized testing procedure. https://www.ashrae.org/news/ashraejournal/measuring-range-hood-capture-efficiency-values

Source: California Energy Commission

- For downdraft and continuous kitchen exhaust requirements, the Energy Code and ASHRAE Standard 62.2 are the same.

The verification protocol for kitchen exhaust systems remains the same. Kitchen range hood fans are required to be verified by a HERS Rater. The verification protocol requires comparing the installed model to ratings in the Home Ventilating Institute (HVI) or Association of Home Appliance Manufacturers (AHAM) directory of certified ventilation products to confirm the installed range hood is rated to meet the required airflow in the Energy Code, as well as the sound requirements specified in ASHRAE Standard 62.2. See the section, *Requirements for Kitchen Exhaust* below for more detail. Kitchen range hood fans that exhaust more than 400 CFM at minimum speed are exempt from the sound requirement.

Limiting the sources of indoor pollutants is an important method for protecting IAQ. The United States Environmental Protection Agency (EPA) provides information and resources on improving IAQ. For more information, see the EPA's Indoor Air Quality webpage: www.epa.gov/indoor-air-quality-iaq.

* * *

Florida

Florida Building Code 8th Edition (2023) is available for free on the ICC site.[24] The Florida State Building Code Part IV, Chapter 11 Energy Efficiency includes several sections on ventilation including Section N1109.ABC.1 "Buildings operated at positive indoor pressure." It states, "Residential buildings designed to be operated at a positive indoor pressure or for mechanical ventilation shall meet," the design air change per hour minimums in ASHRAE 62, that "no ventilation or air-conditioning system makeup air shall be provided to conditioned spaces from attics, crawl spaces, attached enclosed garages or outdoor spaces adjacent to swimming pools or spas." In a hot, humid climate such as Florida, positive pressure ventilation

---

24. https://codes.iccsafe.org/content/FLRC2023P1

can prevent that humidity from entering the home through cracks and leaks in the home because the structure will be slightly "inflated".

The Eighth Edition of the Florida Building Code became effective on December 31, 2023. It is based on the 2021 IRC with sections amended. Mechanical ventilation has been moved to Chapter 15 Exhaust Systems (Section 1507 Mechanical Ventilation). It doesn't vary significantly from the 2021 IRC.

Most of Florida is in climate zone 2 except down in the southeast corner, which is climate zone 1.

* * *

Massachusetts

The ventilation requirements in the Tenth edition of the Massachusetts[25] Residential Code includes section N1103.6 (R403.6) that is similar to the ASHRAE 62.2-2016 requirements. There are **no** provisions in the code that state that ventilation is only required if the tightness of the building is less than 5 ACH_{50} or some other threshold.

N1103.6 (R403.6) Mechanical Ventilation (Mandatory). Each dwelling unit of a residential building shall be provide with continuously operating exhaust, supply, or balanced mechanical ventilation that has been site verified to meet a minimum airflow per:

1. the Energy Star Homes' Version 3.1;
2. ASHRAE 62.2-2013; or
3. The following formula for one- and two-family dwellings and townhouses of three or fewer stories above grade plane:

$$Q = .03 \times CFA + 7.5 \times (N_{br} + 1) - 0.052 \times Q_{50} \times S \times WSF$$

Where:
CFA is the conditioned floor area in sq ft

---

25. https://www.mass.gov/doc/bbrs-10th-edition-building-code/download

N_{br} is the number of bedrooms

Q_{50} is the verified blower door air leakage rate in cfm measured at 50 Pascals

S is the building height factor determined by this table:

Stories Above Grade Plane	1	2	3
S	1.00	1.32	1.55

WSF is the shielded weather factor as determined by this table:

County	WSF
Barnstable	0.60
Berkshire	0.52
Bristol	0.54
Dukes	0.59
Essex	0.58
Franklin	0.52
Hampden	0.49
Hampshire	0.59
Middlesex	0.55
Nantucket	0.61
Norfolk	0.52
Plymouth	0.53
Suffolk	0.66
Worcester	0.59

N1103.6.2 (R403.6.2) through N1103.6.6 (R403.6.6) Add the subsections as follows:

N1103.6.2 (R403.6.2) Testing and Verification. Installed performance of the mechanical ventilation system shall be tested and verified by a HERS Rater, HERS Rating Field Inspector, or an applicable BPI Certified Professional, and measured using a flow hood, flow grid, or other airflow measure device in accordance with either RESNET Standard Chapter 8 or ACCA Standard 5.

N1103.6.3 (R403.6.3) AIR-MOVING EQUIPMENT, Selection and Installation. As referenced in ASHRAE Standard 62.2-2013, Section 7.1, ventilation devices and equipment shall be tested and certified by AMCA (Air movement and Control Association) or HVI (Home Ventilating Institute) and the certification table shall be found on the product. Installation of systems or equipment shall be carried out in accordance with manufacturers' design requirements and installation instructions. Where multiple duct sizes and/or exterior hoods are standard options, the minimum size shall not be used.

N1103.6.4 (R403.6.4) Sound Rating. Sound rating for fans used for whole building ventilation shall be rated at a maximum of 1.0 sone.

Exception: HVAC air handlers and remote-mounted fans need not meet sound requirements. There must be at least 4 feet of ductwork between the remote mounted fan and intake grille.

N1103.6.5 (R403.6.5) Documentation. The owner and the occupant of the dwelling unit shall be provided with information on the ventilation design and systems installed, as well as instructions on the proper operation and maintenance of the ventilation systems. Ventilation controls shall be labeled with regard to their function, unless the function is obvious.

N1103.6.6 (R403.6.6) Air Inlets and Exhausts. All ventilation air inlets shall be located a minimum of ten feet from vent openings for plumbing drainage systems, appliance vent outlets, exhaust hood outlets, vehicle exhaust, or other known contamination sources; and inlets shall be covered with rodent screens having mesh openings not greater than ½ inch. A whole house mechanical ventilation system shall not extract air from an unconditioned basement unless approved by a registered deign professional. When wall inlet or exhaust vents are less than seven feet above finished grade in the area of the venting, including but not limited to decks and porches, a metal or plastic identification plate shall be permanently mounted to the exterior of the building at a minimum eight of eight feet above grade directly in line with the vent terminal. The sign shall read in print size no less than ½ inch in size, "MECH. VENT DIRECTLY BELOW. KEEP CLEAR OF ALL OBSTRUCTIONS."

Exceptions:

1. Ventilation air inlets in the wall ≥ 3 ft. from dryer exhausts and contamination sources exiting through the roof.
2. No minimum separate distance shall be required between local exhaust outlets in kitchens/bathrooms and windows.
3. Vent terminations that meet the requirements of the National Fuel Gas Code (NFPA 54/ANSI Z223.1) or equivalent.

* * *

Minnesota

Minnesota[26] amended the requirements of the International Mechanical Code to comply with the requirements of ASHRAE 62.2. The ventilation system "shall be designed to supply the required rate of ventilation air continuously during the period the building is occupied, except as otherwise stated in other provisions of the code. 1346.0404 Section 404 Garages amends IMC 404.1 to require, "Mechanical ventilation systems for enclosed parking garages shall provide a minimum exhaust rate of 0.75 cfm per square foot (0.0038 m3/s) of floor area." It does not define whether this is both commercial and residential garages.

There is a lengthy description of makeup air systems and pressure equalization. For example: 501.4.3 paragraph 4 states, "When an exhaust system with a rated capacity greater than 300 cfm (0.144 m3/s) is installed in a dwelling constructed during or after 1994 under the Minnesota Energy Code, Minnesota Rules, chapter 7670, makeup air quantity shall be determined by using IMC Table 501.4.3(1) and shall be supplied according to IMC Section 501.4.2. Exception: If powered makeup air is electrically interlocked and matched to the airflow of the exhaust system additional makeup air is not required." The table requires 135 cfm of makeup air for clothes dryers under all conditions.

. . .

---

26. http://www.dli.mn.gov/business/codes-and-laws/2020-minnesota-state-building-codes

MINNESOTA ENERGY CODE (Minnesota Administrative Rules):[27]

R403.5 Mechanical ventilation (mandatory).

The building shall be provided with a balanced mechanical ventilation system that is +/-10 percent of the system's design capacity and meets the requirements of Section R403.5.5, which establishes the continuous and total mechanical ventilation requirements for dwelling unit ventilation. All conditioned unfinished basements, conditioned crawl spaces, and conditioned levels shall be provided with a minimum ventilation rate of 0.02 cfm (0.000566 m^3/m) per square foot or a minimum of 1 supply duct and 1 return duct. The supply and return ducts shall be separated by 1/2 the diagonal dimension of the basement to avoid a short circuit of the air circulation. Outdoor air intakes and exhausts shall have automatic or gravity dampers that close when the ventilation system is not operating.

Exception: Kitchen and bath fans that are not included as part of the mechanical ventilation system are exempt from these requirements.

R403.5.1 Alterations.

Alterations to existing buildings are exempt from meeting the requirements of Section R403.5.

R403.5.2 Total ventilation rate.

The mechanical ventilation system shall provide sufficient outdoor air to equal the total ventilation rate average for each 1-hour period in accordance with Table R403.5.2, or Equation R403.5.2, based on the number of bedrooms and square footage of conditioned space, including the basement and conditioned crawl spaces.

FOR THE PURPOSES of Table R403.5.2 and Section R403.5.3, the following applies:

a. Equation R403.5.2 Total ventilation rate: Total ventilation rate (cfm) = (0.02 × square feet of conditioned space) + [15 × (number of bedrooms + 1)].
b. Equation R403.5.2.1 Continuous ventilation rate: Continuous ventilation rate (cfm) = Total ventilation rate/2.

---

27. https://up.codes/viewer/minnesota/imc-2018/chapter/4/ventilation#403

Conditioned space[1] (in sq.ft.)	1 Total/ Continuous	2 Total/ Continuous	3 Total/ Continuous	4 Total/ Continuous	5 Total/ Continuous	6[2] Total/ Continuous
1000-1500	60/40	75/40	90/45	105/53	120/60	135/68
1501-2000	70/40	85/43	100/50	115/58	130/65	145/73
2001-2500	80/40	95/48	110/55	125/63	140/70	155/78
2501-3000	90/45	105/53	120/60	135/68	150/75	165/83
3001-3500	100/50	115/58	130/65	145/73	160/80	175/88
3501-4000	110/55	125/63	140/70	155/78	170/85	185/93
4001-4500	120/60	135/68	150/75	165/83	180/90	195/98
4501-5000	130/65	145/73	160/80	175/88	190/95	205/103
5001-5500	140/70	155/78	170/85	185/93	200/100	215/108
5501-6000[2]	150/75	165/83	180/90	195/98	210/105	225/113

TABLE R403.5.2 NUMBER OF BEDROOMS

1. Conditioned space includes the basement and conditioned crawl spaces.

2. If conditioned space exceeds 6,000 sq. ft. or there are more than 6 bedrooms, use Equation R403.5.2.

R403.5.3 *Continuous ventilation rate.*

Continuous ventilation rate (CVR) is a minimum of 50 percent of the total ventilation rate (TVR). The CVR shall not be less than 40 cfm (1.13 m3/m) and shall provide a continuous average cfm rate according to Table R403.5.2 or according to Equation R403.5.2 for every 1-hour period. The portion of the ventilation system that is intended to be continuous may have automatic cycling controls to provide the average flow rate for each hour.

R403.5.5 BALANCED AND HRV/ERV *systems.*

All balanced systems shall be balanced so that the air intake is within 10 percent of the exhaust output. A heat recovery ventilator (HRV) or energy recovery ventilator (ERV) shall meet either:

1. The requirements of HVI Standard 920, 72 hours minus 13°F (-10°C) cold weather test; or

2. Certified by a registered professional engineer and installed per manufacturer's installation instructions.

An HRV or ERV intended to comply with both the continuous and total ventilation rate requirements shall meet the rated design capacity of the continuous ventilation rate specified in Section R403.5.3 under low capacity and meet the total ventilation rate specified in Section R403.5.2 under high capacity.

Exception: The balanced system and HRV/ERV system may include exhaust fans to meet the intermittent ventilation rate. Surface mounted fans shall have a maximum 1.0 sone per HVI Standard 915.

R403.5.6 INSTALLATION REQUIREMENTS.

All mechanical systems shall meet the requirements of Section R403.5.6. The mechanical ventilation system and its components shall also be installed according to the Minnesota Mechanical Code, Minnesota Rules, Chapter 1346, and the equipment manufacturer's installation instructions.

R403.5.6.1 AIR DISTRIBUTION/CIRCULATION.

Outdoor air shall be delivered to each habitable space by a forced air circulation system, separate duct system, or individual inlets.

R403.5.6.1.1 Forced air circulation systems.

When outdoor air is supplied directly through a forced air circulation system, the requirements of this section shall be met using one of the following methods:

- a. When an outdoor air supply is not ducted to the forced air system, controls shall be installed to allow the forced air system to provide an average circulation flow rate each hour of not less than 0.15 cfm (0.00425 m3/m) per square foot of the conditioned floor area; or
- b. When the outdoor air supply is ducted to the forced air system, the mixed air temperature shall not be less than the heating

equipment manufacturer's installation instructions. The controls shall be installed to allow the forced air circulation system to provide an average flow rate not less than 0.075 cfm (0.00212 m3/m) per square foot of conditioned floor area.

R403.5.6.1.2 DIRECTLY DUCTED *and individual room inlets.*

When outdoor air is supplied directly to habitable spaces with an airflow of 20 cfm (0.57 m3/m) or greater, the system shall be designed and installed to temper incoming air to not less than 40°F (4°C) measured at the point of distribution into the space.

R403.5.6.1.3 AIRFLOW VERIFICATION.

All mechanical ventilation system airflows greater than 30 cfm (0.85 m3/m) at the building exhaust or intake shall be tested and verified. The airflow verification results shall be made available to the building official upon request.

R403.5.7 *Fans.*

When used as part of the mechanical ventilation system, fans shall be capable of delivering the designed air flow at the point of air discharge or intake as determined by Section R403.5.2 and according to HVI Standard 916. Fans shall be designed and certified by the equipment manufacturer to be capable of continuous operation at the maximum fan-rated cfm. Surface mounted fans used to comply with the continuous ventilation requirement of the mechanical ventilation system shall have a maximum 1.0 sone, according to HVI Standard 915. Fans used to comply with the intermittent ventilation requirement of the mechanical ventilation system shall have a maximum 2.5 sone, according to HVI Standard 915. Mechanical ventilation system fans shall meet the efficacy requirements of Table R403.5.l.

Exception to sone requirements: Sone requirements do not apply to forced air circulation systems and remotely mounted fans. If the remotely mounted fan is not in a habitable space and there are at least 4 feet (1219 mm) of ductwork between the fan and grille, then the fan sone rating shall be 2.5 sone or less. Where mechanical ventilation fans are integral to tested and listed HVAC equipment, the fans shall be powered by an electronically commutated motor.

R403.5.8 *Multifan systems.*

When two or more fans in a dwelling unit share a common duct, each fan shall be equipped with a backdraft damper to prevent recirculation of exhaust air into another room.

R403.5.9 Connection to forced air circulation systems.

When air ducts are directly connected to the forced air circulation system, the outdoor air shall be supplied directly to the forced air circulation system, or the exhaust air shall be drawn directly from the forced air circulation system, but not both. To meet the mechanical ventilation system requirements, the air duct shall be installed according to the manufacturer's installation instructions.

Exception: Both outdoor air and exhaust air may be connected to the forced air circulation system only if controls are installed to operate the forced air circulation system when the mechanical ventilation system is operating or other means are provided to prevent short circuiting of ventilation air in accordance with the manufacturer's recommendations.

R403.5.10 Dampers.

The mechanical ventilation system supply and exhaust ducts shall be provided with accessible backflow dampers to minimize flow to or from the outdoors when the ventilation system is off.

R403.5.11 Intake openings.

Exterior air intake openings shall be accessible for inspection and maintenance. Intake openings shall be located according to the Minnesota Mechanical Code, Minnesota Rules, Chapter 1346, and shall be covered with a corrosion-resistant screen of not less than 1/4-inch (6.4 mm) mesh. Intake openings shall be located at least 12 inches (305 mm) above adjoining grade level.

Exception: Combination air intake and exhaust hoods may be approved by the building official when specifically allowed by the equipment manufacturer's installation instructions.

R403.5.12 Filtration.

All mechanically supplied outdoor air shall have a filter with a designated minimum efficiency of MERV 4 as defined by ASHRAE Standard 52.2. The filter location shall be prior to the air entering the thermal conditioning components, blower, or habitable space. The filter shall be installed so it is readily accessible and facilitates regular service.

R403.5.13 Noise and vibration.

Mechanical ventilation system components shall be installed to minimize transmission of noise and vibration. The equipment manufacturer's installation instructions shall be followed and any materials provided by the equipment manufacturer for installation shall be used. In the absence of specific materials or instructions, vibration dampening materials, such as rubber grommets and flexible straps, shall be used when connecting fans and heat exchangers to the building structure. Isolation duct connectors shall be used to mitigate noise transmission.

R403.5.14 Controls.

Balanced mechanical ventilation system controls shall comply with all the following:

1. When the mechanical ventilation system is not designed to operate whenever the forced air circulation system is operating, the mechanical ventilation system shall incorporate an accessible backflow damper to prevent flow from the outside when the mechanical ventilation system is off.
2. Controls shall be compatible with the mechanical ventilation system, its components, and the manufacturer's installation and operating instructions.
3. Controls shall be installed to operate the mechanical ventilation system as designed.
4. Each control shall be readily accessible to occupants and shall be labeled to indicate the control's function.

R403.5.15 Labeling.

All ventilation intake and exhaust outlets shall include permanent, weather-resistant identification labels on the building's exterior.

R403.5.16 Documentation.

Documentation, which includes proper operation and maintenance instructions, shall accompany all mechanical ventilation systems. The documentation shall be in a conspicuous and readily accessible location.

* * *

Vermont

Revisions to the Fifth Edition of the Vermont[28] Residential Building Energy Code[29] that took effect September 1, 2020, required all newly constructed homes to be mechanically ventilated. "All newly constructed homes to be mechanically ventilated with a whole-house ventilation system." The whole house or primary ventilation system must be capable of supplying "the specified amount of air during all periods of occupancy automatically without the need for anyone to turn it on or off."[30] The Handbook has descriptions of basic ventilation terms and criteria such as sones and building pressures.

The whole-house mechanical ventilation requirement can be met:

1. ASHRAE 62.2-2016
2. Building Science Corp. (BSC) Standard 01-2015 (Ventilation for New Low-Rise Residential Buildings)
3. Passive House ventilation requirements (PHI or PHIUS)
4. Prescriptive method

The Handbook in Section 3.1e Capacity states that the fan used can either be rated to meet the flow requirement or tested on-site and provide "a minimum of 15 cubic feet per minute (CFM) plus 15 CFM for each bedroom."

Number of Bedrooms	Minimum Rated Capacity (CFM)	Minimum Number of Fans
1	50	1
2	75	1
3	100	1
4	125	Centrally ducted systems: 1, All other systems 2 or more
5	150	Centrally ducted systems: 1, All other systems 2 or more
Homes over 3000 sq. ft.	0.05 x sq. ft. of conditioned space	Centrally ducted systems: 1, All other systems 2 or more

Table 3.2 Capacity Requirements for Whole-House Ventilation Systems

---

28. https://publicservice.vermont.gov/content/building-energy-standards
29. https://publicservice.vermont.gov/sites/dps/files/documents/2020-VT_Residential_Energy_Code_Handbook_v8.pdf
30. http://publicservice.vermont.gov/energy-efficiency/ee_resbuildingstandards.html

* * *

Washington State

Washington has a detailed ventilation code, which can be found on the Washington State Building Code web page under "Ventilation Code".[31] Washington's codes has provisions for installed system testing to verify performance, it limits fan noise for "Whole House Ventilation Systems" to 1.5 sones, and that the "whole house ventilation fan shall be controlled by a 24-hour clock timer with the capability of continuous operation, manual and automatic control." The code includes a table for ventilation rates from homes from 500 square feet to more than 9000 square feet and up to 8 bedrooms. It also includes a "Prescriptive Exhaust Duct Sizing" table.

Note that the Washington Ventilation code has been superseded by the requirements in the International Mechanical Code and International Residential Code.

* * *

Safety Testing and Performance Certification

Products are safety tested by a variety of organizations. None of these organizations are government controlled. Most are privately held, not-for-profit underwriting companies. HVI and AMCA are performance certification organizations, verifying to the consumer that similar products will perform in similar, certified ways. Since there are no government agencies that control manufacturer's claims of performance, organizations like HVI and AMCA are vital in assuring the consumer that products with these marks will indeed perform as advertised. Some government programs like Energy Star and California's Title 20 require performance as well as safety testing by a recognized laboratory.

Home Ventilating Institute (HVI)[32]

HVI "represents a wide range of home ventilating products manufactured by companies in the United States, Canada, Asia, and Europe, producing the

---

31. https://sbcc.wa.gov/state-codes-regulations-guidelines/state-building-code/energy-code
32. http://www.hvi.org/

majority of residential ventilation products sold in North America". HVI's Certified Rating Program was created to provide a credible, third party means for comparing the performance of similar products. "Not only are products Certified, but a random verification program ensures that those products still meet their original performance." Performance Certification is required for Energy Star recognition. HVI has five different certification procedures all of which are downloadable in PDF format on the HVI website[33]:

915 Procedure for Loudness Rating of Residential Fan Products - This is the procedure that is used to rate the sound or sone level of fans.

916 Air Flow Test Procedure - The procedure and set-up and equipment that is used for certifying the airflow rate.

920 Product Performance Certification Procedure - This is the procedure that is used to actually record the certification and to document challenges to the results.

921 Performance Verification Procedure for Product Not Certified by HVI - This procedure is designed to verify products that are not HVI certified to protect the safety and interest of the general public.

925 Label and Logo Requirements - These procedures are designed to protect the HVI brand.

Air Movement and Control Association International, Inc. (AMCA)[34]

AMCA is a not-for-profit international association of related air system equipment manufacturers, primarily commercial systems. Their Air Movement Division certifies the performance of residential ventilation products.

The Heating Refrigeration and Air Conditioning Institute of Canada (HRAI)[35]

HRAI is a non-profit national trade association of manufacturers, wholesalers, and contractors in the Canadian heating, ventilation, air-conditioning, and refrigeration industries. They provide excellent system training.

---

33. https://www.hvi.org/hvi-certified-ratings-programs/hvi-certification-program-policies-and-procedures/
34. www.amca.org
35. www.hrai.ca

· · ·

UNDERWRITER LABORATORIES (UL)

UL is the most-recognized U.S. product safety underwriter, testing a very wide variety of products. "UL is an independent product safety certification organization that has been testing products and writing Standards for Safety for over a century. UL evaluates more than 19,000 types of products, components, materials and systems annually with 21 billion UL Marks appearing on 72,000 manufacturers' products each year." UL has 62 laboratories and certification facilities serving customers in 99 countries.

A product that has a **UL Listing** has been tested as a whole. It is a stand-alone product. A product that has been **UL Recognized** is used as a component of another product. "A product is UL Listed if the UL Listing Mark is on the product, accompanied by the manufacturer's name, trade name, trademark or other authorized identification."[36] Further, "The UL Listing Mark on a product is the manufacturer's representation of that complete product has been tested by UL to nationally recognized Safety Standards and found to be free from reasonably foreseeable risk of fire, electric shock and related hazards and that the product was manufactured under UL's Follow-Up Services program."

The UL Recognized mark means that the component alone meets the requirements for a "limited, specified use".

UL Standard 705 for "Power Ventilators" has a limited impact on residential "fans intended for heated and conditioned air and for connection to permanently installed wiring systems in accordance with the National Electrical Code, NFPA 70." Alternatively UL Standard 507 covers a high percentage of residential fan products. Products are subjected to a thorough array of safety checks from the flammability of any plastics to electrical safety to the design of the labels.

Once a manufacturer begins producing the product with the UL listing, UL inspectors regularly visit the manufacturing facility to verify that the product continues to be manufactured as it was initially submitted to UL for testing and that the materials used are the same coming from the same suppliers. If changes are made to materials or suppliers, the manufacturer is

---

36. www.ul.com

required to notify UL of those changes and have the alternatives added to their "Follow-up" procedure.

The addition of a "C" in the UL logo circle indicates that the product has been tested to both U.S. and Canadian safety standards.

Canadian Standards Association International (CSA Group)[37]

CSA provides a similar and competing testing service. UL and CSA have "harmonized" many of their standards to make them less onerous to manufacturers wishing to sell products on both sides of the border. CSA has a similar follow-up service.

Intertek (ETL)

Intertek (using the ETL mark)[38] "specializes in electrical product safety testing, EMC testing, and benchmark performance testing." They have more than 70 offices and laboratories on six continents. Intertek provides a wide variety of safety testing and other services.

Maryland Electrical Testing (MET) Laboratories[39]

Eurofins MET Laboratories is a product testing and safety laboratory. They have been certifying, listing, and labeling products for electrical product safety for more than 60 years. They are qualified to NRTL (Nationally Recognized Testing Laboratory) certify products. They test residential fan products under the UL 507 Standard, and they require a follow-up service. The MET circle mark indicates if the product has been tested to both Canadian and U.S. standards.

---

37. www.csagroup.org
38. www.intertek.com
39. www.metlabs.com

Chapter 13

Program Requirements and Opportunities

Residential ventilation is a single component of residential building science, and although there are specific skills and knowledge and expertise that can be applied, the fact is that the "house is a system". There are few educational programs that concentrate solely on residential ventilation. On the one hand, that is a bad thing because there is a lot to know. On the other hand, it is a good thing, because the science of residential ventilation must be a part of the building as a whole.

The strategy should be the same whether you are working on a new or existing building: build a tight house and ventilate it. The space must be comfortable, safe, and healthy. It must be designed to last a long time, keeping the water and the weather out. It must be serviceable and maintainable or nature will reclaim the space.

There are programs for a doctorate in building sciences that take years. There are conferences in building science that last for four days. There are weeklong courses in residential ventilation.

For example, the Massachusetts Institute of Technology (MIT) includes mechanical ventilation in their HVAC course content[1]. They delve into psychrometrics, HVAC system types, indoor air quality, and environmental indices. "The methods cover from simple degree-day and bin methods to advanced computer analysis." MIT also has a "Natural Ventilation Work-

---

1. https://web.mit.edu/4.427j/www/syllabus.html

shop"[2] that digs into natural (non-mechanical) air movement systems for passive building design.

Many of the degree programs in building science fall into the architecture or Civil Engineering departments. The University of Southern California (USC) describes an applicant for their program as an "individual [who] probably pictures himself as becoming the master builder—the person who builds the structures which are symbols of our civilization."[3]

The basic science of structures is well known. Artisans learned why buildings stand up or why they fall down many years ago. Populations have learned how to create homes that are remarkably well adapted to their environments, from cliff dwellers to adobe structures to igloos to thatched homes to New England saltboxes and high-tech modulars. As we have improved the indoor environment by sealing ourselves off from the outdoor environment, the amount of technical knowledge required has increased dramatically. When breezes blew through wall structures, they got wet and they dried continuously. Materials and tools have changed, making it almost impossible to build a house that is loose enough to provide adequate, natural ventilation. Codes have demanded that homes be constructed better. Economics and concerns about the long-term conditions on the earth have demanded that energy loads be reduced.

Many of these conditions bring out the opportunists that will take advantage of popular concerns with "snake-oil" solutions that at best don't work and at worst do significant harm. Honest knowledge is the best way to avoid these problems.

The knowledge base is changing every day. Although we have been building homes for thousands of years, the new conditions and technologies have given us tools we can use to measure building performance, "look" into existing walls, "see" building pressure, temperature, and humidity differences, and tests houses and ducting for air leaks. These tools and technologies are only a few decades old at most. We are just learning how to use them effectively and what the information means.

Although energy use has been a pressing concern for a long time, the impact of the 2019 Novel Coronavirus (COVID-19) exploded the need for effective mechanical ventilation in homes. Large amounts of research were

---

2. http://coolvent.mit.edu/natural-ventilation-workshop-mit/
3. https://cee.usc.edu/academics/undergraduate-programs-civil/bsce-building-science/

done on air borne virus transmission, clearly linking mechanical ventilation and health.

Contractor Training and Certification Programs

Because building science training is a relatively new field, the certification programs are confusing and organizations are still jockeying for position. Contractors have always been locally controlled, and building science professionals continue in that vein. All the renewed interest in energy saving, the cost of conditioning, and the health impacts have explosively affected the industry and the training and knowledge base. Consequently, the information included here will change, but the resources should serve as a place to start.

Two primary building science organizations in the U.S. are RESNET[4] (Residential Energy Services Network), which operates the HERS program (Home Energy Rating System) and BPI[5] (Building Performance Institute). Residential ventilation is a component, but not the focus of their programs. Many other organizations use HERS or BPI ratings as templates or integral parts of their own programs.

There is one primary resource for learning about residential ventilation in the U.S. or Canada. The Heating Refrigeration and Air Conditioning Institute's (HRAI) (the Canadian national HVACR industry association) Skill-Tech Academy[6] is an intensive course on residential ventilation skills. This is an in-depth program that covers the fundamentals of building science that particularly relate to residential ventilation and the details of ducting design, installation, and testing. It provides checklists, charts, sizing, commissioning and maintenance lists. The course provides an in-depth component of duct design for HRV/ERV systems.[7] These systems are considerably more complex than throwing a bathroom fan in the ceiling and venting it to the outside. The duct design for an independent HRV/ERV installation is equivalent to the detailed duct design work that is required for a ducted HVAC system. Once it has been installed, the flows should be reasonably balanced between supply and exhaust and require only minor adjustment. Design criteria include the location of the grilles and the connections to the air handler if the two systems

---

4. http://www.resnet.us
5. http://www.bpi.org
6. www.hrai.ca
7. See Appendix H: Manual BV

are combined. The course also details combustion safety issues concerning depressurization of the building and other building pressure issues.[8] HRAI describes their two-day certification program in "Residential Mechanical Ventilation Installation" as:

The Residential Mechanical Ventilation Installation Course is designed for contractors and building professionals who may be interested in developing opportunities in the growing residential ventilation market, besides those currently involved with designing and installing residential mechanical ventilation systems, including Energy Recovery Ventilators. The course covers the fundamentals of air quality assessment, system requirements, and focuses specifically on system design and installation. Course participants receive the complete HRAI Residential Mechanical Ventilation Manual, as endorsed by the Home Ventilating Institute (HVI).

The Home Ventilating Institute (HVI)[9] is the U.S. counterpart to HRAI, but they do not offer training programs. HVI's Certified Products Directory is useful in providing 3rd party performance testing of ventilation products. HVI's website has connections to resources for sizing and specifying systems and provides downloads of the "Fresh Ideas" ventilation guide.

Some product manufacturers, including Panasonic, offer extensive information on their websites, including Panasonic's Ventilation University.[10] The information is very detailed for design, sales, and installation professionals.

North American Technician Excellence (NATE) is an organization that certifies heating, ventilation, air conditioning, and refrigeration technicians. It is an independent, third party, non-profit certification organization. They say, "NATE tests technicians; others train."[11] Although NATE does not supply training, other organizations offer courses that are NATE recognized. The HRAI, Residential Mechanical Ventilation Installation course, for example, qualifies for sixteen hours of continuing education credits toward NATE recertification.

The Building Performance Institute (BPI)[12] also provides certification of building science knowledge, recognizing other training programs. BPI accredited professionals have had to pass a BPI examination, including both class-

---

8. HRAI also offers an in-depth course on Indoor Air Quality
9. www.hvi.org
10. https://go.bluevolt.com/Panasonic/s/
11. https://natex.org/contractor/nate-training-academy
12. http://www.bpi.org

room and field testing, and they have to maintain that certification through ongoing education and training. (The HRAI ventilation course is BPI-Recognized and qualifies for 16 hours of continuing education for individuals certified as a BPI Heating Specialist.)

BPI only provides certification testing. But as of this writing, BPI has more than a hundred organizations that offer training on building performance issues that follow BPI education templates. Many of these organizations list and certify professionals under their own banners. You'll find a listing of many of these in Appendix E. Several of them are described here.

In Person Training

Hands-on ventilation training is a component of HERS Rater, BPI, and weatherization training. The only stand-alone, in-depth residential ventilation courses that I know of are presented by HRAI. Although most of the HRAI courses take place in Canada, HRAI offers on-site training of day-long courses at organizations such as the Maine Indoor Air Quality Council[13] Since these are in-person training programs with committed trainers, check the dates and schedules as courses listed here may have already happened, but most programs will repeat courses that they have previously developed.

BPI TEST CENTERS: https://www.bpi.org/test-centers/ Even if you don't intend to get BPI certified in one of their many credentials, most of these test centers have extensive models, props, and other tools and contacting them for group training outside of the credential might be an option.

RESNET (RESIDENTIAL ENERGY Services Network) HERS (Home Energy Rating System) Rater Training Providers: https://www.resnet.us/providers/accredited-providers/accredited-rater-training-providers/ You may not want to become a HERS rater, but if there is a rater training provider in your neighborhood, they might use their training center for a ventilation class. This has been mainly for new construction, moving toward a Zero Energy home, but the auditing technique applies as well to existing buildings. The

---

13. https://maineindoorair.org/

HERS rater certification program offers building science training that has a ventilation component to it. The program has a thorough quality control element, and detailed records are maintained.

MAINE INDOOR AIR QUALITY COUNCIL https://maineindoorair.org/ventilation-installation/ "The Maine Indoor Air Quality Council is dedicated to creating healthy, productive, and environmentally sustainable indoor spaces where you can live, work, play, and learn."

NATIONAL COMFORT INSTITUTE[14]: "National Comfort Institute, Inc. (NCI) is an organization that provides heating, air conditioning, plumbing, and electrical contractors with a focused offering of services and tools to help them improve their businesses, differentiate themselves, grow, and become more profitable." The National Comfort Institute provides HVAC training programs.

PA CONSTRUCTION CODES ACADEMY:[15] PCCA's mission is the professional development of code officials through certification and education.

SLIPSTREAM[16] (Formerly Wisconsin Energy Conservation Corporation) "Slipstream is a nonprofit on a mission to combat climate change with a focus on equity."

SOUTHFACE ENERGY INSTITUTE[17]: Southface (in Atlanta, GA) offers HERS certification preparation and LEED training events and offering their Earth-Craft House training and their Homebuilding School and training for contractors to meet the Home Performance with ENERGY STAR guidelines.

---

14. https://www.nationalcomfortinstitute.com/
15. https://www.paconstructioncodesacademy.org/residential-mechanical-systems-whole-house-ventilation-and-forced-air-distribution
16. https://slipstreaminc.org/education
17. https://www.southface.org/training/

. . .

WEATHERIZATION TRAINING CENTERS[18] The network of weatherization training centers spans the country and offers in depth training on all aspects of home and multifamily weatherization. Along with their courses on air sealing and insulation, they provide training on furnaces, boilers, and ventilation systems. Some interesting videos, documents, and state documents: https://nascsp.org/energy-education/

THE ENERGY OUTWEST site includes a listing of all the regional training centers in the western U.S.: https://www.energyoutwest.org/Tech-Info/Resources/Regional-Training-Centers

AEA, NYC: Providing weatherization, health, and safety improvements for low-income New Yorkers: https://aea.us.org/ **Association of Energy Affordability, Inc.**: AEA is "committed to using energy efficiency to maintain affordable and healthy housing for low and moderate-income families and communities." AEA offers BPI template training and certification in weatherization, energy efficient building operations, multifamily building analysis, hydronic heating system design, building analyst, and envelope specialist.

ALASKA HOUSING AND FINANCE CORPORATION: "Alaska Housing Finance Corporation (AHFC) is a self-supporting public corporation with offices in 16 communities throughout Alaska." Through a wide variety of workshops, AHFC offers training for professionals on building science, the use of blower doors, cold climate retrofits, and airtightness. They also provide workshops for the general public on energy and indoor air quality and to builders, inspectors, lenders, and real estate professionals on home inspections and financing.

https://www.ahfc.us//efficiency/education-and-events/energy-efficiency-now-conference

---

18. https://nascsp.org/wap/waptac/weatherization-training-centers/

EnergySmart Academy at Santa Fe Community College: https://www.energysmartacademy.com/ The EnergySmart Academy offers both in-person and on-line training.

The Indoor Climate Research and Training program at the University of Illinois at Urbana/Champagne has comprehensive building science training including an in-depth course in ASHRAE 62.2. https://ccrpc.gitlab.io/icrt/training/training-home/

Montana State University Weatherization Training Center: Located in beautiful Bozeman, Montana: https://www.montana.edu/extension/weatherization/

Southwest Building Science Training Center: https://swbstc.org/ SWBSTC is operated by FSL Home Improvement division in partnership with the Arizona Governor's Office of Energy Policy providing highly specialized technical weatherization and energy efficiency continuing education to Arizona weatherization agency personnel.

Energy OutWest has a page listing regional training centers: https://www.energyoutwest.org/Tech-Info/Resources/Regional-Training-Centers

On-line Training

The internet is a wonderful thing, a place where you can get information about just about anything, delivered by many people. That is a blessing and a curse. I have listed on-line courses here that come from authoritative sources with believable information.

AECDaily. Introduction to Residential Ventilation (Sponsored by Panasonic Eco Systems North America): https://www.aecdaily.com/course.php?node_id=2023918

. . .

BUILDING SCIENCE FIGHT CLUB: Fundamentals of Residential Ventilation for Architects and Builders: https://www.buildingsciencefightclub.com/courses/fundamentals-of-residential-ventilation-for-architects-and-builders

THE BUILDING PERFORMANCE WORKSHOP: https://buildingperformanceworkshop.com/ventilation

COLORADO ENERGY OFFICE: Building Code Training: Residential Ventilation Strategies: https://www.youtube.com/watch?v=ZwLshmU4zPo

GREENTRAININGUSA HTTPS://WWW.GREENTRAININGUSA.COM/ASHRAE-622-VENTILATION-TRAINING.HTML

HEATSPRING: ASHRAE 62.2 Ventilation for Single Family Dwellings: https://www.heatspring.com/courses/ashrae-62-2-ventilation-for-single-family-dwellings

EFFICIENCY VERMONT: Introduction to Residential Ventilation: (Sponsored by Zehnder): https://www.efficiencyvermont.com/online-trainings/introduction-to-residential-ventilation

SATURN RESOURCE MANAGEMENT[19]: Whole Building Ventilation Systems (Mini Course): https://srmi.biz/courses/whole-building-ventilation-systems-ceu/ Saturn Resource Management, Inc. delivers online courses for building energy professionals from BPI's Building Analyst to RESNET's Home Energy Rater, as well as a series of continuing education courses. They offer

---

19. Saturn has a Technical Brief called Residential Ventilation Systems by John Krigger https://srmi.biz/product/residential-ventilation/

overview courses to "provide training for those just starting in energy auditing" as well as certification and proficiency courses to provide training for career-oriented professionals.

COMMUNITY COLLEGE PROGRAMS offer incredible opportunities to learn more about more topics than almost any other resource. The programs are too varied and too fluid to describe here, but they are certainly worth investigating.

Many equipment manufacturers have expanded their websites to provide in-depth product selection information (these naturally direct potential customers to their own equipment, but they still provide a substantial amount of useful information. Test equipment manufacturers also provide training in using their test equipment. These often occur at conferences and trade shows.

Some conferences focus on the trade show component and some on the educational aspect of the program. ASHRAE incorporates the largest U.S. trade show for HVAC equipment—AHR Expo (Air-Conditioning, Heating, and Refrigerating). Although it focuses on commercial equipment, there are interesting exhibits that relate to residential applications. The associated conference also has a primarily commercial focus.

More residential building science training can be found at such conferences as the Home Performance Coalition Conference, the Energy and Environmental Building Association (EEBA) conference, NESEA (Northeast Sustainable Energy Association) Building Energy Conference, and Southface's Greenprints conference among others. These conferences feature a body of dedicated, volunteer teachers and building scientists. The conferences often include HERS or BPI training as well as providing hands on experience with equipment, and they are available over a wide geographic area.

> IREC is the Interstate Renewable Energy Corporation. Training organizations and trainers who have been accredited or certified have gone through a significant amount of scrutiny. Although there are not accreditation categories for all subjects, a training program, or trainer with IREC credentials indicates an excellent program or trainer.

Green Building Programs

Green Building programs are developing and changing at an astounding rate. What's listed here are just a few of the national and state programs. Virtually all of these programs recognize that when the house is tightened up for energy efficiency that mechanical ventilation is required and most of them connect their ventilation requirements to ASHRAE 62.2. This listing is provided for a "taste" of what is going on, and it is important to do some local research. Building an energy efficient structure makes consummate sense and creates a structure that will be more comfortable to the occupants both physically and economically, and make it more salable. But it is important to carefully follow the guidelines, particularly regarding mechanical ventilation because as the building gets tighter, the margin for error decreases, and there is nothing worse than callbacks and unhappy building owners!

The United States Green Building Council (USGBC), LEED for Homes, administers the best-known, national, Green Building program. LEED is a comprehensive program that includes much more than just ventilation. There are eight different areas of which Environmental Quality (EQ) which includes ventilation, is just one.

The EQ requirements can be met by following the steps for ENERGY STAR with Indoor AirPlus whose ventilation requirements follow ASHRAE 62.2. Alternatively, EQ4 prescribes the requirements for Outdoor Air Ventilation, which also requires ASHRAE 62.2[20] be followed as a prerequisite or a passive ventilation system that is verified by a licensed HVAC engineer. These systems can be enhanced through the use of a variety of controls or third party testing.

The NAHB has developed a "Green Building Standard" that has been ANSI recognized and can be purchased from ICC as ICC/ASHRAE 700-2015 National Green Building Standard™ (NGBS). The Standard provides points for various ventilation system configurations, although no ventilation system is mandatory.

The Green Communities[21] building criteria for green building serves as an excellent resource for all aspects of green building above and beyond ventilation. They recommend the use of ASHRAE 62.2 and 62.1. They have

---

20. The ASHRAE 62.2 Standard is updated every 3 years. As of this writing it is version 2025.
21. http://www.greencommunitiesonline.org

references to the ENERGY STAR web sites and provide "Things to Consider" referring to LEED for homes requirements and HVI references and the Building Science Corporation's "Residential Ventilation Technologies" which link to a 2005 paper on residential ventilation systems.

One local program, Wisconsin's Green Built Home,[22] includes points for installing heat or energy recovery ventilators, two, properly supported ceiling fans, and a high efficiency whole-house fan installed with an R-38 insulated cover. The program also gives points for attached garages ventilated to "neutral pressure" and ENERGY STAR rated bath fans.

University Programs

Universities around the world offer building science degrees. The Society of Building Science Educators[23] is an international group representing training programs and universities. "The Society of Building Science Educators (SBSE) is an association of university educators and practitioners in architecture and related disciplines who support excellence in the teaching of environmental science and building technologies."

The International Network for Information on Ventilation and Energy Performance (INIVE)[24] is an international ventilation organization that "was set up as a worldwide acting network of excellence in knowledge gathering and dissemination." It includes AIVC (Air Infiltration and Ventilation Centre) which produces publications and holds conferences on ventilation issues. INIVE also includes TightVent Europe and Venticool, which is focused on using ventilation for cooling.

ASHRAE Standards

ASHRAE (The American Society of Heating, Refrigeration, and Air Conditioning Energy) is the U.S. national professional HVAC association. ASHRAE has developed Standard 62.2 for residential buildings and Standard 62.1 for all other multi-purpose residential structures. ASHRAE offers

---

22. https://weigogreener.org/g_bh.php
23. http://www.sbse.org/
24. https://www.inive.org/

on-line training courses on ventilation and HVAC systems, although their emphasis is on commercial buildings.

ASHRAE offers Guideline 24-2015 to assist in implementing the ASHRAE 62.2-2016 Standard. The Guideline also offers extensive amplification of IAQ issues, international thresholds, system design and commissioning. Some of this information is included in the Informative Appendices at the end of the 62.2 Standard. The Standard is in continuous maintenance and ongoing changes and amplifications are made and reflected in Addenda.

Standard 62.2-2025[25] consists of several parts including Purpose, Scope, and Definitions, but the heart of the Standard is the definition of the Dwelling Unit Ventilation system sizing and design, a description of "Local Exhaust" systems, and "Other Requirements" such as "transfer air", system instructions, clothes dryer installation, and garages (among others).

Using the Standard is straightforward:

- Select a Primary or Whole Building Ventilation System that matches the size of the house and the number of bedrooms;
- Run this system continuously (if intermittent operation is preferable, the system has to be more powerful);
- Add local exhaust to the bathrooms and kitchen;
- Make sure that make-up or transfer air is coming directly from the outside and not from polluted sources like garages and crawl spaces;
- Make sure clothes dryers are vented to the outside and that combustion and fuel burning appliances have adequate combustion and ventilation air;
- Make sure the house/garage interface is carefully sealed and that HVAC systems in the garage have little to no leakage;
- Provide a filter for supply ventilation system with a minimum efficiency of MERV 6 and that inlets are at least 10 feet (3 meters) from known contaminant sources and won't be obstructed by snow or plantings;
- Use equipment that has been tested and certified by HVI to HVI 915 for sound (1.0 sone or less for continuously operated fans and

---

25. ASHRAE 62.2 is updated every 3 years.

3.0 sones or less for intermittently operating fans) and HVI 916 for airflow;
- Install the equipment so that it performs correctly.

Ideally, according to 62.2-2025, the dwelling unit ventilation system should run continuously at a relatively low rate, changing all the air in the building. The ventilation rate for this system is defined by the table (ASHRAE 62.2-2025 Table 3.1a and Table 3.1b) or by using the formula described in Chapter 3 of this book. If the system cannot be run continuously, a more powerful fan will have to be used to reach an "equivalent" ventilation rate. For example, if a 50 cfm rate is required, running it half the time would double the flow rate required, i.e. a 100 cfm fan running for thirty minutes each hour.

Standard 62.1 includes a great deal of information on indoor air issues and should be directly referred to for application details.

Standard 119-1988—Air Leakage Performance for Detached Single-Family Residential Buildings is to establish the performance requirements designed to reduce the air infiltration load and classify the air tightness of residential buildings.

Standard 136-1993—A Method of Determining Air Change Rates in Detached Dwellings is for use in evaluating the impact of air change range in detached dwellings on indoor air quality. This Standard has been combined with Standard 62.2.

ASHRAE Standard 241-2023 Control of Infectious Aerosols "establishes minimum requirements for control of infectious aerosols to reduce risk of disease transmission in occupiable space in new buildings, existing buildings, and major renovations to existing buildings including requirements for both outdoor air systems and air cleaning system design, installation, commissioning, operation, and maintenance." This Standard was developed after the Covid-19 pandemic shook up the world.

Ventilation & Health: Healthy Housing Programs

BPI provides a Healthy Housing Principles[26] certification. The BPI HHP

---

26. https://www.bpi.org/certificates/healthy-housing-principles/

certification connects home energy with health professionals. This certification does not require in depth building science training.

BPI also offers Healthy Home Evaluator certification. In order to acquire HHE certification, the candidate must hold a BPI Building Analyst, Energy Auditor, or Quality Control Inspector certification. This is a wonderful blend of physical building science knowledge - how houses work - with medical knowledge to keep the occupants safe and healthy. This training helps to open the eyes of the evaluator who may understand combustion safety or zonal pressure from an energy standpoint and now can connect that knowledge to occupant health and safety.

Healthy and Efficient Homes is a program developed by the American Lung Association (ALA).[27] The ALA program provides a list of healthy air initiatives, support documentation, and extensive guidance on making homes healthier.

Housing and Urban Development's Healthy Homes Program:[28] This program was launched in 1999 to protect children and their families from housing-related health and safety hazards. "The Healthy Homes Program addresses multiple childhood diseases and injuries in the home. The Initiative takes a comprehensive approach to these activities by focusing on housing-related hazards in a coordinated fashion, rather than addressing a single hazard at a time." Ventilation is a component to the program for improvement of indoor air quality, particularly addressing allergens, asthma, carbon monoxide, pesticides, and radon.

Improving Ventilation in Your Home:[29] The Centers for Disease Control (CDC) has a lot of suggestion on improving ventilation in homes. This post-COVID-19 site focuses on reducing virus particles and suggesting preventive actions to help prevent the spread of Covid-19 and other respiratory viruses.

Healthy Housing Solutions was established by the National Center for Healthy Housing in November 2003 to provide federal, state, and local agencies and the private sector organizations with professional services related to residential environmental and safety issues. Healthy Housing Solutions teams up with other organizations, such as the Building Performance Association (National Home Performance Conference) to provide training in such areas

---

27. https://www.lung.org/policy-advocacy/healthy-air-campaign/healthy-efficient-homes
28. http://www.hud.gov/offices/lead/hhi/index.cfm
29. https://www.cdc.gov/coronavirus/2019-ncov/prevent-getting-sick/improving-ventilation-home.html

as lead abatement, ventilation, and mold mitigation. Healthy House Institute (HHI) "provides consumers information to make their homes healthier. HHI strives to be the most comprehensive educational resource available for creating healthier homes."[30] HHI provides extensive information on many aspects of healthy homes (including ventilation) on their site.

---

30. http://www.healthyhouseinstitute.com/

Chapter 14

Fan Types and Applications

There are a lot of different fan designs, each suited to particular applications. Most of them are hidden inside their systems, like the blowers in the bath fan in the ceiling or the motorized impeller in the in-line fan. Some of them are pretty obvious, like the big paddle fan in the ceiling or the oscillating propeller fan, twisting back and forth in the hot summer afternoon air. Fan product designers don't just randomly select a fan design because they like the way it looks. A great deal of engineering thought goes into even the least expensive ventilation product. For a while, residential ventilation products didn't change much. But as homes become tighter and mechanical ventilation becomes a common thread by design and by code, residential ventilation system manufacturers are aggressively competing to produce the quietest and most energy efficient products with the greatest economic value possible. All ventilation fans move air, but some are better at pushing or pulling air through ducts and some are better at gently stirring up the air in a room. Neither would do the other's job well. Selecting the wrong product for the application means that the job won't get done efficiently and may not work at all.

Fan Laws

It is useful to have some familiarity with Fan Laws in designing a ventilation system, as they provide a means for predicting the effects of altered operating conditions. The mechanical efficiency of a fan remains constant throughout its range of operating speeds (revolutions per minute or rpm). The performance of fans and their relationship to the system in which they are installed is governed by the principles of fluid dynamics.

Fan law variables are the fan size, the rotational speed, the density of the gas being moved, the volume of gas being moved, pressure, power (in watts), and the mechanical efficiency. Fan Law 1 describes the effect of changing the fan size, the rotational speed, or the density of the gas on the cubic feet of gas moved, the pressure, and the power. Fan Law 2 describes the effect of changing the fan size, pressure, or density on cubic feet of gas moved, the rotational speed, and the power. Fan Law 3 describes the effect of changing the fan size, volume of gas flow, and gas density on rotational speed, pressure, and power. For all the fan laws, the fans being considered must be aerodynamically similar. The fan laws may also apply to the same fan at different speeds when all the other flow conditions are the same.[1]

Fan Law 1 says that the volume of air moved will vary directly with the change in rotational speed.

Air volume (cfm) varies directly with the speed:

$$CFM_2 = CFM_1 \times \left(\frac{RPM_2}{RPM_1}\right)$$

Formula 14.1 Fan Law Number One

Fan Law 2 says that the system pressure will vary with the square of the change in rotational speed.

$$SP_2 = SP_1 \times \left(\frac{RPM_2}{RPM_1}\right)^2$$

Formula 14.2 Fan Law Number Two

Fan Law 3 says that the power of the system will vary with the cube of the change in rotational speed.

---

1. See ASHRAE Handbook: HVAC Systems and Equipment for the complete Fan Law listing

$$HP_2 = HP_1 \times \left(\frac{RPM_2}{RPM_1}\right)^3$$

So if a 10" diameter fan that was spinning at 1,500 rpm moving 500 cfm at 0.15 iwg and 50 watts had its speed decreased and had a new measured airflow of 400 cfm, its new rpm would be 1,200. The air volume (cfm) varies directly with the fan speed. The resulting pressure would drop to 0.096 since the pressure varies at the square of the fan speed. And the power would drop to 25.6 watts.

Also, the air volume will vary with the cube of the fan diameter. So if the 10" diameter fan blade were replaced by an 8" diameter fan blade of exactly the same design, the flow would drop 256 cfm.

For most residential ventilation applications, the density of the gas and the mechanical efficiency of the system are not variables of great concern. Most installers will rely on the product measurements made by the manufacturer, but it is interesting to understand why manufacturers choose the products they choose for various applications. Understanding what happens to the power consumption when the size of the fan increases or how the rpm can be reduced to quiet the system down helps to analyze and resolve problems.

Axial Fans

The most familiar type of fan is the axial. They are fans we see all the time in windows, on pedestals, oscillating back and forth in hot summer weather. They are used in cooling computers and other electronic products, any place where they don't have to work too hard to move the air in, under, around, or through some resistance. An axial flow fan is a fan the air flows through in an axial direction, from one side directly or straight through to the other side, parallel to the shaft of the fan blade. They consist of a direct drive or belt drive motor, a hub or central "spider", a series of blades, a venturi housing, and a mounting platform for the motor. In residential applications, the belt driven fans are most commonly found in whole house comfort ventilators mounted in the attic floor or as attic exhaust fans.

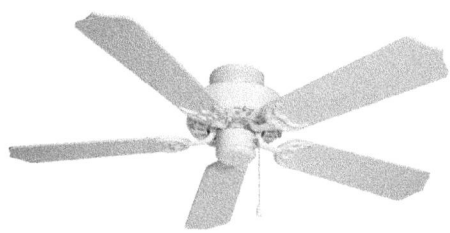

Figure 14.1 Ceiling Mounted Axial Fan (Broan)

The belt drive adds some flexibility to the fan design as the speed of rotation of the fan blade can be varied and high-speed motors are less expensive than slower ones of the same horsepower. They need to have their belts checked as a part of regular maintenance and they are less efficient than direct drive systems since the belt drive consumes 10 to 15 percent of the brake horsepower of the system.

The direct drive approach puts the fan motor directly in the middle of the airstream behind the hub of the blade, where it doesn't restrict the airflow. This makes it a more compact design that is more suitable for restricted space. It also makes it less expensive because there are fewer parts, which also reduces maintenance issues.

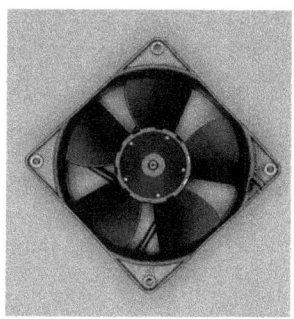

Figure 14.2 Small Axial Fan (Muffin Fan) (EBM-papset)

The efficiency of airflow delivery depends on optimizing all the elements of the fan design. Sound level, for example, can be reduced by using a bigger blade but rotating it more slowly. The pitch and curvature of the blade, the number of blades relative to the number of motor mounting struts, the proximity of the end of the blade to the inside of the venturi all effect efficiency, sound level, and delivered air. Because the end of the rotating blade is where much of the noise is generated, some manufacturers "feather" or notch it.

The optimum design may not be robust enough for a residential application if all the elements of the delivery of the product from the manufacturer to the retailer to the installer are considered. A blade that is perfectly located in the Venturi housing for optimum performance may shift just enough to rub the housing after installation, causing the fan to be discarded.

A propeller fan is the simplest of axial fans commonly used as a panel or box fan in a window or a "man cooler" fan, oscillating back and forth. It is a direct drive arrangement with the motor in the air stream, a number of fairly large blades, and limited components for smoothing or directing the airflow.[2]

A tubeaxial fan is an axial fan in a tube or cylinder. They are known for high airflows at relatively low operating pressures. The efficiency of a tubeaxial fan can be as high as sixty-five percent. The outsides of their housings do not have to be cylindrical. Square tubeaxial fans are the fans found in electronics. Larger tubeaxial fans are used in industrial and commercial applications like paint booths, where they may be subjected to contaminated or corrosive materials.

A vaneaxial fan is a tubeaxial fan with guide vanes to improve the efficiency by straightening and directing the airflow. The vaneaxial design allows for high performance in a minimal space. The efficiency of vaneaxial fans can be as high as seventy-five percent. They are used in applications requiring high-volume airflows at moderate to high pressures.

Axial fans can be installed in a side-by-side configuration to increase the volume of the air that they move or they can be installed in series, one behind the other to increase their strength, their ability to push the air through a duct. In some configurations, in a series arrangement, the blades can be spinning in the same rotational direction and sometimes in opposite directions. When they spin in the same direction, they increase the rotational "twist" of the air through the duct. When they spin in opposing directions, the air stream spin is reversed by the second fan or fan blade and straightened. Stacking the fan blades or mounting them in series on the motor shaft can have somewhat the same strengthening effect, although adjustments have to be made to the fan motor selection to allow the blades to spin at an effective rate.

Centrifugal Fans

Centrifugal fans suck the air into the middle, spin it around, and fling it out centrifugally into the ducting, essentially making the air execute a ninety-degree turn. Small centrifugal fans are the most common design for ceiling mounted bath fans. A large percentage of centrifugal fans allow air to enter on

---

2. Fan Handbook, McGraw-Hill, 1998 by Frank P Bleier provides extensive information on fan design

only one side (a single inlet), which is a typical arrangement in a ceiling mounted bath fan. Some allow air to enter on both sides (double inlet). The motor spins the wheel in a housing that is shaped to collect and guide the air around the perimeter of the wheel and force it out through a duct opening. In most residential ventilation system designs, this housing is called a "scroll". The scroll is carefully shaped to optimize the air pressure of the air, leaving the fan housing and entering the ducting. The velocity of the air at the blade tips is considerably higher than the velocity at the housing outlet. The scroll is a spiral shape governed by a series of proportions, starting with a relatively narrow passage to the wide-open space at the housing outlet. (See the Scroll Housing description in "Fan Handbook".)[3]

Centrifugal fans come in six basic versions:

1. Centrifugal fans with airfoil (AF) blades;
2. Centrifugal fans with backward curved (BC) blades;
3. Centrifugal fans with backward inclined (BI) blades;
4. Centrifugal fans with radial-tip (RT) blades;
5. Centrifugal fans with forward-curved (FC) blades;
6. Centrifugal fans with radial blades (RB).

The first of these, the centrifugal fan with an airfoil blade, has the best mechanical efficiency. Each stubby blade shaped like an airplane's wing is located around an open circle, standing between a flat plate and a curved inlet plate.

For all the centrifugal fans, the air located between the blades and rotating with them is subjected to the centrifugal force. That force has a greater effect on the air movement than the shape of the blades, with the exception of the forward curved blades. Because of the centrifugal effect, centrifugal fans produce more static pressure than axial fans of the same wheel diameter and running speed because the centrifugal effect adds that additional force to the air movement. In the airfoil bladed version, the shape of the blades does not serve as an airfoil since there is no "lift". It is simply a backward curved blade with a blunt leading edge that improves the structural strength of the blade and allows it to move smoothly and quietly through the air. Airfoil blades can be 92% efficient, whereas the typical straight, radial bladed design has an

---

3. Fan Handbook, Blier, page 7.11

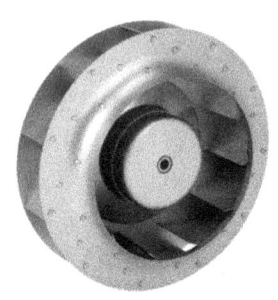

Figure 14.3 *Backward Curved (BC) Motorized Impeller (EBM-papst)*

approximate efficiency of 60%.[4] The other blade designs fall between these two. The fan system designer has to select the fan blade and housing design that best suits the application for efficiency, sound level, cost of manufacture, and ease of assembly and service.

Forward curved blades deliver considerably more air volume and a higher static pressure than airfoil, backward curved, or backward inclined blades but at lower efficiencies. Forward curved blades can run at about half the speed needed for a comparably sized blade, moving the same volume and static pressure. This makes them particularly suitable to the smaller fans in a ventilation system and for cooling electronic equipment where the slower rotational speed will minimize noise and vibration.

The number of blades is governed by compromising between providing a large enough channel to minimize the resistance to the airflow but tight enough to effectively guide the air through the blade and out through the outlet. The passages between the multitude of blades in the forward curved centrifugal fans are relatively narrow. The edges of the blades are the principal cause of turbulence in the fan, and turbulence means noise and inefficient air movement.

The height of the blades is governed by efficiency and available space, and the length of the blade may slightly overlap the leading edge of the following blade. The space between the inlet and the rotating blade should be as small as possible for the best performance. (This is another area where there must be a compromise between fan performance, structural integrity, and product delivery to the installed site. Any shift in a tight clearance will cause the blade to rub on the inlet, which will produce unacceptable noise and product rejection.)

The highest relative air velocity occurs at the leading edge of the fan blade. That is the point of most concern for noise issues. Noise is less of a concern for centrifugal fans than for axial fans because the air entering the centrifugal fan has experienced turbulence, making the ninety-degree turn entering the fan, whereas the axial fan's straight-through configuration intro-

---

4. Fan Handbook, Blier, page 7.2

duces the turbulence inside the fan. Some additional turbulence created by the fan blade tips is therefore less noticeable in a centrifugal fan. These are relative observations, of course. As the fan "noise" in room mounted bath fans drops below 1 or even ½ sone, every sound-generating element becomes critical to the design. The beauty of minimizing the sound is that it includes optimizing the efficiency.

Motorized impellers

The difference between a standard fan motor and a motorized impeller is that, in a standard fan motor, the rotor is internal and doesn't move. In a motorized impeller, the rotor is external, spinning with the fan blade. This means that all the heat from the rotor is dissipated into the air stream, keeping it cooler. Simpler adjustment of the speed of a motorized impeller is possible because of the effective heat dissipation.

Motorized impellers are commonly used in residential ventilation as remote mounted or in-line duct fans. They combine the qualities of tubeaxial fans for pulling air through ducting, the compact efficiency and power of centrifugal blowers, and the unique speed adjusting option of the design. They use backward curved blades to optimize their static pressure capabilities, working against the resistance of ducting and fittings like hoods and grilles. They are the workhorse fans that can be applied to dragging radon-polluted air out from under slabs or operating quietly enough to be used with kitchen range hoods.

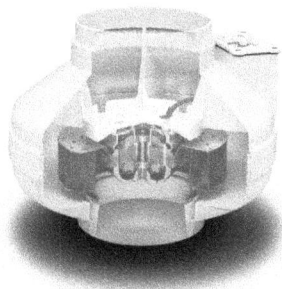

Figure 14.4 Motorized Impeller in an In-Line Fan (Fantech)

Motorized impellers are available with permanent split capacitor (PSC) motors, electronically commutated motors (ECM), or direct current (DC) motors. Both ECM and DC motors are particularly well suited to speed adjustment.

Tangential Blowers

In tangential or "cross-flow" blowers, the air passes through the forward curved blades of the rotating wheel twice, both on the intake and on the exhaust. Tangential blowers are the long, narrow blowers that are commonly used in devices like copiers, mini-split heads, or fireplace inserts where the air enters and exits from the blower through long, narrow slots. They can be made to virtually any width desired. The air is induced to make a ninety to almost a one hundred and eighty degree change in direction. The maximum efficiency of a cross-flow blower is much lower than for a similarly sized, forward curved centrifugal blower because of the air moving twice through the fan wheel and the ensuing rapid changes R403.5of direction.

They produce relatively large volumes of air, but their structural strength is limited, restricting rotational and blade tip speed. And they can be expensive because of manufacturing costs of assembly and balancing.

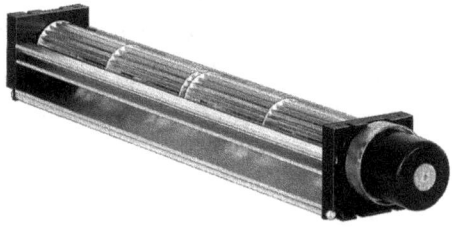

Figure 14.5 Tangential Blower (EBM-papst)

Chapter 15

Special Application Ventilation

The controlled movement of air in a house is not all just for air for the occupants to breathe, and not all air movement in homes happens mechanically. There are areas of particular pollutant concern like garages, the radon gas under the slab, crawl spaces, or attics. Clothes dryers and central vacuums are also ventilation systems, but they have their own, built-in exhaust fans. Balancing the make-up air for these devices is something else you have to be concerned about.

Fireplaces and wood stoves

Fireplaces also serve as exhaust systems. They are particularly difficult to deal with because the flow rate up the chimney changes as the heat of the fire changes. The airflow through the chimney is of particular concern at the beginning and the end of the burning cycle. When the fire first starts, the chimney is cold, leading to a poor draft and sometimes causing the fire to smoke or backdraft. At the end of the fire, the chimney cools and the smoldering embers may not generate enough heat to encourage the combustion gases to flow up the chimney. Those incomplete combustion gases include Carbon Monoxide (CO), which can be deadly. If there are backdrafts at this point in the combustion cycle, the effects can be extremely serious for the health of the occupants.

Fireplace insert manufacturers have come a long way in improving the doors and the combustion chambers, but none of these systems are completely airtight. (Note that many of them will function even without an outside air intake. That can't occur unless there is an air connection to the house.) Fans are available that install on the top of a chimney that can be speed controlled to ensure that air is moving up and out. These systems can be used for single family or multi-family buildings.

Then there is the damper in the flue. The chimney goes all the way up through the house and through the roof. It's a purposeful "stack". (They call them smoke stacks on ships.) Polluted air is supposed to move up through it when there is a fire, but the air doesn't care. It's like a teenager. It does what it wants. It will move up the chimney whenever the pressure conditions push up, whether or not there is a fire burning. Closing the damper helps to block that flow and consequential heat loss. If the damper is directly over the firebox, the chimney is full of cold air, and it's all sitting on top of that damper and that cold air will ooze into the house whenever the pressure in the house is lower than the pressure in the flue. Dampers are not very tight. The average effective leakage area of a closed fireplace damper is 30 square inches.

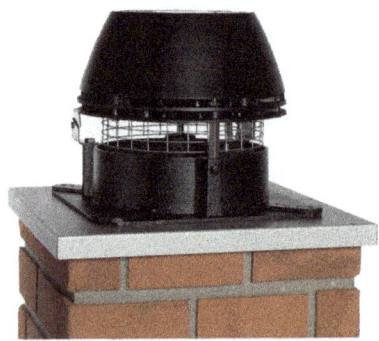

Figure 15.1 Chimney Top Fan (Exhaust)

Dampers are available that mount on the top of the chimney. They close tightly, and they keep the air in the chimney warmer because it is full of house air as opposed to being full of outside air. There are also inserts that can be installed in the fireplace when it is not in use that can be inflated to seal up the opening.

A source of intake air balances out the system during combustion. That air should be ducted from the outside. There should be a means for closing off this "hole" in the house, when the fireplace or stove is not being used. Even though the opening in the house may be in the fireplace or stove, it will still be open to the house. If the house is under negative pressure, air will be sucked in through that pipe from the outside, air that will need to be conditioned.[1] A round exterior opening for a four-inch duct is a 12 ½ square inch hole in the side of the house, letting air in and out, twenty-four hours a day, seven days a week.

Radon ventilation systems

Radon is a naturally occurring gas that can seep into homes and cause cancer. According to the Environmental Protection Agency (EPA), "Radon is the leading cause of lung cancer among non-smokers. It is the second leading cause of lung cancer in America and claims about 20,000 lives annually."[2] Homes should be tested for radon. It appears to be indiscriminate in terms of location. Just because none of the other homes in the neighborhood have a radon issue, it doesn't mean that your home doesn't. Testing should also take place over a period of time rather than a quick "snapshot". If the test is short term—only a day or so — the house may be under positive pressure and the radon gas will be kept out. There are many sources of information and products and services for testing for radon.[3]

- National Radon Proficiency Program[4] certifies radon professionals.
- National Radon Safety Board[5] is a formal recognition of radon professional excellence.
- AARST–Indoor Environments Association[6] is a professional nonprofit organization dedicated to hazard identification and abatement of radon.
- Kansas State University[7] Radon program offers on-line and in-person radon courses.

---

1. www.hoyme.com
2. www.epa.gov/radon/
3. www.radon.com
4. https://nrpp.info/certification/types-of-certification/
5. https://nrsb.org/
6. https://aarst.org/
7. https://radoncourses.com/

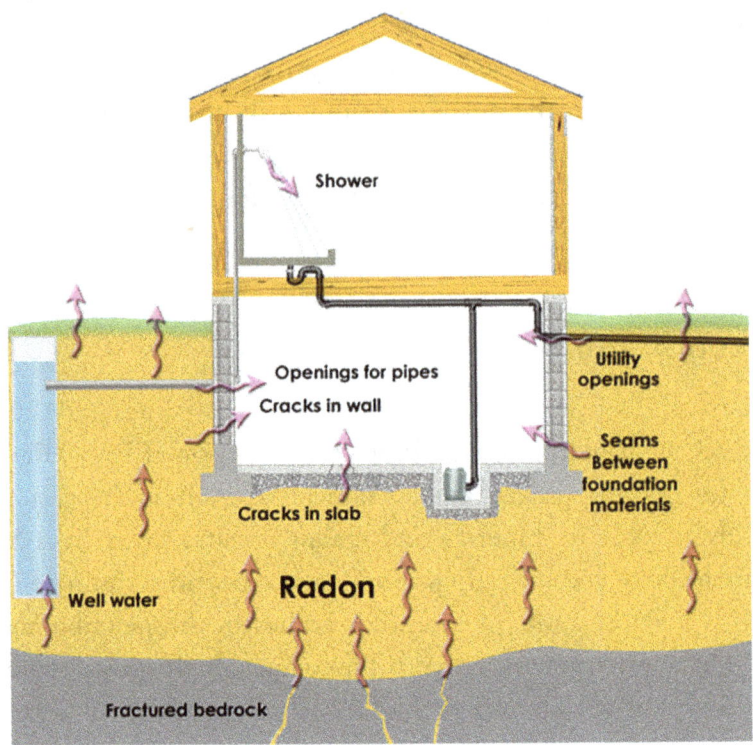

Figure 15.2 Radon Sources (Panasonic/Morrissey)

No level of radon is safe. The EPA lists 4 picocuries per liter (pCi/L) as an action level. The levels will be different in different levels in the home, but since most radon gas enters the home from the ground, it is best to test in the lowest level where people spend time. But since radon enters the home as a gas, it will move around, flowing up from the basement through interstitial spaces like interior wall cavities.

The goal is to provide a means for the gas to by-pass the living areas of the house. Think of it like a lightning rod in reverse. Lightning strikes the rod and is conducted around the house through a wire to the ground where it dissipates. A radon mitigation system sucks the air out of the ground and ducts it up and out into the atmosphere.

Different states have different radon construction codes. Sometimes information is available through the local Department of Public Health. There is a great deal of information about radon issues at the EPA website: www.epa.gov/radon.

If the house is under construction, there are radon resistant construction techniques that will help to air seal the foundation from a ground connection and that form an air chamber under the slab of the house that is connected to a pipe that runs all the way up through the house and through the roof. By "dumping" the polluted air out through the roof, it is less likely to flow back in through open windows or other inlets. An in-line fan that can run continuously and strong enough to suck the air out from under the slab can be added to the duct. The system should also include a "fan-proving" indicator that clearly alerts the occupants if the fan system fails. This is usually a simple and inexpensive 'U' tube manometer with a tap into the ducting that monitors the pressures on either side of the fan. Also note that since the radon stack pipe is likely to look like a standard plumbing pipe, it must be clearly labelled so that it is not mis-purposed.

In an existing house, sub-slab depressurization can still be achieved. A channel can be formed around the perimeter of the basement if there is a gap between the slab and the basement walls. That channel can then be connected to the pipe that runs out through the roof. If there is a sump pump, the sump can be capped and air from the chamber can be tapped into the radon riser pipe. Some existing homes have drain tiles or perforated pipe that directs water away from the house. Suction from these tiles can be effective in reducing the radon gas that gets into the home.

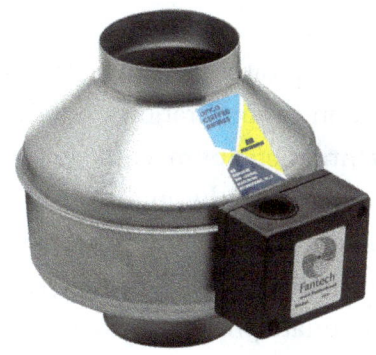

Figure 15.3 In-line Fan for Radon Mitigation.

If the house has a crawlspace instead of a basement, the ground or floor of the crawl space can be carefully covered and sealed with a high-density plastic sheet. (This will also keep the humidity down in the space.) The air under the sheet can then be attached to the vent pipe and fan, providing "sub-membrane suction".

It is best if the piping and fan system not be installed in and through the house since any air leaks in the piping will allow radon gas to leak back into the living spaces. The piping should be run outside of the house. This simplifies finding a continuous path from the basement or crawl space all the way up through the roof. The fan that is selected must be suitable for installation in ambient conditions. The fan also must be quiet and not near a window since it will run continuously.

There is a great deal of discussion of the best way to handle the air in a crawl space. Many building scientists feel strongly that a crawl space should be sealed and insulated. But many building codes require that they be vented. All the issues of pipes and ducts and mechanical equipment in the crawl space must be considered for either approach. Power venting the crawl space to the outside for radon can effectively remove the radon gas before it migrates up into the house. However, putting the crawl space under negative pressure may suck more radon gas into the space. Balancing the increase in gas with a flow rate to the outside is difficult at best. If there is mechanical equipment and ductwork in the crawlspace, it is advisable to carefully seal the space up, and use a sub-slab or sub-membrane system to vent all the way out through the roof.

A positive pressure ventilation approach in the house may protect it from radon gas infiltration from the crawl space or basement. But as is true with all ventilation approaches, it is best to try to effectively remove the pollutant at its source, like the moisture in a bathroom or the cooking smoke over a stove. There are so many variations forces in pressure in and on the house that it is virtually impossible to guarantee that the living space will always be under adequate pressure to keep the radon gases where you want them to be.

If a radon mitigation system is installed, it must be clearly marked. Once again, this is going to be one of those systems that runs all the time with no operator involvement. The "out-of-sight, out-of-mind" syndrome applies. The homeowner will not be interacting with the system at all. Even if there is an alert system on the fan, it needs to be clearly marked as to what it is and what a warning means. If the alert light or buzzer is behind a stack of boxes full of old clothes in a corner of the basement, the homeowner will never know what it is or why it is buzzing (if they can hear it). If they don't know why it is important to do something about it, they will probably just defeat it entirely.

Ideally, maintenance on the radon system should be on the list of other regular maintenance procedures. There is no filter to replace. It essentially consists of making sure that the fan is still running and that the alert system is connected.

> The EPA site refers to using an HRV as an approach to radon reduction. All the ventilation approaches discussed in this book, including HRVs and ERVs,

will dilute the pollutants in the home, including radon gases. But the dwelling unit ventilation systems for improving the general air quality in the house are not directly coupled to the radon gas source. As such, an HRV or ERV will remove the smoke from the hearth fire if the chimney was eliminated, but it wouldn't be as effective! Radon is a serious health risk and radon gas should be vented directly with an independent system. See the radon section in Chapter 18.

Installed cost and operating cost will vary by the location and the system and by the house. The electrical cost of running the fan continuously is small. Most of the in-line fans consume less than 50 watts, many less than 20 watts. Some systems will take air from the house, which will need to be replaced with conditioned air, but the flow rates are extremely small. Total operating costs of $50 to $200 per year are pretty inconsequential if it reduces the risk of cancer.

Crawl Space Ventilation

Codes require crawlspaces to be ventilated under most conditions. It would seem illogical to bring warm, humid air into a cold, dark crawlspace and not expect there to be condensation and mold problems. Techniques have been developed and approved for sealing or encapsulating crawl spaces, making them a part of the living space, serving as a very short "basement". Many homes have their ducting and other mechanical equipment in the crawl, which requires careful attention to combustion air.

Codes allow crawl spaces to employ mechanical ventilation in place of simple passive vents. Replacing passive crawl space vents with mechanical ventilation that draws air from the house and vents the crawl space air to the outside can reduce moisture problems and increase energy efficiency, but attention must be paid to the design of the system.

The International Residential Code § R408.3 (see Chapter 12) specifically allows an unvented crawlspace design with mechanical exhaust. To comply, the crawl space must have a continuously sealed, vapor retarding ground cover, have no passive openings to the outside, and employ a continuously operating exhaust fan. For the code minimum, mechanical ventilation must be provided at a rate of 1.0 cfm per 50 square feet of under floor space. The code does not specify what sort of fans should be used, but Colorado amended the IRC to require a fan rated for 44,000 hours (5 years) of continuous operation with flex connections to reduce any fan vibration and resulting noise. There must also be some sort of indicator to alert the occupants if the fan should fail.

The system must also include transfer air openings, one per 250 square feet of crawlspace floor area that are installed in the decking between the crawlspace and the conditioned rooms above. To meet the Colorado Code (and a practical guide for other locations), the transfer air openings should comply with the following table:

Amount of Air required	Minimum Hole Size square inches	Maximum Hole Size square inches
0 – 10 cfm	1.5	2.4
11 – 15 cfm	2.4	3.6
16 – 20 cfm	3.6	4.4

Table 15.1 Sizing Crawlspace Transfer Air Openings

The crawlspace exhaust fan airflow (typically 30 to 60 cfm) would be divided by the required number of openings to determine the flow per hole. The fan will exert a slight negative pressure on the house above. If there is an atmospherically vented appliance in the crawl space, the openings should be large enough so that the appliance will never experience a negative pressure condition of over 2 Pascals (and the installation MUST be in accordance with all local codes for atmospherically vented appliances).

Passive Ventilation

Passive ventilation is ventilation without the benefit of a mechanical device like a fan. Opening the windows is passive ventilation when the air moves through them. Using windows for ventilation requires the right ambient conditions on both sides of the window, creating the pressure differentials that will force the air through the opening.

Passive inlets work with exhaust only or supply only ventilation systems to balance them out. There are passive inlet devices that have been dubbed "smart holes" that purposefully let air in more predictably. These devices have been described in Chapter 8.

Natural or passive ventilation strategies have been around since they put a hole in the house's roof to let the smoke out. It was logical to take advantage of the stack effect or cross ventilation to get the pollutants out of the building. Central courtyards with fountains, so-called airshafts between city buildings, "solar chimneys", and building shapes have all taken advantage of prevailing natural conditions to passively compel air to move through buildings. To get passive or natural ventilation to work, it must be incorporated into the design of the building—the true house as a system approach. From that standpoint, considering a natural ventilation approach will enhance the overall building design and prevent it from working against itself. It is more difficult to design aggressive natural ventilation strategies into a traditionally designed home than it is to add a glass-enclosed stairwell or solar chimneys or ventilation stacks into a commercial or industrial building.

There can be a thermal penalty for adding natural ventilation to a residence. Adding a space like a sunroom on the south side of the house can provide an "engine" to drive air circulation, but it will add heat at the same time. Strong temperature differentials can generate strong airflows, but it is not just for fresh air ventilation.

Early passive ventilation systems relied heavily on heat to provide the necessary buoyancy forces necessary to drive the airflow.[8] Natural or stack ventilation systems are extremely common in the United Kingdom, Northern European countries and Canada although U.S. homes are built to generally lower tightness levels than homes in the other areas except for the U.K. This unintentional passive ventilation is known more commonly as infiltration and exfiltration. The potential advantage of passive ventilation is that using natural forces could avoid the energy that is required for mechanical ventilation. The challenge is achieving an adequate level of control in all seasons while avoiding the multitude of issues of dust and moisture, occupant intervention, potential drafts, and loss of conditioned air.

The European Building Research Establishment (BRE) has assumed the lead role in developing and promoting Passive Stack Ventilation (PSV) systems. Their best practices system is concerned (as we are) with removing the pollutants at their primary sources in the home—bathrooms and kitchens. The systems consist of fresh air inlets and an exhaust stack that runs up

---

8. Axley, "Residential Passive Ventilation Systems: Evaluation and Design", AIVC, 2001 https://www.aivc.org/sites/default/files/members_area/medias/pdf/Technotes/TN54%20RESIDENTIAL%20PASSIVE%20VENTILATION.pdf

through the roof with circulation openings in doorways or interior walls (Chapter 8).

According to the Axley article[9], the BRE best practices PSV system includes:

- A service room inlet vent with a free area opening of 6.2 square inches (4,000 square mm), intended to provide a low, continuous flow of inlet air, essentially a "trickle" ventilator;
- An outlet ventilator placed in the ceiling plane or high on the wall above the primary moisture source having a free area equal to or greater than the stack cross sectional area;
- A ventilation stack duct, 5 inches (125 mm) in diameter for kitchens and 4 inches (100 mm) for bathrooms that conducts the air from the space all the way up to above the roof line;
- A stack terminal fitting that allows the air to flow out, maintains suction pressure, and prevents the infiltration of rain, insects, animals, and leaves and other debris.

Control and adjustment of the system have been traditionally left to the occupant through the use of adjustable louvers, but because the driving forces are in constant flux, this requires frequent if not continuous intervention and awareness by the house's occupants. Passive inlet devices are available that automatically respond to pressure or humidity, or both, restricting the amount of incoming air to a prescribed level. These can make the PSV system far less dependent on occupant intervention.

On average, these systems have been shown to work effectively. Moment to moment ventilation requirements, however, are not well served. A sudden smoky event in a kitchen will be more quickly removed through the use of a local, well-designed and installed kitchen exhaust fan. People don't live in homes on an "average" basis. They live there all year 'round, in various conditions. But thinking again on a whole systems basis, a carefully designed combination of passive and active ventilation systems, a hybrid system, may satisfy both average and immediate condition. PSV systems can be designed and installed to meet the constant, low flow, background ventilation requirements of ASHRAE 62.2, although PSV rates will never be truly constant as wind

---

9. Axley, page 8

and changing house pressures drive them. They demand effectively addressing air circulation throughout the building, which has been a key element in diluting pollutants. And they are particularly suited to tighter homes, as they provide controlled rather than random "leakage".

North American building codes have no specific provisions for passive ventilation systems beyond minimal window opening regulations for rooms that are not required to be mechanically ventilated. Because passive ventilation systems rely on pressures to function correctly, they will interact with other pressure reliant systems like fireplaces and atmospherically vented water heaters, boilers, and furnaces. Implementation of passive ventilation strategies needs to consider possible interactions including code provisions that define the location on the lot, light, and ventilation, dwelling unit separation, protection against radon, wall constructions, chimneys, and fireplaces, mechanical exhaust systems, combustion air for chimneys and vents, and plumbing vents and traps.

Passive ventilation systems could be a useful tool in whole house systems integration, a means to cut one more piece out of the home's energy load. But without careful forethought and design, they are "delicate" systems in that they must be more carefully balanced than a mechanical ventilation approach. For example, when a thermostat turns on a heating system, the temperature and the amount of air delivered to the house is a known entity (all the maintenance issues set aside). As far as the thermostat is concerned, the air delivered to the house will warm the house. Working with an alternative source of energy, such as solar heat, the amount of energy is variable—it might be hot, it might be warm, or it might be cool. The driving forces in a passive ventilation system depend on the weather and on the occupants, variables that make it difficult to maintain control of the flow.

Testing, verifying, and balancing the performance of passive ventilation systems on an average basis is virtually impossible, as the flows are constantly changing. The occupants have to be well informed about the operation of the system and able to pass that information along to the next occupant of the home.[10]

---

10. William Paton Buchan wrote a ventilation text book in 1891 call Ventilation: *A Text-book To The Art of Ventilating Buildings* that was entirely passive ventilation. It describes some unique approaches to solve ventilation problems before the advent of electric fans. https://www.google.com/books/edition/Ventilation/wfwJAAAAIAAJ?hl=en&gbpv=1&printsec=frontcover

Garage Ventilation

Attached garages are effectively just another room on the house where we put all the stuff that we don't want in the house. If it is included in the house's structure and seems to be outside the living space, unless careful steps are taken, what's in the air in the garage will be in the air in the house. There isn't much difference between the average garage and those big glass doors that they open in automotive showrooms to drive the new cars in. Garages are commonly located beside and underneath homes. There are rooms over them and, often these days, rooms under them. As houses have gotten bigger, garages have gotten bigger. They have room for more cars and sometimes boats. Mechanical equipment is located there—furnaces, boilers, air handlers. Ducting runs through them with all their associated gaps and leaks and pressure issues.

If the garage is not attached to the house, ventilation issues center on maintaining conditions in the garage for any activities that are pursued there. If, for example, there is a workshop in a detached garage, keeping it cool and keeping the air fresh by venting the fumes from a hobby or from the cars is a good idea. Any cooling system should be vented directly to the outside and not into an attic area, and it must not overpower any combustion device in the garage. A means must be provided for supply air. The same is true for any "spot" venting system to remove the fumes over a workbench, for example.

To work on vehicles in the garage, careful consideration of venting exhaust fumes and providing make-up air must be made for the health of the garage occupants. These measures may be as simple as an exhaust fan or as complex as a commercial exhaust fume ventilation system. As in other buildings, consideration of the interaction of other ventilation/exhaust system should be kept in mind. If there is a dust collector, for example, it will draw air out of the garage, working against a garage exhaust fan.

Attached garages are far more of a problem because they are ... attached. Building components join the garage to the living spaces in the house. Wall and ceiling cavities conduct air just as they do in other parts of the house. Moving air carries pollutants, and the garage is a haven for pollutants that are not good for human health. Ninety-three percent of the one million houses built in the United States in 2003 had one-, two-, or three-car garages.[11]

---

11. U.S. Bureau of the Census

Multiple studies and tests have been done in both the U.S. and Canada to determine the extent of carbon monoxide and benzene transfer into the house and determined that the pattern of carbon monoxide in the house mimicked the pattern in the garage.

> Note that the 2021 International Mechanical Code (IMC) includes a provision for in Table 403.3 for 0.75 cfm per 100 square feet in residential garage applications. "Mechanical exhaust required and the recirculation of air from such spaces is prohibited." IMC Table 403.3.

Responding to many CO alarms, fire departments often have a difficult time determining the source of the CO and blame faulty detectors or the furnace because it's the most obvious combustion source. CO infiltrating from the garage is a slow process, commonly taking an hour or more with a low pressure differential between the two spaces. An elevated level in the garage can continue for four to six hours after the car has been removed. (Note that UL 2034 approved CO alarms may not alarm if the CO level exceeds 70 ppm continuously for an hour but must alarm at that level before four hours have passed.) When a car is started in the garage, the engine is cold and it produces a huge amount of carbon monoxide, as much as 80,000 parts per million (ppm). Even if the garage door is open, the garage can fill with deadly CO within two minutes. The car should not be allowed to run for any length of time in the garage, even with the door open.

Go back to the pressure discussions in Chapter 7. When the house is heated, a hole at the lowest point will allow the most air in. A hole near the top of the house will let the most air out. (This naturally depends on wind loading, temperatures, etc.) A garage door is a very large hole, and it is always located close to the ground. Unfortunately, it is difficult to locate the garage entrance near the middle of the building! Homes and garages that are leaky have less of a problem with CO because of their elevated air change rates. (They also have a higher energy cost.) CO is slightly lighter than air and moves easily throughout the house, but it will not attach itself to surfaces in the garage and a complete air change will remove all the CO.[12]

Mild CO poisoning feels like the flu. More serious CO poisoning can lead

---

12. For a free CO modeling tool, go to https://energytools.com/ Select Garage to House Pollutant Transfer Model

to breathing difficulties, lack of reasoning and death. It is likely to have the most serious effects on the young, the sick, and the elderly.

Before adding any sort of mechanical exhaust to an attached garage, the building system should be carefully analyzed. If the pressure in the garage is higher than the pressure in the house, air will flow toward the house carrying all the garage pollutants with it. Different configurations will require different ventilation approaches.

- What part (if any) of the mechanical systems for the house is located in the garage? Is the air handler in the garage? Are there duct runs beyond the basic connections to the air handler?
- Is there a gas fired water heater in the garage? Is it a sealed-combustion system?
- Are there rooms above the garage? Below?
- Is there a stairway that leads to a basement door?
- How much of the house's infiltration comes from the garage? Sealing all the openings between the house and the garage will eliminate or significantly reduce that infiltration. (It is common for 25% of the total house leakage to come through the garage.)[13] That may impact the ventilation and combustion appliances in the house.
- Consider the climate. (A garage in a cold climate may suffer from excessive condensation in the winter when a wet car is driven into the garage. In a hot climate, overheating may be a more important issue.)

The goal of any approach to improving the garage/house connection is to remove the garage from the house. This is difficult to do with an existing house, unless the garage can be converted to another room and a new garage built away from the house. This may not be an acceptable option because homeowners like the ability to walk from the garage to the house without going out in the inclement weather. So the next best step is to do everything possible to seal the connections between the house and garage (the House/Garage Interface) with the goal of disconnecting the air connection of the two but leaving them physically attached. Because some gases will move

---

13. Wilber & Klossner, 1997 "A Study of undiagnosed carbon monoxide complaints"

by diffusion through some building materials (like block), it will be almost impossible to eliminate all the transfer, but if it can be significantly reduced, the rest can be vented more easily.

Every crack, gap, or hole between the house and garage must be sealed. Be merciless! Seal them up and get the house tested with a blower door. You could even get one of those theatrical smoke generators that they sell at Halloween and fill the garage with smoke and see where it goes. (Be sure to alert your neighbors first in case they think your house is on fire when smoke pours out of soffits and the chimney and other unexpected places.) The primary leakage spots include:

- Basement headers;
- Pipe penetrations from the basement into the garage;
- Forced air heating supply duct chases in common walls;
- Plumbing penetrations in walls of laundry rooms or powder rooms next to the garage;
- A lowered ceiling abutting the house/garage common wall;
- Cold air returns passing through stud spaces in the common walls;
- Un-taped or damaged drywall joints on the garage side of the common walls;
- Pocket doors in the partition abutting house/garage common walls.[14]

It is difficult to find the leaks without a blower door or other specialized equipment, but the following symptoms may show that there is a problem that needs to be addressed:

- The carbon monoxide alarms in the house go off frequently when the car is started;
- Exhaust fumes are noticeable in the house and cause headaches or general, noxious smells (Note that CO has no odor);
- Cold drafts are felt in spaces adjacent to the house/garage common walls;
- The floors in the living space over the garage are commonly cold.

---

14. CMHC, Garage Performance Testing, The Sheltair Group, 2004, page 26

If there is combustion equipment in the garage, make sure that it has adequate combustion air. Newer, more efficient furnaces and boilers send less waste products up their flues, creating a low stack pressure. It is ironic that more efficient combustion equipment is more susceptible to backdrafting simply because of their efficiency. Even more care has to be taken in not overpowering these devices with competing exhaust equipment.

If the air handler fan is used for ventilation or continuous air circulation, sealing the house/garage interface may have little effect. The air handler fan can significantly reduce the pressure in the HVAC system if it will suck in and circulate any of the pollutants that are in the garage.

Passive, through wall vents between the garage and the outside will reduce the pollutants in the garage because they make the garage "leakier", but like other passive inlets and outlets, they don't always work in the desired direction, and they can't be controlled to work when there is a pollutant level in the garage. If they are located high in the wall, they are more likely to serve as outlets than inlets. The passive vent approach works better if the house is tight and the house/garage common walls are sealed.

Finally, an exhaust fan can be an effective solution, bearing in mind the issues of combustion air, etc. The question is how big should the fan be? It partially depends on the tightness of the garage. Very tight garages can be effectively ventilated with very small fans (as low as 10 cfm) running almost continuously. In most garages, 50 cfm is about as small as the airflow can be to have any impact. 100 cfm per car is working its way into local building codes. (Note that is a fully delivered, installed measurement, not 100 cfm marking on the box.)

The size of the fan depends also on how it is controlled. If the purpose is to remove the high level of CO that is generated when a cold car is started in the garage, activating the fan when the garage door opens is a reasonable control strategy. The fan should continue to run for at least 30 minutes after the door closes.

A CO control can activate the fan whenever the carbon monoxide exceeds the set point, whether the car is in the garage and running or has been removed and the CO is lingering in the air. It will also activate the exhaust fan if there is an elevated CO level from a barbecue grille or generator (as long as there's power!) or leaf blower. It's not always just CO that is a problem with the air in the garage, however.

A differential pressure control can sense the pressure difference between the house and the garage and activate the exhaust fan to keep the garage at a lower pressure than the house. In that condition, the pollutants can be kept out of the house, essentially flowing "downhill" from the garage to the outside.

Moisture is also a problem in a tight garage, particularly in a cold climate. Pulling a car or truck covered with snow into a garage that is above freezing will bring a great deal of moisture into the space. That moisture can cause the windows to fog and mold to grow.

Because of all these conditions, a continuously operating, low power fan in the garage is worth considering. If the fan is only drawing 20 watts, at $0.13 per kilowatt hour, it would cost less than $25 per year to operate the fan continuously. There isn't a conditioning penalty as there is for household air. This is another of those continuously running fans like the radon mitigation system that is definitely worth its operating cost.

Displacement Ventilation

Displacement ventilation is a strategy for introducing ventilation air near the floor, ideally at a temperature that is lower than the air in the room and allowing it to rise to the ceiling where it is exhausted. The room is purposefully stratified, the warmer air "sitting" on the cooler, denser air providing cooler, fresh air into the area where people sit and work. Stale air polluted with carbon dioxide (CO_2) is pushed up to the ceiling.

This ventilation strategy can work effectively in school classrooms or office spaces. Stale air is not recirculated. 100% outdoor air can be supplied. Cooling capacity can be reduced because of the thermal stratification. Often, less fan horsepower is needed and there is less room noise because the air velocity is so low.

Some applications for displacement cooling in residential applications have been tested and found to reduce cooling loads. Introducing conditioning air of any type near the floor in a house, however, risks having furniture put in front of it, blocking the flow. If the vents are in the floor, things cover them, stuff falls in them. The volume of air moving into and out of the room requires relatively large ducting, raising installation costs and requiring a sacrifice of space. There may be proven benefits in the future for residential applications if ventilation is combined with other conditioning functions.

Chapter 16

Ventilation for Cooling

There was a time not that long ago that "ventilation" in the common vernacular meant a cool breeze wafting through the house, or simply a way to disperse the warm and stuffy air in the room. Home occupants smell some pollutants, but they certainly feel overheated air. And while the nose gets acclimatized to smells, the body doesn't stop feeling the heat. More and more homes in all climates are installing central air conditioning. That technology has allowed us to move into areas that were previously considered uninhabitable for much of the year. As long as there is a temperature difference between the inside and the outside of the house, ventilation can cool down the house and cool down the people. It can get rid of excess heat in the attic.

There is some controversy about ventilation that is used for cooling, particularly if we start at the top of the house. Is it necessary to remove the heat from the attic? Does it accomplish anything in terms of the cooling load? Should the same rules to cooling the attic be applied in all climates? Attics are one of those simple spaces that have become complicated, like garages and crawl spaces. Before tight building materials and high levels of insulation, the attic was just an empty space at the top of the house. If life got crowded, one kid moved up

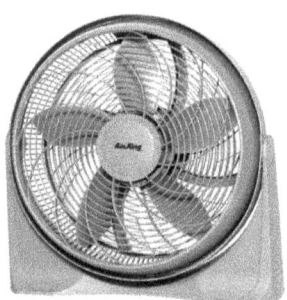

Figure 16.1 Room Fan (Air King)

there. Ice dams and humidity are attic issues, but they are not directly "cooling" issues, which is what this chapter is about. But when considering an attic, air motion for cooling is also air motion for removing moisture.

Attic ventilation has two distinct purposes: 1. Controlling the temperature of the roof primarily for ice dams and roofing material manufacturer requirements, (the passive ridge and soffit ventilation system) and 2. Cooling the attic for stuff stored there and reducing the temperature of the blanket of air that sits at the top of the house (powered attic ventilators (PAV) or attic fan and passive gable vent systems). These are two different systems with two distinct purposes.

Ridge and Soffit Vents

Soffits are the underside of the overhangs at the bottom of the roof. The ridge is the top or peak of the roof. The object of the combination of these two vents is to allow air to enter at a low point and flow passively to the high point, allowing the roof deck to be at the same temperature from the bottom to the top. For it to work effectively, the path for entry and exit must be clear. If insulation or other attic detritus is jammed down on top of the soffit vents, the airflow path will be blocked. Since the point is for air to blow through the soffit vents, loose insulation piled there will be blown back. This is known as "wind washing". Air moving through insulation significantly reduces its ability to prevent conductive heat loss. At the ridge, often the roof has not been cut open and there is no way for the air to leave.

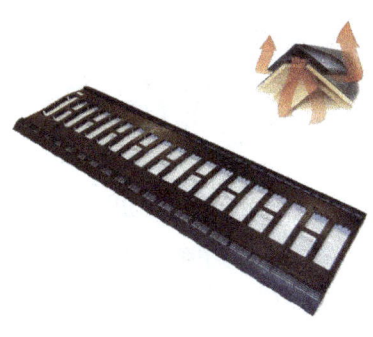

Figure 16.2 Ridge Vent Insert (Heartland Industries

It is difficult to know what the ridge or soffit vent can do as a product. Its performance will change as the pressures change. How much air should be able to move through it if the conditions are right? How much of an opening does it provide? Product manufacturers calculate the area of the openings and arrive at what they call the Net Free Area (NFA). That doesn't provide the whole picture. The configuration of the product will affect its flow resistance, as it does with fans or grilles. The best way to determine the ability of the product to allow air to flow through it is to measure the flow of air through the product!

The Home Ventilating Institute (HVI) has a procedure for testing what they call "Static Vents"[1]. A test stand is set up that imitates how the product will be installed on the roof. Air is pushed or drawn through the product at four separate static pressures. The rate of flow is plugged into the equation:

$$NFA = (0.0592 \times Q) / \sqrt{\Delta P}$$

Formula 16.1 Net Free Area

NFA is the effective net free area.

Q is the airflow in cfm.

ΔP is the difference in pressure (in this case the static pressure measurement point at standard atmospheric density).

Manufacturers of HVI Certified products can put their products through this procedure to provide an accurate indication of the effective Net Free Area. This is what should be stamped on the product and used to determine the adequacy of meeting the 1:300 attic ventilation standards for attics with a vapor diffusion retarder separating them from the living space. Tests have been established by the International Conference of Building Officials (ICBO) and the University of Illinois and HVI to determine what they call an Equivalent Net Free Area or ENFA. But the protocols are different and the manufacturers aren't willing to promote the resulting lower performance number, so unfortunately consumers are stuck with what in many cases is erroneous performance data.

In terms of temperature change, what effect does the ridge/soffit venting approach have? There is about a 30°F difference in attic temperature between an attic with no vent cap—just shingled over—and an open ridge vent slot (not a real world, practical approach because of weather issues!)

Attic ventilation was added to building codes to prevent roof damage

---

[1]. There is no code requirement for HVI Certified static vents. As of this writing, there are no static vent products listed in the HVI Product Directory.

caused by moisture laden air migrating from the living space during the winter when that warm moist air hits cold surfaces, condenses, freezes, and causes mold problems. The change was implemented after the introduction of indoor plumbing and central heating systems. With the introduction of increased attic insulation, ventilation proved valuable in preventing ice dams. If the entire roof deck can be kept at the same temperature, snow will melt off it uniformly and not cause a problem. But if the edges of the roof, hanging out beyond the attic area, are colder than the middle, the snow melt will freeze there and form a dam, pushing the water up under the roof shingles. Keeping a flow of air moving up the underside of the roof sheathing will keep it at close to a uniform temperature.

As with many technologies, layered in tradition, eventually these original purposes were forgotten, particularly in cooling climates where ice dams are not an issue. The thought was that attic venting could lower the attic temperature, which would reduce the cost of cooling and prolong shingle life even though there was no research to support those concepts. Adding an active cooling system or fan was assumed to amplify the effect, but field testing has shown that the "temperature of roof sheathing of an unvented roof will rise by a few to no more than 10F more than a well-ventilated attic."[2] Despite this, shingle manufacturers insist on the vented deck design and most codes require it.

If the deck is to be ventilated, there should be a minimum 2" clearance between the bottom of the deck and any insulation or other air blocking materials. This will effectively allow for a 2" x 22.5" "duct" in each cavity (if the rafters are 24 inches on-center), "open" at the bottom and top, forming an effective solar chimney, passively venting each cavity. Baffles must be used to prevent "wind washing" of the insulation at the eaves, which reduces the thermal resistance of the insulation. Choose your soffit and ridge vents carefully, looking for HVI Certification. Compare the actual openings in soffit vents. Visually, you can often tell if one is more open than the other, despite the claims. Neither may be accurate, but a visual inspection can provide logical clues. The more open it is, the easier it will be for the air to flow through it. So called "button-louvers" are almost impossibly restrictive to the airflow.

---

2. "Understanding Attic Ventilation", Joseph Lstiburek, Building Science Digest 102, 2006 https://buildingscience.com/documents/digests/bsd-102-understanding-attic-ventilation

Some ridge vents include baffles to prevent the air from blowing through from one side to the other. Winds and breezes will drive the air up the outside of the roof and over the ridge, creating positive pressure on the side facing the wind (the windward side) and negative pressure on the opposite side (the leeward side). By adding the baffles, more air may be forced over the top, creating more negative pressure, and sucking more air out of the attic. Although this may have some effect on performance, the clear openings are the most important performance factor.

Attic Fans (Powered Attic Ventilators)

If passive vents work so well, why not add some mechanical assistance and put fans in? Once again, a simple and logical ventilation approach is not as simple as it appears. There are many articles about why it is so important to use power attic ventilators (PAVs) or attic exhaust fans. Companies that make PAV products have produced most of these, but they can't all be discounted. Manufacturers get a lot of feedback about their products—both good and bad. How much they listen is another question.

There is no doubt that attics get hot. Ridge and soffit vents are not there to significantly reduce the temperature in the attic. If it is important to reduce the attic air temperature, something more is needed.

If the attic is completely sealed off from the house, then the problem is limited to the attic, and adding more airflow will affect only the attic. But in most homes, the top floor ceiling plane is not well sealed. There are a myriad of holes from recessed lights, wiring boxes, wall stacks, plumbing stacks, chimneys, etc. Lowering the pressure in the attic with an attic exhaust fan will draw air from the house up into the attic. If the fan is powerful enough and the house is closed up, that could depressurize the house enough to back-draft combustion appliances or draw radon or soil gas in from the crawl space. This is just another of those "house-as-a-system" issues that you have to think about. Air sealing the ceiling plane solves a lot of problems in both warm and cool weather. Keeping the mechanical equipment out of the attic solves another pile of issues like servicing and limiting duct leakage to the outdoors.

Another air conflict may arise between the passive ridge/soffit system and a powered attic ventilator. The PAV will draw its balancing air from the closest place, which may be the ridge or soffit vent, short-circuiting the path up the underside of the roofing material. Adding any PAV requires adding an adequate, intentional source of balancing air. (Remember: one cfm in equals one cfm out.) HVI recommends 1 square foot for each 300 cfm of airflow. Remember that these are "clear" openings to the outside. Weather louvers will reduce the opening size because they block some of the opening area. Insect screens will severely reduce the openings, so the overall hole size will have to be bigger than these numbers.

Exhaust airflow cfm	Inlet area in square feet
300	1
600	2
1200	4
1650	5.5
3000	10
3900	13

Table 16.1 Exhaust Fan Inlet Hole Sizes

The tighter, better sealed the attic space relative to the outside, the larger the hole needs to be to balance the airflow exhausting through the PAV. PAVs are generally axial fans and don't work well against back-pressure or flow resistance. Most of them will operate at about half the flow rate printed on the box once they have been installed because of the added resistances of grilles, louvers, and inlet openings.

In terms of the effect of the cost of cooling the air in the house, reducing the attic air temperature has only a small effect. Warm air flows upward. The hot air in the attic will not flow down into the house. In terms of conduction, if the floor of the attic is poorly insulated, the ceiling of the house will reach the same temperature as the attic, that heat will be conducted and radiated into the house. You can feel it if you stand under a poorly insulated attic hatch. If the floor of the attic is well sealed and insulated, then the attic temperatures will be isolated from the house, and the large temperature swings up there are less important.

If the mechanical equipment and the ducting are in the attic, reducing the air temperature is much more important than if it is just empty space. The floor of the attic may be covered by R30 insulation, but the ducting is only wrapped in R4, R6, or at most R8. If the attic air temperature is 140°F and the house temperature is 72°F, that is a 68°F temperature difference across R30 insulation. The air temperature in the ducting may be 60°F, providing an 84°F temperature difference across R8 insulation. Ducting may cover 25 to 30% of the attic floor area, but the total surface area of the ducting exposed to the attic temperatures is much greater than that. Every 5 degrees of temperature drop will save 1.6 BTUs per linear foot of R8, 10" diameter ducting, per hour the air conditioning is running. (Assuming that the entire perimeter is exposed to the attic air temperature.)

5°F reduction in temperature per linear foot per AC operating hour	12" Flex Duct	10" Flex Duct	8" Flex Duct
R8 insulation	2 BTUs	1.6 BTUs	1.3 BTUs
R6 insulation	2.6 BTUs	2.2 BTUs	1.7 BTUs
R4 insulation	3.9 BTUs	3.3 BTUs	2.6 BTUs

Table 16.2 Attic Temperature Effect on Duct Insulation

With 200 linear feet of 10" R6 ducting in the attic of an 1800 square foot house and the AC runs 30% of the time or 8 hours per day: 200 x 8 x 2.2 BTUs = 3,520 BTUs per day per 5 degree temperature reduction. At an optimistic sensible EER (Energy Efficiency Ratio) for the AC system of 10 BTU/Wh, this would be a daily savings of 0.35 kWh. At $0.129 per kWh the savings would be approximately $0.045 per day. Adding that to the saving through the R30 insulation on the floor of the attic of another $0.093 would show savings of about $0.14 per day for each five degrees, the attic temperature was reduced. Although these are approximate numbers, they provide a scale. As the attic temperature approaches the outside temperature, the attic's ventilation system's affect will be reduced. It will take more and more air to remove the last few degrees.[3]

If the attic space is used for storage, it will be important to maintain a reasonably temperate environment. Moisture as well as temperature is a factor in maintaining the integrity of personal treasures. Moisture will come primarily from air leaks between the house and the attic (or the practice of

---

3. Danny Parker of the Florida Solar Energy Center (FSEC) noted that "attic ventilation can make a difference but not nearly so great as that achieved from a light colored roof." See "Comparative Evaluation of the Impact of Roofing Systems on Residential Cooling Energy Demand in Florida" on the FSEC website www.fsec.ucf.edu/en/

ventilating bathrooms into the attic, or laying the bathroom ducting outlet "near" a gable or soffit vent hoping it will find its way outside). Roof or chimney leaks are another potential source of moisture and obviously need to be sealed/fixed.

Passive vents offer an alternative to PAVs. Most of these are like tiny dormers or "eyebrows" that are mounted on the roof. They are larger and far more open to airflow than ridge or soffit vents because they are cooling the temperature of the air in the attic, not just reducing the temperature of the roof deck. There are also "wind spinners" that are more commonly found in commercial buildings, the top spinning around in the response to breezes, establishing a vortex in the air inside their pipes that sucks the air out of the attic.

One company[4] has a passive vent cap that employs directional louvers to establish the vortex flow inside the pipe. These can be effective in low wind speeds to establish low exhaust flows that exceed passive stack effect ventilation rates.

There are a number of solar powered attic exhaust fans. The beauty of these is that the fan runs when the sun is shining and the attic is heating. (It is also the period of highest ambient relative humidity.) Different sized photovoltaic (PV) arrays produce a different amount of power, producing a variety of airflows from the fans. The power of the PV array is directly related to the air movement capability of the fan.

It is important to remember that the attics are part of the house. Negative pressure in the attic developed by exhaust fans of any type will impact the pressure in the house to varying degrees, dependent on the house/attic interface.

Whole House Comfort Ventilators (Whole House Fans)

A Whole House Comfort Ventilator, or what is commonly referred to as a whole-house fan, is a fan that moves the air from the living space for cooling. They are not used for improving the air quality in the house except for reducing the temperature by exchanging the existing warm house air with cooler outside air. They have no mechanical cooling capacity beyond their air

---

4. Active Ventilation Products roofvents.com

moving capabilities, so if it is hotter outside than it is inside, they shouldn't be used.

Whole House Fans are NOT the same as attic fans or PAVs, even though several knowledgeable web pages identify them that way. Attic fans (as discussed previously) are for reducing the temperature of the air in the attic. Whole House Fans or Whole House Comfort Ventilators are for reducing the temperature of the air in the house.

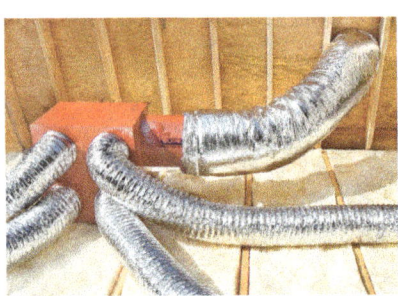

Figure 16.3 Duct Whole House Comfort Ventilator

The traditional design is a large axial fan mounted in the top floor ceiling between the house and the attic. The ceiling side is covered by a grille and/or passive louver that is sucked up and open when the fan is turned on. They have been very large fans, two to four feet in diameter that can move thousands of cubic feet of air per minute, changing all the air in the house four to six times per hour. The point of these large airflows is to create a breeze that moves through the house to convectively cool the people. Unfortunately, fans that are strong enough to move that large a volume of air are, as a rule, big, noisy, and power hungry, probably not the sort of thing you want running all night long in your bedroom. To have the maximum effect on the largest volume of the house, they are commonly mounted in a central location, like in the hallway. Bedroom doors and windows need to be left open to admit the balancing air to circulate properly, keeping the convective cooling going. Opening first-floor windows allows the air to be drawn in and pulled through much of the house. The fan pushes the house air into the attic, reducing the temperature of the attic air and pressurizing the attic. If there are adequate relief vents from the attic, the air will be forced to the outside. If the attic relief vents are too small, air will find its way through any opening, sometimes into wall cavities, pushing attic air and dust back down into the house, creating that sort of "burnt", stuff odor. The effectiveness of the fan will be reduced because it will work against a higher pressure and its airflow will be reduced.

Whole House Comfort Ventilators work by depressurizing the house. They will draw air from any opening, always taking the biggest, easiest path. They are designed to be powerful and move a lot of air. NEVER operate a whole house comfort ventilator with the windows closed. The fan will almost certainly suck the air down a chimney for a combustion appliance. The switch for the fan should be clearly labeled. If an automatic control, like a timer or thermostat, is used, be sure windows are open before leaving the fan unattended.

As the air in the house warms up during the day, all the materials in the house warm up, absorbing and holding heat. (Heat moves toward cold.) Circulating cooling air through the house allows the heat flow from the materials to reverse, and the materials give up the stored heat to the cooler air, warming the air. The greater the temperature differential, the more quickly the materials give up the heat. "Eat your supper before the food gets cold!" Moving more air across the materials will cause it to give up its heat more quickly (which is why people blow on hot soup before they put it in their mouth). But the air is not all that good at holding heat. A kitchen match produces about 1 BTU (British Thermal Unit) of heat. One cubic foot of air can only hold about 0.018 BTUs for each degree of temperature change. So if it is only one degree cooler outside than inside the house, you need a lot more air to bring the temperature down than if it is 30 degrees cooler. Turn on the whole-house fan when it is 40°F outside and you'll cool the house down pretty quickly! But if it is 70°F inside and 69°F outside, it will take a lot of air to cool the mass of the house.

You can use a really big fan and move the air quickly or you can use a smaller fan running over a longer period. It is common for the outside air temperature to drop over the course of the evening and night, and a smaller, quieter fan can take advantage of the increasing thermal effect.

As houses become more energy efficient, smaller fans work even more effectively. Because of higher insulation levels, the temperature inside the house will not rise as much in warm weather as less well insulated homes. A smaller fan working over a longer period can produce a gentle flow of air through the house, cooling the mass and making the occupants comfortable.

When thinking about the installation of a whole house comfort ventilator, think about the complete system and how you will use the product. Because these products rely on outside air for cooling, windows will need to be open when the fan is running. That means that whatever is in the outside air will be pulled into the house. Window screens will be the primary filtration system.

You will also want to carefully consider the exhaust side of the system. If the fan is venting into the attic, the attic pressure will be raised. Providing adequate exhaust openings from the attic is critical to the performance. Dividing the listed airflow of the fan by 765 will provide a good approximation of an opening from the attic space to the outside to minimize the back-pressure on the fan. For example, if the whole-house fan is rated at 4,000 cfm, the exhaust opening: 4000/ 765 = 5.23 square feet. Again, note that this is "free area" opening. Insect screening will cut the open area of 20% to 30%. Louvers may cut another 20%. Since whole house comfort ventilators will only be used in hot weather when ice dams are not a concern, including the ridge and soffit vents in the opening calculation is acceptable.

How quickly a whole house comfort ventilator reduces the temperature in the space depends on the size of the house, the temperature of the "mass" of the house, and the temperature difference between the inside air and the outside air. As the temperature in the house approaches the outside temperature, it will take longer and longer to cool those last few degrees. It's the old question of, "How many steps will it take to walk to a wall if you walk half the distance each step?" Each step becomes smaller and smaller.

As long as it's cooler outside than inside, a whole house comfort ventilator can provide essentially free cooling. For example, if it is 65°F outside and 75°F inside for an hour, a temperature difference of 10°F and the fan moves 1,800 cfm: 1200 x 10 x 1.08 = 19,440 BTUs, more than a ton of cooling (1 ton of cooling equals 12,000 BTUs). Small central air conditioners deliver 2 tons of cooling. The cooling ability of a whole house comfort ventilator is not as predictable as an air conditioner, of course, but a ton or more of free cooling is not something to scoff at.

In terms of airflow, dividing the volume of the house by the cfm capacity of the fan provides the number of minutes per air change. A 2,000 square foot house with 8-foot ceiling would have a volume of 2,000 x 8 = 16,000 cubic feet. A 4,000 cfm fan would move all the air in 4 minutes. A 1,800 cfm fan would move all the air in 9 minutes.

When the weather cools and the whole house comfort ventilator isn't needed anymore or when the weather is really hot and the central air conditioning is running, the opening for the fan needs to be closed. The gravity louvers on a typical whole house comfort ventilator have a lot of "edges". Each one of those edges is a potential air leak. Stack pressure in the house will constantly push up on the louvers, and there will be a continuous trickle of air leakage. Providing a winter cover for the fan is an important seasonal step. Any control system needs to be defeated or carefully marked so that the system can't be activated with the winter cover in place, otherwise the fan will be burned out.

Some smaller, whole house comfort ventilators have motorized and insulated covers that automatically close when the fan is turned off. These will provide a positive air-tight and insulated seal. Make sure the edges of the fan are insulated as well as possible, adding loose fill insulation around the perimeter. Some of these small units blow the air out of the sides, horizontally. Loose fill won't help those units. They will need to be installed high enough above the insulation.

There are several ducted versions of whole house comfort ventilators. Some of these use large, 14" diameter flexible ducting attached to a panel fan in the attic. As described in Chapter 14, axial fans are not good at moving air against any kind of resistance. Flexible ducting has a high resistance, which will degrade the performance of the fan. Be sure that the complete whole house comfort ventilator system—including the grille, the ducting, the fan, and the backdraft louvers—has been Certified for performance by a third party like HVI. Otherwise the manufacturer may be just citing the "free air" (no resistance) performance of the panel fan. One nice thing about these products is that the fan is located remotely from the living space and they can be very quiet.

Another version of this product is a multi-port approach using a motorized impeller that pulls air through flexible ducting. It is also designed to vent directly to the outside so that it is not relying on attic openings and will not interfere with ridge and soffit ventilation. With multiple ports, it can draw air from multiple, individual rooms, meaning that bedroom doors can be closed at night, allowing for privacy and maximizing the cooling performance in the bedrooms where people are sleeping. The bedroom window can be opened a few inches, making the total volume of air to move through a smaller opening, increasing the velocity of the airflow.

Some issues in deciding on the use of a whole house comfort ventilator:

Pros	Cons
Enhances "natural" cooling by accelerating the transfer of cooler outside air through the house to the outside	Brings in large amounts of outside air and all the things that are in it including dust, pollen, and humidity
Less expensive to operate than air-conditioning systems	Depressurizes the house and may interact with other air sourced appliances like water heaters
Uses natural, outside air (not everyone likes air-conditioning)	Uses natural, outside air
Can be quiet enough to provide a background white noise that can mask outside traffic noises	Can be noisy (minimized by using smaller or remotely mounted fans)
Big fans can provide a rapid dump of overheated air to reduce the air-conditioning load	Big fans are generally not well sealed and heat from the attic will radiate down through them
House air is considerably cooler than attic air so pushing attic air out means the whole house comfort ventilator is serving two purposes	Should never be used when the outside air is hotter than the inside air, and if the fan vents into the attic, the pressure can force attic air back down into the house.

Table 16.3 Whole House Comfort Ventilator Variables

In selecting a whole house comfort ventilator, be sure that the fan is safety tested by Underwriter Laboratories (UL), Intertek (ETL), the Canadian Standards Association (CSA), or another recognized independent safety laboratory. If you want to be sure that the airflow the manufacturer is claiming is real, it also needs to have been performance tested by a 3rd party laboratory like HVI or AMCA.[5] Sound level will be an issue for the larger fans. Some of them offer multiple speeds that will allow some flexibility in how the fan is used. Even some of the smaller fans are noisy and generally don't offer speed control capabilities.

> Not all fans have been tested for use with solid-state speed control devices. In fact, some installation instructions will specifically state "Not for use with solid state speed controls" if they have not been safety tested. (If they haven't been tested, you won't know.) Speed controls can also create motor hum and may burn out the motor.

---

5. https://cacertappliances.energy.ca.gov/Pages/Search/AdvancedSearch.aspx Note that the performance of whole house comfort coolers listed on the CA site are generated by the manufacturers: "Fan Airflow CFM is derived by method of test with measurement equipment in accordance with AMCA International. Home Ventilation Institute (HVI-916) Standard CFM Specifications are derived by method of test recognized by CA Title 24 for use in Residential New Construction (RNC) new home modeling by energy consultants and builders."

If you want to -	Consider -
Change all the air quickly, creating a breeze and "flushing" the house out before turning on the air-conditioning...	A large, traditional design, whole house fan, something that will change the air every 4 or 5 minutes.
Cool the mass of the house over an extended period of time and push the air out through the attic vents...	A smaller, centrally located fan or a number of smaller fans located in individual rooms.
Cool the mass of the house over an extended period of time, push the air out through the attic vents, and sound level is a major concern...	A ducted, attic mounted fan with a central or multiple vents.
Cool the mass of the house over an extended period of time, sound level is a major concern, vent from a number of rooms, and not pressurize the attic...	A multi-port attic mounted system, with a direct vent to the outside.

Table 16.4 Whole House Comfort Ventilator Decision Tree

Sizing, determining the cfm rate of the fan depends on what you want the fan to do as described in table 16-4. The traditional approach was to calculate the volume of the house and then multiply that by ½ to 1. So if the house has 1500 square feet of floor area with 8-foot high ceilings: 1500 x 8 = 12,000 cubic feet. Half of that would be 6,000 cubic feet per minute. That fan size would change all the air every minute and would require almost an 8 square foot, free area opening from the attic! It would be difficult to store anything in the attic with that much air moving through it. One builder stated that fans that big put so much pressure on the attic space it will push the nails out of the roof! That may have been an exaggeration, but that is the sizing method the government flyer on whole house fans suggests and is repeated in many informational pieces. As described previously, selecting a fan with a lower airflow rate just extends the cooling time and allows the house to cool down more naturally.

Pedestal and Box Fans

Smaller, whole house comfort ventilators do a great job of cooling down the mass of the house. Pedestal fans or desk fans or hassock fans provide a portable means of convectively cooling people. They can be set up in any room. They are almost always capable of multiple speeds and many of them oscillate, turning back and forth, blowing air throughout the room. They are made in many sizes and styles, from inexpensive units you can find in a drugstore to solid industrial types that are used in factories, known as "man coolers". They all have the common characteristic of being designed to circulate air in the room without any ducting resistance, sucking the air in one side and blowing it out on the other.

> Pedestal or oscillating fans move air around inside a room. They do not change the temperature of the air. Leaving a pedestal fan running when the room is unoccupied will not change the room's temperature unless there are other sources of conditioning like a room air conditioner or space heater.

Unless it is an industrial or commercial application where the fan will be subjected to fairly polluted air and run almost continuously, these products are remarkably durable. Most of the variations are cosmetic, and there are certainly variations in the quality of the materials and the assembly. The grilles may come loose and the base may become wobbly, but for the most part, they seem to last a long period of time.

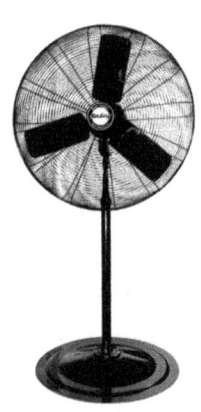

Figure 16.4 Pedestal Room Fan (Air King)

Most of these fans have height adjustments. Be sure that the range adjustment works for your application. You may not want it blowing on you all the time. Some fans also have an angle adjustment, allowing you to tip the fan back so the airflow sweeps across the ceiling, again limiting the direct draft.

The weighted base versions help to keep the fan from getting knocked over easily, but also making them less portable. If you want to put your fans away up in the attic in the fall when the cooling season is over, you want a version with a lighter, un-weighted base. Some products come with wheels on the base, but that probably means that the fan is heavy. The wheels will help to maneuver the fan around a limited area.

The more industrial grade versions can be noisy. In a factory setting, the sound level isn't important. In your living room where you are trying to have a conversation or watch TV, noisy fans are unacceptable. Having multiple speeds can quiet most of the fans down to a reasonable level, but it is worth reading some reviews before making a purchase. The speed controls that have a limited number of settings mean the fan has a number of "windings" on the motor, providing fixed points for the speed selector to connect to. That means that whatever setting you select, the motor will operate normally. If the speed settings are infinite, then the controller will be reducing the energy supplied to the fan. The fan may hum and its life may be reduced. Having a handful of settings is probably enough to satisfy most people.

The descriptions of these products do not always tell you how much air the fan moves. This is probably because most people don't know what cfm means and whether it is 750 cfm or 1000 cfm doesn't matter. The fans are commonly sized by the diameter of the blade: 16 inch, 20 inch, 22 inch, 30 inch. Larger blade diameters will move more air. For most household applications, the smaller diameter fans are more than adequate. A 30 inch fan may move as much as 10,000 cfm at high speed, a 24 inch 8,200 cfm, and a 12 inch fan may move 1,000 to 1,200. That's still enough air motion to push the pages of magazines around on your coffee table. What is needed in a residential application is enough air motion to provide a gentle, barely noticeable, continuous breeze.

Box fans are commonly used as window fans. Commonly they are square, box-like, with a handle on the top to make them portable. Installed in a top-floor window, they can serve as a portable whole house comfort ventilator. They should be adjusted so that they are blowing out of the house when they are used on the second floor. That way, they will draw air up from the first floor and cooling the whole house. For the best effect, the room door should be left open, allowing the air to flow both into and out of the room. (One cfm in equals one cfm out!)

Some of these fans are less "boxy" and may actually be two fans, side-by-side, but whatever the design, they are more often used as space coolers or space ventilators than "man coolers", like the pedestal fans.

Ceiling Fans

There are so many variations of ceiling fans on the market that it is difficult to describe them. There are wooden ones, plastic ones, stainless steel ones, fans with lights, fans with heaters, and fans that clean the air, but the basic, common purpose is air movement—slow, gentle, pushing the air around in the room.

They are available at a wide range of costs. The motor grade is a major cost factor. The least expensive ceiling fans are not designed to run for over 8 hours per day. All motors have a life expectancy, so you should figure on replacing the fan in the future depending on how much it is used. Some motors have sealed bearings that require no maintenance. Other will require periodic lubrication.

Most ceiling fans are relatively low power—between 50 to 75 watts. Some have aerodynamically optimized blade design to minimize power consumption and maximize performance.

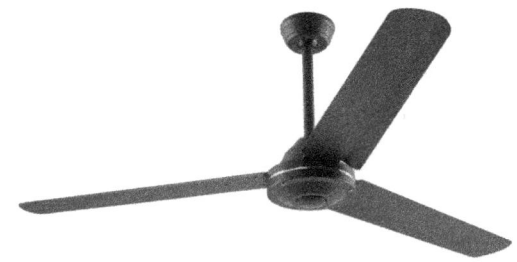

Figure 16.5 Ceiling Fan (Broan)

All Energy Star rated ceiling fans include the use of a control that allows the ceiling fan to be used throughout the year. In hot weather, the fan should rotate counter-clockwise, pushing the air down and causing the occupant to feel a minimal warm breeze. In cool weather, the fan should operate clockwise at a low speed, creating a gentle upward flow, accelerating the natural upward movement of warm air. The fan causes the airflow to impact the ceiling, sweeping the air back down into the room. (Note that ceiling fans have no mechanical cooling component. Leaving them running in an unoccupied room will not cool the room.)

The Environmental Protection Agency, ENERGY STAR program, makes the following sizing recommendations:

Room Dimensions	Suggested Fan Size
Up to 75 square feet	29" – 36"
76 to 144 square feet	36" – 42"
144 to 225 square feet	44" – 50"
225 to 400 square feet	50" - 54"

Table 16.5 Energy Star Ceiling Fan Sizing

ENERGY STAR[6] rates ceiling fans for efficiency based on how much air the fan moves for the amount of electricity that it uses or cfm per watt. All things being equal, the efficiency increases as the blade length increases. This chart's suggestions won't get you the most efficient size fan to get the job done. Consider getting the biggest, most efficient fan you can afford. Fans that are listed as ENERGY STAR have a minimum 30 year warranty and many of them include Lifetime warranties.

Ceiling fans provide an effective means to make the room occupants more comfortable by getting the air moving. In the cooling season, raising the thermostat by just one degree can reduce the air-conditioning bill by approximately four percent over the course of the cooling season. Lowering the set point by one degree in winter results in approximately three percent savings in overall heating cost. Many energy efficiency programs give credit for having ceiling fans for just this reason. When the air isn't moving, the room can feel stuffy. However, if the air is too cold, moving it around can make it feel drafty at which point the ceiling fan will need to be turned off. It is not one of those automatic products. It requires operator involvement to be effective and reduce energy costs.[7]

Cooling Tubes

Earth tubes or cooling tubes are an unusual cooling/ventilation strategy that was explored in the late 1970s that seems of interest once again. The concept

---

6. https://www.energystar.gov/products/lighting_fans/ceiling_fans/ceiling_fan_basics
7. Sonne, J. and Parker, D., 1998, "Measured Ceiling Fan Performance and Usage Patterns: Implications for Efficiency and Comfort Improvement," Presented at the
   1998 ACEEE Summer Study on Energy Efficiency in Buildings, Vol. 1, pp. 335-341

is that air is drawn through pipes that are run through the ground, six to twelve feet below the surface. Since the ground temperature can be relatively stable and cooler than the above ground temperatures, the air is "conditioned" as it moves through the pipe into the house.

Experiments were done at the Passive Solar Research Test Facility at the Omaha campus of the University of Nebraska in 1982 that produced a significant volume of data on 9 tubes of different sizes and length and buried at different angles. They confirmed that the maximum cooling effect for any tube is "heavily dependent upon the difference between the ambient outdoor temperature and the soil temperature surrounding the tube."[8] They also determined that the depth of the tube and night ambient conditions played a role in maximizing the cooling effect.

As the air passes through the tubes over the course of the cooling season, the surrounding ground temperature will rise as it absorbs the heat from the air moving through the pipes. The diameter of the pipes, the number of pipes, and the length of the runs all impact the effectiveness of this strategy. Lower airflow velocity at the mouth of the inlet allows the slower moving air to give up more heat to the ground. Sophisticated control strategies were developed that varied the fan speed with the changing temperature.

There are numerous reasons the strategy is not more commonly used today. Running warm, humid air through pipes underground will naturally cause condensation to occur on the walls of the pipe. Moist surfaces in dark spaces will grow mold. Insects, animals, and soil gases can all enter the pipe in both the short term and the long term. And installing long length and circuitous paths of pipe in the ground can be an expensive process.

Yet the experiments continue.

Evaporative Coolers

This is a topic that should fall under a space-conditioning text, but the evaporative cooling process relies on pressurizing the house, pushing a lot of air in and allowing it to "leak" out. They are sort of like whole house comfort ventilators in reverse with a mechanical cooling component.

---

8. Bing Chen, Tseng-Chan Wang, John Maloney, James Ennenga, Mark Newman, "Measured Cooling Performance of Earth Contact Cooling Tubes", Passive Solar Research Group, University of Nebraska, 1982

Evaporative coolers, or "Swamp Coolers", rely on the fact that as water evaporates, it removes heat from the surrounding air. They rely on low ambient relative humidity. Dry air can absorb a significant amount of moisture. A large volume of air is pushed or pulled through a wet medium and as the water evaporates, the air is cooled. The cooler air flows into the house and is allowed to escape through open windows or openings into the attic. They use less energy than most mechanical cooling systems. The pads, which are often made of wood shavings, from wood like aspen that resists mold growth, have to be replaced every season or two.

The systems can work effectively at fairly high ambient temperatures as long as the relative humidity is low. When the relative humidity (RH) is as low as 2%, an evaporative cooler can drop 105°F air to 72°F. But if the RH rises to 40%, the 105°F air can only drop to 89°F. An advantage evaporative coolers have over whole house comfort ventilators is that they work best during the hottest time of the day because the RH drops as the temperature rises.

Evaporative coolers are not designed to carry away the heat stored in the mass of the materials in the house. They cool the air and cool the people, so the sizing "rule of thumb" is to calculate the volume of the house and divide it by two (the traditional formula for whole house comfort ventilators). So a 2,000 square foot house with 8 foot ceilings that have a 16,000 cubic foot volume would require an evaporative cooler with an 8,000 cfm capacity.

The technology is evolving as the price of energy and interest in the impact on the planet increases. There are maintenance issues with the pads, the effects of all the moisture on the system, and the security concerns with leaving windows open. Pushing a lot of air into the attic without adequate relief vents is as much of a concern for evaporative coolers as it is for whole house comfort ventilators. Thinking through all the aspects of the system remains an important design and installation consideration.

Chapter 17

Humidifiers, Dehumidifiers, Filters, and Ventilation Accessories

Humidity is a major pollutant in homes, and it is carried on air currents. This is not meant to be an exhaustive treatment of dealing with humidification and dehumidification issues in the home. There are many in-depth resources for that. Care should be taken in selecting and installing any system that essentially may add a pollutant (moisture) to a home.

Relative Humidity (RH) and Dew Point

Air can hold moisture. Warm air can hold more moisture than cold air. The moisture holding capacity of 100 °F air is ten times the moisture holding capacity of 30 °F air. If it is snowing, the relative humidity of the air is going to be quite high - close to 100% RH! Drawing that air into a house will warm it, giving it the capacity to hold more moisture, consequently lowering the relative humidity. Think of a shot glass 100% full of liquid. The entire capacity of the shot glass is full. Now pour all of that liquid into a big beer stein. It's the same amount of liquid, but it will fill only a small percentage of the volume of the stein. As the air is warmed, its relative humidity or RH goes down.

The dew point is the temperature below which the air can't hold any more moisture and the water vapor changes from a gas to a liquid form. If the temperature of the surface of a blade of grass is below the dew point temperature, moisture will form. An air conditioner or dehumidifier uses that fact to cool a component in the machine to force water out of the air. If the temperature of a wall surface is below the dew point, moisture will form on it, providing nourishment for mold. That spot could be cold because of missing insulation or because the cold air from an air conditioning supply was blowing on it. Moisture condenses on cold water pipes, toilet tanks, ducting, and any place that is below the dew point.

Before adding a mechanical device to solve a humidity problem, be sure you understand the root cause of the problem, not just the observable symptom.

Humidifiers and dehumidifiers

Humidifiers add moisture to the air. Dehumidifiers remove moisture from the air. But why the air is too humid or too dry is not always obvious, and adding one of these devices is definitely not always the solution. It is key to the durability of the house and the comfort and health of the occupants to determine why the air is too dry or too humid before deciding on the best approach to resolving the problem. Not to belabor the point, but moisture causes many indoor air quality problems, and it is not something to be treated casually.

In a cold climate, a house may be too dry because it has too many air leaks. The cold outside air is very dry relative to the air in the house. If the house is drafty, all that outside air leaking in will make the air in the house uncomfortably dry. The best solution is to tighten up the house, air-seal the leaks. It will save lots of money on the heating bills and is bound to raise the relative humidity in the house. It may get to where better mechanical ventilation is required to remove some of the humidity. Adding a humidifier to a central HVAC system can cause serious problems if the house is too leaky because that warm, humid air striking a cold surface will condense, and the moisture will grow mold and that's not good for either the building or the occupants. It is critically important to understand why the house is too dry before adding a humidifier to address the problem rather than the symptom.

And that's the other side of the problem: the house is too humid. The problem might be solved with better ventilation, making sure that there are adequate air changes and that the fans are working properly, that the ducting goes all the way to the outside, etc. Certain areas like basements or rooms housing priceless antiques may need dehumidifiers.

Remember that the house is a system. Make sure you understand the cause of the humidity issue before proceeding to resolve it.

Both heating and cooling systems will dry out the air. A major function of an air conditioning or cooling system is to remove the excess humidity from the air. Adding a humidifier to an air conditioning system is asking the two systems to work against each other: one adding humidity and one taking it away. If the AC system is not effective enough at removing the moisture, there may be system design issues that should be remedied before adding a secondary dehumidifier to the system, which would certainly increase the operating cost.

> Note that most mini-split air conditioners run the internal fan continuously even after the temperature setting has been satisfied. Some of the residual moisture on the coil can be blown back into the room, significantly raising the relative humidity and requiring supplementary dehumidification. That setting can be adjusted during installation.

A portable room humidifier may need to be added to the room of a child that is suffering from winter colds and whose sinuses are laboring with the dry air. Portable devices should be selected carefully and cleaned regularly. Blowing humidity into the air, whether it has been aerated acoustically or through an evaporative medium or by some other method (other than boiling) is bound to carry anything else in the water or in the system with it. Ultrasonic systems create a white dust that settles on surfaces in the room. Ultrasonic and impeller humidifiers disperse the greatest amount of microorganisms and minerals into the air. It is important with any humidifier to clean it regularly and thoroughly.

The ideal humidity levels in the home in winter vary between 35% RH and 50% RH. Dust mites enjoy relative humidity above 50%. If air conditioning is not needed, a good dehumidifier should be able to keep the humidity under control. Dehumidifiers can be stand-alone units, units attached to the HVAC ducting to dehumidify the air circulating in the house, or units that are used to dehumidify incoming, fresh air for ventilation.

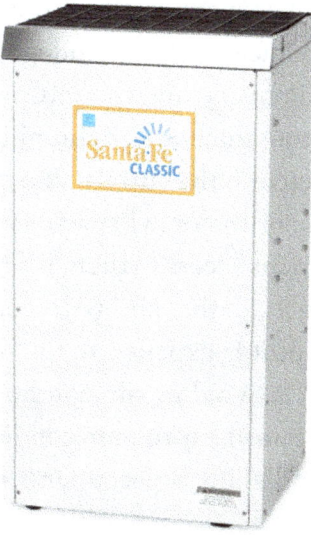

Figure 17.1 System Dehumidifier (Thermastor)

The EPA's ENERGY STAR program does rate dehumidifiers. These models are 10% to 20% more energy efficient than unrated models. ENERGY STAR rated dehumidifiers are qualified by the amount of water they remove per kilowatt-hour of electricity used: 1.20 to 1.80 L/kWh (2.53 pints/kWh to 3.8 pints/kWh) for standard capacity units and greater than 2.5 L/kWh (5.28 pints/kWh) for high-capacity units. ENERGY STAR units range in capacity from just over 11 pints per day to over 144 pints per day.

There are stand-alone dehumidifiers that are available for basements, primary living spaces, or individual room applications. If the dehumidifier is to be used in the basement, it is important to use a unit that is rated for colder temperatures because the coils can start freezing on many units if the temperature drops below 65°F. Some units have an anti-frost sensor that will cycle the unit off. Many portable units have collection tanks that need to be manually emptied, although most have gravity drains with an option for a condensate pump.

Beyond the decision on how much water you want to remove from the space, there are energy use and durability (life cycle) considerations. If you purchase an inexpensive unit that has to be replaced in a year, has it saved you any money? There are calculators on-line available through ENERGY STAR that will help determine the energy and dollar savings of ENERGY STAR versus non-ENERGY STAR units.

Whole house dehumidifiers need to effectively circulate their conditioned air throughout the house. Some of them include high efficiency filters and can be installed in between the outside and the return side of the HVAC system. If the system is taking air from the house, dehumidifying it, and returning it to the house, it can be connected to the supply side of the HVAC system. Units can be installed in the attic or the crawl space. (Wherever they are installed, be sure that there is convenient access to them for maintenance and cleaning.)

Dehumidifiers add heat to the air. (Air conditioners using the same process add heat as well, but it is expelled to the outside with either a central air conditioning system or a window air conditioner.) The lower moisture level of the air reduces the load on the air conditioning system, making the home more comfortable, and allowing occupants to raise the set point on the thermostat (and save energy).

Room Air Filters

Homes that use central air systems include a filtration element. Originally, that filtration was included to limit the dust build-up on the air handler blower. The one-inch thick filters were effective at keeping 'Arizona Road Dust' off the blower wheel, but had little effect on the particulates circulated throughout the house. It is important to recognize that the system filters do insert resistance to the airflow. During system design that flow resistance is included with other back-pressure elements such as ductwork bends, increasers, decreasers, and grilles and registers. All of those elements impact the delivered airflow and are based on the capability of the air handler blower. Adding a more restrictive filter, such as a HEPA filter, will impact system performance.

This book is focused on ventilation. Central air systems are dedicated to delivering comfortable amounts of conditioned air. Making them perform other tasks such as delivering humidified, filtered, and ventilation air to the home is a compromise and is best achieved when designed in from the beginning.

Rather than clean all the air moving through an air handler, individual room sized devices can effectively play an IAQ role. There are products that are identified as room air filters and products that are identified as room air purifiers. The primary difference is that air purifiers add extra elements to the filtration process, which may or may not be a good thing.

Stand-alone, single-room air filter devices are available in a wide variety of types and sizes. Indoor air quality is a major concern, and manufacturers and retailers have jumped on that fear offering all sorts of approaches to cleaning the air—some valid and some bordering on dangerous. The Covid-19 pandemic brought on a flood of room air filtration products.

The EPA offers a comprehensive booklet, "Guide to Air Cleaners in the Home"[1]. This booklet details the choices for both room and furnace air cleaners.

The room systems are rated by their Clean Air Delivery Rate (CADR) which indicates the volume of filtered air an air cleaner delivers. The higher the CADR number for tobacco smoke, pollen, and dust, the faster the unit filters the air. AHAM (Association of Home Appliance Manufacturers) recommends that the CADR of the air filter should equal at least two-thirds of the room area.[2]

The simplest and most straight-forward of these is a box fan drawing air through an array of furnace filters, known as the Corsi-Rosenthal Box or Comparetto Cube[3].

Fundamentally, all these approaches, from the least expensive to the most expensive, draw air through a filtration system. Some filtration devices stack a series of filters of various types, including charcoal (for odors) and HEPA filters. The replacement filters can be expensive, and they will need to be replaced regularly—at least once a year.

Room filtration systems pull the air in through a filter or series of filters and then push it back out into the room. They come in a wide variety of prices and styles. Keeping the system simple and ignoring all the sales hype is probably the best approach. Look for a system that is made well and well supported.[4]

Room Air Cleaners/Purifiers

Negative-ion generators emit negatively charged ions into the air that attach

---

1. https://www.epa.gov/indoor-air-quality-iaq/guide-air-cleaners-home
2. https://ahamverifide.org/ahams-air-filtration-standards/
3. https://en.wikipedia.org/wiki/Corsi%E2%80%93Rosenthal_Box
4. The EPA's Indoor AirPlus program states, "Where provided, UVGI or other electronic air cleaners (e.g., plasma generators, PCOs, etc.) must not exceed ozone concentration limits of 0.005ppm."

themselves to dust particles, causing the dust particles to have a negative charge. The dust is attracted to positively charged surfaces, like walls and ceilings, which serve as massive dust collectors. So they remove the particles, at least temporarily, from the air, creating dirty walls and ceilings in the process. They also produce ozone.[5]

Ozone generators generate ozone that may react with VOCs (volatile organic compounds) in the air and may convert a few to harmless water vapor, carbon dioxide, and oxygen. Ozone generators can also increase the level of VOCs in the house when the ozone reacts with some non-volatile and semi-volatile VOCs. Health Canada concluded in January 1999 that ozone generators pose a risk to the health and safety of the public.[6] The California Air Resources Board states that "some devices that are advertised as 'air purifiers', air cleaners, or ozone generators purposely emit large amounts of ozone, the main component of smog!"[7] They include a continuously updated list of over 60 manufacturers of devices that have not been tested to the required test protocol regulation. The Environmental Protection Agency describes ozone as "a toxic gas with vastly different chemical and toxicological properties from oxygen."[8] With all the evidence against them, devices that claim to clean the air, adding ozone in the process, are not an acceptable alternative.

Ventilation and furnace filters

Any ventilation system that brings air in from the outside also brings in the dust, pollen, and other particulates that are floating in the outside air. Filters in HVAC systems filter the air circulating about the house, but they also protect the mechanical equipment. The equipment doesn't mind really small particles, particles that are less than 2.5 microns in size. The filters on many HVAC systems remove only larger particles, coarse dust in the 2.5 to 10

---

5. Be very careful seeking the magic solution to IAQ. Products which tout the benefits of "hydroxy (OH) radicals" which are harmful chemicals. Not all the products from a reputable company are reputable products.
6. Health Canada, Consumer Product Safety, https://www.canada.ca/en/health-canada/services/air-quality/indoor-air-contaminants/ozone.html
7. California Environmental Protection Agency, Air Resources Board, http://www.arb.ca.gov/research/indoor/o3g-list.htm
8. EPA, "Ozone Generators that are sold as Air Cleaners", http://www.epa.gov/iaq/pubs/ozonegen.html

micron range. Furnace filters are filters for the furnace, not filters for the occupants (unless the system is running all the time).

There are a wide range of filtration systems available, including electrostatic, media, pleated, HEPA, and activated carbon air filters. Note that all filtration systems require maintenance. They remove and hold air borne junk! They have no way to get rid of the stuff they collect. As the air passes through the filter and collects, the air passages gradually clog, increasing the efficiency of the filter but blocking the airflow, reducing the efficiency of the air moving system. Until the filter is cleaned or replaced, all the air borne stuff it has collected will remain trapped and are still in the air stream.

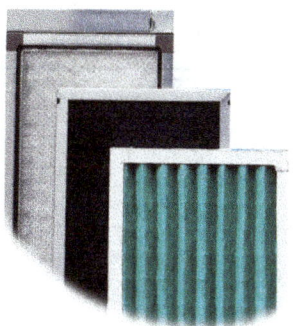

Figure 17.2 Various filter styles (Venmar)

ASHRAE, through Standard 52.2, has developed a filter rating system known as MERV (Minimum Efficiency Reporting Value) that simplifies filter ratings. The higher the MERV rating, the more effective the filter is at removing smaller particles. The period at the end of this sentence is about 400 microns across. Fine human hair is about 40 microns in diameter. House dust can range from 100 microns to less than 0.01 microns. Skin flakes fall into the 10 to 25 micron size range, bacteria 0.25 to 10, and viruses in the 0.001 to 0.1 micron range. So if the system uses a MERV 6 filter, it will not be at all effective at removing the small particles, and it will be 35% to 49.9% efficient at removing pollen, mold spores, skin flakes, lint, and some animal dander. It's not until you put in a MERV 13 filter that you will reduce the full range of particulates.[9]

---

9. In most circumstances MERV 11 filters are adequate.

MERV Rating	Particle Size		
	0.3 – 1.0 microns	1.0 – 3.0 microns	3.0 – 10.0 microns
1 – 4	-	-	Less than 20%
5	-	-	20 – 34.9%
6	-	-	35 – 49.9%
7	-	-	50 – 69.9%
8	-	-	70 – 84.9%
9	-	Less than 50%	More than 85%
10	-	50 - 64.9%	More than 85%
11	-	65 – 79.9%	More than 85%
12	-	80 – 89.9%	More than 90%
13	Less than 75%	More than 90%	More than 90%
14	75 – 84.9%	More than 90%	More than 90%
15	85 – 94.9%	More than 90%	More than 90%
16	More than 95%	More than 95%	More than 95%

Table 17.1 MERV Filter Effectiveness

The problem is that most of the higher-level MERV filters increase the resistance to the flow of air through the air handler. It is important to check with the system manufacturer to determine the highest level MERV filter that will work with the system. Unfortunately, not all filter manufacturers make it easy to find the MERV ratings on the packages. System manufacturers don't make it easy to determine the maximum filtration level either. That's partially because the performance of an air handler depends on its installation. The manufacturer can provide a maximum airflow resistance level, but much of that may be taken up by the ducting and other installation components, leaving an unknown amount of tolerance for the resistance of the filter.

3M, for example, on their Filtrete™ filters have their own rating system called the Microparticle Performance Rating (MPR). In order to address particles between 0.3 and 1.0 micron in size 3M developed the MPR scale. 1250 on the MPR scale is approximately equivalent to MERV 12, 1000 MPR is approximately equivalent to MERV 11, and 600 MPR is approximately equivalent to MERV 8.

There are several test methods other than ASHRAE's that manufacturers may choose to reflect in their advertising. Stating that a filter is 90% efficient without relating what test was used or the size of the particles is essentially useless information. The weight-arrestance test, for example, was developed to measure the efficiency of a filter's ability to capture Arizona road dust over 8 microns in size! This might be helpful to the blower in the HVAC system, but is not very effective at improving health for the occupants of the home.

Filters that are in the HVAC system will remove particulates from the air as the air circulates through the system and through the house. The filtering efficiency will improve as the air moves around and around the system, passing multiple times through the filter. Filters work best on the inlet side of the air-handler with the air being pulled through them. The airflow is more uniform and passes through more of the filter surface. Located on the inlet side, the filter also helps to protect the equipment. If the filter is located on the outlet side, the airflow can be quite turbulent and the particulates are not easily removed. When the HVAC system is not running, airborne particles will settle throughout the house where they can't be removed by air filtration. For maximum effectiveness, the air should pass through the filter 2 to 4 times per hour. So if it is desirable to use the HVAC system as the whole house filtration system, long, or even continuous, operation of the system is required.

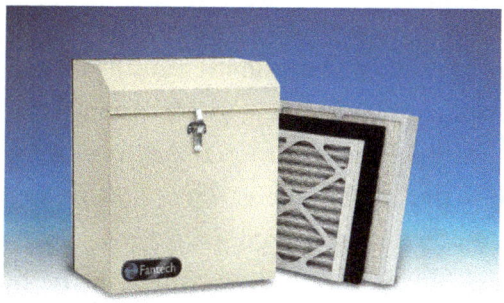

Figure 17.3 HEPA By-Pass Filter (Fantech)

Bringing the ventilation air in on the return side of the air-handler allows the outside air to pass through the furnace filter. This system can include its own filtration to further protect the occupants. A "filter-box" can be added to the ductwork that will allow for the use of a reasonably high MERV level filter in the line. These boxes consist of a sheet metal box with duct adaptors on both sides. The box must include the ability to be opened, and a filter inserted. The size should be relative to the ducting dimensions and a common filter size so that replacements can be easily found. It should be located in such a way that replacing the filter can be done as regularly as the air handler filters.

> Washable media filters should not be washed multiple times, as the moisture in the filter can provide an enhanced growth medium for mold and bacteria. Filters that can be replaced and thrown-away are the safest approach.

Many HRVs and ERVs have only minimal filtration. Filter boxes can be added to the intakes of these devices as well. The additional filtration will not only help the occupants breath better, it will also keep the heat exchanger elements cleaner and more efficient. (It is important that the filters be matched to the capabilities of the equipment. The increased filtration may increase the airflow resistance beyond the capability of the fans.)

HEPA (High-Efficiency Particulate Air) filters exceed ASHRAE's 52.2 Standard testing. All HEPA filters must meet a minimum efficiency of 99.97% at 0.3 microns. They were originally developed during World War II by the Atomic Energy Commission to filter out deadly plutonium particles in nuclear laboratories. Until recently, they were most commonly used in commercial applications—electronics laboratories and "clean" rooms. Stand-alone room filtration devices can handle HEPA filtration.

In residential applications to keep the frequency of replacement down, most of these systems include pre-filters that remove the largest particles before the air reaches the HEPA filter. They can be installed on the return side of the air-handler, being activated each time the blower turns on. The internal blower in the filtration unit draws some of the house air through the filters and then returns it to the HVAC air-stream. Without the additional blower in the filter housing, the air would bypass the filter, seeking the easiest path through the system. Unfortunately, because it only filters part of the air, the overall effectiveness of these "by-pass" filters is very limited.

In most cases, HEPA filtration may be more than is needed in a residential application unless there are specially sensitive occupants in the house, particularly in a tight house where the air is infrequently circulated through the HVAC system. If the HEPA filter is a by-pass system that filters 10% to 20% of the air moving through the system and if the system were perfectly effective and cleaned only the dirtiest air on each pass, it would take 5 to 10 complete passes through the system to clean all the air.

Electronic filters need frequent cleaning. Manufacturers recommend four times a year, but in many applications, monthly cleaning is required to maintain effectiveness. Although they start out at close to 90% efficiency, the plates fill with dust quickly, dropping the efficiency to 40% or less in a few days. Because of the high voltage used in these systems, they also produce low levels of ozone that can dissipate quickly if the system is run continuously. If the system includes a humidifier, it should not be located upstream of an electronic filter because the aerosolized moisture will land on the charged plates and reduce the filter's efficiency further.

It's hard not to go for all the marketing hype on filters because occupant health is important, the information is unclear, there will always be confusing claims, and people are different with different sensitivities.

- The basic furnace filters you can hold up to the light and see through may be okay for the furnace, but do little for the people;
- Use the highest MERV rated filter your furnace air handler can move air through effectively;
- Clean/replace your filter regularly—at least twice a year;
- SEAL the opening where the filter is inserted with a removable medium such as tape or a cover so that the air handler won't suck in non-system air (this will also improve the system's efficiency).
- ***A coverless filter slot is the worst leak in the HVAC system because it is at the lowest pressure point in the system.***

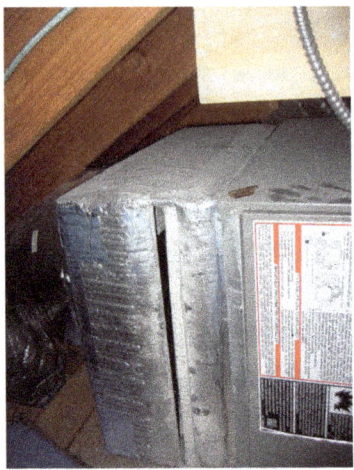

Figure 17.4 Uncovered Filter Slot (PHR)

Be careful using a high tech, whizz-bang IAQ device. Filtration is the simplest and most reliable approach to IAQ.

Chapter 18

Indoor Air/Environmental Quality Concerns

Homes are essentially boxes of air—admittedly fairly complex boxes of air. What they are made of, what we put in them, how we condition them, and how we use them all contribute to the contents of the air inside them. Books, conferences, organizations, and tons of research papers have been created around this subject, so this will not be an exhaustive discussion. However, the point of residential ventilation is to improve the quality of the air in the home. If the junk in the air in the house did not affect people's health, then ventilation systems would not be necessary, but, of course, we would be very different creatures. Humans are generally incredibly tolerant of many of the pollutants we put into our air regularly. The greatest impact is on the very young and the old, and infirm and people with compromised immune systems. Some people are very sensitive or allergic to particular pollutants.

> There are a number of valuable indoor air quality resources for people who suffer from Multiple Chemical Sensitivity (MCS). The National Center for Healthy Housing (NCHH), the American Lung Association (ALA), and the Healthy House Institute, as well as a wide variety of MCS websites, are great sources for information.

> Although the effects of relatively high levels of pollutants are obvious such as death, the onset of cancer, and increased levels of asthma, there is still not a

great deal of information on low-level effects, and it is even more difficult to clearly link health effects and ventilation rates. But these indoor pollutants impact health. Removing the source of the pollutant from the living space is the most effective approach, and diluting the concentration of the pollutant in the air is the next best step in reducing the potential impact. If there is a pile of excrement on the floor of the living room, it doesn't matter much what kind it is. It is more important to remove it!

The most common air contaminants found in buildings:

- Are given off when something is burned. This includes gas stoves, fireplaces, and wood stoves, and candles;
- Enter through cracks and holes from the ground (radon and soil gas) or from outside, including from an attached garage;
- Are out-gassed from building materials and furnishings like cabinets and carpets (formaldehyde);
- Are generated by activities in the house like aerosols and perfumes;
- Result from organisms living off the moisture, the materials, and human skin flakes (mold, dust mites, animals, bacteria, viruses);
- Are the high levels of humidity produced by water generated in the house by human activities, plumbing leaks, moisture, and condensation from the outside?

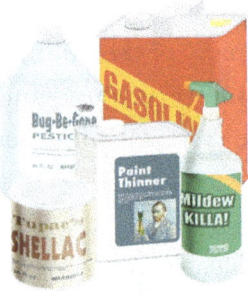

Figure 18.1 Common Household Pollutants (Panasonic/Morrissey)

The simplest and most effective ways of and preventing IAQ problems:

- Don't bring the polluting stuff into the house in the first place. (Verify that the materials used in furniture and carpeting do not include formaldehyde, for example. Don't use unvented kerosene heaters in the house. Using a generator in an attached garage is an invitation to disaster even if the door to the outside is wide open.)
- Isolate any source that is in the house. (Cover or seal asbestos, seal cabinet backs and sides prior to installation, etc.)
- Ventilate near the source of the pollutant. (Bathrooms, kitchens, hobby areas, etc.)
- Use and maintain whole dwelling ventilation systems. (Change filters, clean HVAC cabinets (water sitting at the bottom of the drain pans will grow mold or dry up and become dust that gets air borne), remove central humidifiers, etc.)
- Keep the humidity in the house between 30% and 60% RH. (This will keep down mold and dust mite and other micro-organism growth.)

Pollutant	Typical Source	Equipment & Materials	Ventilation strategy	Occupant maintenance
Radon & Radon daughters	Soil and rock under the house, drawn in through cracks in the foundation	Radon proof construction techniques, EPA's Home Buyer's & Seller's Guide to Radon E-2121	Vent the sump, sub-slab, or basement perimeter crack out through the roof	Maintain fan, periodically verify that it continues to run
Asbestos	Insulation on pipes and old furnaces, also found in siding and "popcorn" ceiling paint	Don't use, cover existing asbestos with a sealant, have removed professionally	Vent the basement or source location	Maintain the ventilation system, don't disturb the asbestos
Formaldehyde and other Aldehydes	Composite wood products like particle board, OSB, foam insulation, paneling, fiberglass insulation	Use low emission materials, seal source materials such as cabinets	Vent the house at a higher rate when introducing these materials; continuous, whole house ventilation	Remove source materials from the house if possible
Suspended combustion particulates	Unvented gas or kerosene appliances; wood stoves & fireplaces; cigarettes, candles; aerosol sprays	Pilotless ignition; proper chimney and combustion air; smoke outside	Ventilating hood; whole house ventilation; provide adequate combustion supply and exhaust	Use range fan; load wood stoves with an updraft; improve insulation & air sealing to limit need for auxiliary heating; read product instructions.
Carbon Monoxide (CO)	Gas stoves; unvented heaters; wood stoves and fireplaces (particularly at the end of the burn); attached garages; backdrafting; cigarettes, etc.	Pilotless ignition; proper chimney and combustion air; carefully seal the house/garage interface; sealed combustion appliances; smoke outside	Functional range hood that vents outside; supply correct combustion air; vent the garage (but don't backdraft any appliance in the garage; isolate house intake air from the garage.	Use the ventilation system; maintain the ventilation system; load wood stoves with an updraft; smoke outside, away from intake openings
Carbon Dioxide (CO_2)	People; unvented heaters; cigarettes; air from attached garages	Can't remove the people; don't use unvented heaters in inhabited spaces; seal the house/garage interface; smoke outside	Central ventilation system; isolate house intake air from garage or driveway	Maintain the ventilation system and HVAC filters; don't run the car in the garage; keep the door between the house and garage closed
Nitrogen Dioxide (NO_2)	Unvented heaters; gas stoves; cigarettes; outside air	Pilotless ignition; don't use in inhabited spaces	Ventilating hoods; smoke outside	Use range fan; improve insulation & air sealing to limit need

Table 18.1 Pollutants and Sources

Adapted from Brennan & Turner, "Indoor Air Quality: Problems & Solutions", Northeast Sun, June, 1985

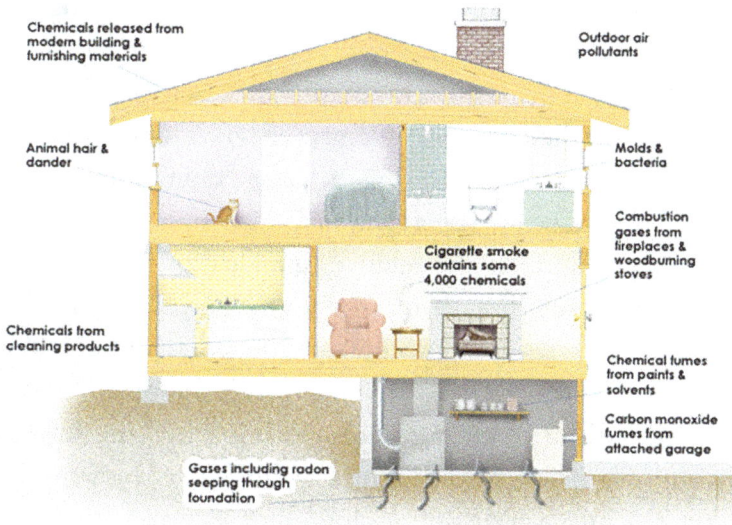

Figure 18.2 Pollutant Sources (Panasonic/Morrissey)

Moisture

Moisture is the principal pollutant in the house. It is the source of many other pollutants, like mold and dust mites. The good thing is that compared to other pollutant sources, it is relatively simple to measure and control. Low-cost digital hygrometers can measure the humidity in a room reasonably accurately. Humidity will vary throughout the house and throughout individual rooms. It may be 30% RH in the middle of the room and 70% RH near a window where it is cooler. Relative Humidity, or RH, is a measure of the amount of moisture the air can hold at a particular temperature. If the air is at 100% RH, it can't hold any more moisture. It is at the dew point so that moisture will condense on any surface that is at a lower temperature. A glass of 76°F water in a 75°F room at 100% RH will not have condensation on it. Lowering the temperature of the water to 74°F will cause condensation to form. If ice is added to the glass, the temperature of the water will drop and, on a very local basis, the temperature of the air surrounding the glass will also drop. The temperatures of all the surfaces and all the materials in the house will not be at exactly the same temperatures. Wherever the temperature is below the dew point of the air, condensation will form. The glass of the mirror in the bathroom may be at the same temperature as the rest of the room before you take your shower, but as the RH in the surrounding air increases to 100%, the mirror may be cool enough for moisture to form on it. Dew forms on blades of grass because they are completely exposed and cooled by the air moving around them. Any surface in the house or in its structure that is below the dew point at any time will have moisture condense on it. Moisture is sustenance and refreshment for mold and dust mites. When the relative humidity rises above 70 percent, mites can grow in dust without added moisture from our bodies. As the relative humidity rises, dust mites "increase their rate of reproduction, intake of skin scales, and defecation."[1] A level of humidity below 30% can cause respiratory problems and dry, cracking skin.

Some building moisture issues are blatant, like a broken water heater tank or an over-filled bathtub. Other moisture issues may hide in the walls and develop over an extended period. Vinyl wallpaper, for example, is a vapor diffusion retarder. In an air-conditioning climate, warm, moist air that gets sucked into the building through the wall systems and strikes the back of the wallpaper, can't get through and condenses there. Peeling the wallpaper away will reveal the mold.

Understanding the role of building pressures is critical in keeping moisture out of the building. In a house with a central return, closing bedroom doors at night without adequate pressure relief to bypass the door will cause the bedrooms to increase in pressure and the rest of the house that is connected to the returns to be depressurized. In air-conditioning climates that depressurization will suck the warm, moist air into the building system. It may not be much, but like a slow drip, it will bring in enough moisture to grow mold and cause serious indoor air quality problems. The opposite effect is also true for a heating climate. Pressurizing the bathroom, for example, may force warm, humid air through any cracks or leaks in the wall system. Mold can also grow in the ducting for the exhaust fan, particularly if it isn't used all that much because it is too noisy or poorly installed.

Supply-only ventilation systems are rarely used in heating climates because of the potential of pressurizing the building and forcing the moisture into the wall system. If the humidity level in the house is low enough (25% RH or less), air that gets forced into the wall system won't reach the dew point and condense. But even at 40% or 50% RH, there can be moisture problems.

For new construction, there are well proven wall construction techniques for every climate that will minimize the potential of hidden mold problems in

---

1. May, Jeffrey C., *My House is Killing Me!*, The Johns Hopkins Press, 2001, p14

the building structure.[2] Available materials, building codes, and heating and cooling systems make it mandatory that builders follow these steps. Construction errors can cause massive mold problems, health issues, and a gaggle of lawyers on your doorstep.

Adding a whole dwelling, continuously running ventilation system to an existing house requires making sure that the existing HVAC system can handle an additional load. Introducing warm, humid air to an air-conditioned home will require the AC system to work harder to remove the additional moisture from the air. The addition of the ventilation systems should not be thought of as isolated components, but rather as part of the system for the house. Are there ways to reduce the cooling/dehumidification load of the house? These may be structural or mechanical issues. It may require the use of an Energy Recovery Ventilation (ERV) system that removes some of the moisture from the incoming air, transferring it to the outgoing air stream.

A well-installed spot ventilation system with an inlet near the pollutant source, such as in a bathroom or kitchen, can remove much of the pollutant before it causes a problem. That's why fume hoods are used in laboratories.

IAQ stands for Indoor Air Quality. IEQ stands for Indoor Environmental Quality. There are issues that affect the health and comfort of the occupants of the house that are not floating around in the air. Sound is one of them. As homes get tighter, noise levels go down. Noises that would have been masked by road noise are more obvious and more annoying. IEQ represents the whole system approach to indoor environmental quality.

Carbon Monoxide

Carbon Monoxide (CO) is an odorless, invisible, deadly gas. It is commonly generated in an incomplete combustion process. As that lovely, romantic fire in the fireplace dwindles down to a few smoldering embers, the chimney cools, and the stack effect, driving the air up the flue becomes weaker and weaker, making it easier for gentle backdrafting to draw the CO into the house.

One drawback of the new, very efficient combustion appliances is that the temperature of the air going up the chimney is lower, making it easier for these

---

2. https://buildingscience.com/

devices to backdraft and draw CO into the house. This makes sealed combustion and powered exhaust systems more necessary.

Underwriter Laboratories (UL) states, "Studies have shown that the severity of CO poisoning is based upon the concentration of CO in a victim's bloodstream. Symptoms may progress from a slight headache to nausea, dizziness, drowsiness, vomiting, collapse and ultimate death as carboxyhemoglobin (COHb) levels increase in the bloodstream and displace oxygen. The level of COHb in the bloodstream may increase relatively slowly because of exposure to low concentrations of CO or more quickly when higher CO concentrations are present."[3] Carbon monoxide reduces the amount of oxygen to the brain, causing CO intoxication, and lack of reasoning. Even if the alarm isn't sounding, low levels of CO can build up in the blood. It is worth investing in a low-level CO alarm to protect your family.[4]

CO is NOT the same as smoke! Don't buy combination smoke/CO detectors.
Waving a towel at a CO detector will not stop the alarm!

CO is measured in part per million (ppm). The short-term maximum exposure allowed by the Environmental Protection Agency (EPA) is 9 ppm over 8 hours or 35 ppm for 1 hour. Typical, UL-2034 listed CO alarms provide no warning below 30 ppm. At 70 ppm, residential detectors must alarm after a required time delay. At 100 ppm, there will be slight headaches, tiredness, dizziness, and nausea after several hours of exposure. Manufacturers warn that people who may be sensitive to lower levels, such as pregnant women, infants, elderly people, and people with compromised immune systems, may need devices that provide audible and visual signals for CO levels below 30 ppm. At present, for a CO detector to receive UL-2034 approval, the detector must not activate the alarm before the level exceeds 30 ppm for 8 hours.

---

3. https://code-authorities.ul.com/wp-content/uploads/2014/04/ul_CarbonMonoxideAlarms.pdf
4. https://www.defenderdetectors.com/ll6170.html

Concentration (ppm)	MUST activate before:	MUST NOT activate before
30	N/A	8 hours
70	240 minutes	60 minutes
150	50 minutes	10 minutes
400	15 minutes	4 minutes

Table 18.2 UL 2034 CO Alarm Activation Levels

Elevated CO levels in the house are often attributed to malfunctioning furnaces, but it can come from other sources, including attached garages. It is often difficult to link the elevated levels starting the car because the two events may be separated by several hours. The pressure in the garage should be lower than the pressure in the house so that any pollutants in the garage flow to the outside rather than into the house.

It is critically important to perform Combustion Appliance Zone (CAZ) testing before and after performing any "air sealing" in the home. Air sealing will reduce the amount of infiltration that would naturally occur, reduce the cost of heating the home, and reduce unpleasant drafts. It may also choke off the combustion air needed for the proper operation of "natural" combustion appliances that rely on infiltration to expel their exhaust fumes.

Concentration of CO in Air	Effects
1-2 ppm	Might be normal, from cooking stoves, traffic, or outdoor air
2-8 ppm	Identify why the CO level is elevated
9 ppm	Maximum allowable concentration for an 8 hour period in any year (EPA, ASHRAE) Typical concentration after the operation of an unvented gas kitchen range. City air
15 – 20 ppm	Impaired performance in time discrimination and shortened time to angina response
20 ppm	Typical concentration in flue gases of a properly operating furnace or water heater
30 ppm	UL standard requires that CO detectors not alarm at 30 ppm unless exposure is continuous for 30 days. Earlier onset of exercise-induced angina
35 ppm	Maximum allowable outdoor concentration for one-hour period in any year, EPA, ASHRAE
50 ppm	Maximum allowable 8-hour work place exposure (OSHA)
70 ppm	UL 2034 listed detectors must sound full alarm between 1 and 4 hours
150 ppm	UL listed detectors must sound full alarm between 10 and 50 minutes
200 ppm	Maximum workplace exposure (NIOSH)
400 ppm	UL listed detectors must sound full alarm between 4 and 15 minutes.
500 ppm	Often produced in a garage when a cold car is started with the door open and run for 2 minutes
800 ppm	Dizziness, nausea and convulsions within 45 minutes. Unconscious within 2 hours. Death within 2-3 hours. Maximum air-free concentration from gas kitchen ranges (ANSI)
1,600 ppm	Headache, dizziness, and nausea within 20 minutes. Death within 1 hour. Smoldering wood fires, malfunctioning furnaces, water heaters, and kitchen ranges typically produce these concentrations
3,200 ppm	Headache, dizziness, and nausea within 5 -20 minutes. Quickly impaired thinking. Death within 30 minutes. Concentration from a charcoal grille used indoors
6,400 ppm	Headache, dizziness, and nausea within 1-2 minutes. Thinking impaired before response possible. Death within 10-15 minutes
12,800 ppm	Death within 1-3 minutes
70,000 ppm	Typical tailpipe exhaust concentrations from cold gasoline engine during the first minute of cold weather start. (Concentrations decrease to 2 ppm after 17 minutes of running.)

Table 18.3 CO Levels

TABLE ADAPTED FROM TOM GREINER, Ph.D., P.E. Iowa State University[5]

---

5. Greiner, "The Silent Killer: Carbon Monoxide", Iowa State University, January, 1998

PM 2.5 Particles

PM$_{2.5}$, or fine particulate matter, is a mixture of solid and liquid particles that are 2.5 micrometers or less in diameter. This is about 30 times smaller than the width of a human hair. Particles with diameters smaller than 10 microns are inhalable and can induce adverse health effects. Fine particulates are less than 2.5 microns in diameter, small enough to pass through the barrier between the lungs and the bloodstream. Larger particles are heavier and will drop out of the air stream more quickly while great air flows will carry them further.

Adverse effects are greatest among the most vulnerable populations — infants, children, and older adults with preexisting heart or lung disease. Of all the common air pollutants, PM$_{2.5}$ is associated with the greatest proportion of adverse health effects related to air pollution, in both the United States and world-wide based on the World Health Organization's Global Burden of Disease Project[6].

Particle Diameter (microns)	Primary PPE	Engineering Controls	Transmission Characteristics
0.1 - 2	N95 respirator, Level II surgical mask, powered air purifying respirator	Building ventilation with MERV 14 filters, HEPA filters, UV sterilization	Indoor exposure over many hours, spatially uniform, multi rooms
2 – 8	Well-fitted mask with decent filtration efficiency	Building Ventilation, MERV 12 – 13	Transmission uniform within rooms; exposure ~ hour
8 – 15	Any mask as long as it fits well	Local air extraction/filtration	Transmission <hour, non-uniform within room
15 – 30	Any mask if it fits; possible some protection from face shields	Important to avoid strong drafts from fans and HVAC	Transmission follows air pathway in room; exposure in minutes; close range outdoor contact starts to become a risk
30 – 100	Face shields & distance	Avoid strong drafts and install partitions	Transmission within a few meters of subject or direct air current; exposure of <min.
> 100	Face shields & distance	Barrier and physical distancing	Indoor or outdoor transmission with very brief contacts within 6.5 feet.

Table 18.4 Particle Size and Engineering Controls[7]

---

6. https://www.thelancet.com/journals/lancet/article/PIIS0140-6736(15)00128-2/fulltext
7. https://www.aerosol.mech.ubc.ca/what-size-particle-is-important-to-transmission/

ASHRAE's Standard 241 Control of Infectious Aerosols establishes minimum requirements to reduce the risk of disease transmission by exposure to infectious aerosols in new buildings, existing buildings, and major renovations.[8]

Other Pollutants

There are certainly other pollutants that affect indoor air quality.

Radon (See Chapter 15) is a radioactive gas that is a natural decay product of radium, which is found in varying quantities in the ground virtually everywhere. Neighboring houses can have very different radon levels. It is an invisible and odorless gas that decays to progeny or daughters that can lodge themselves in the lungs and cause cancer. The Surgeon General has warned that radon is the second leading cause of lung cancer in the United States today, with over 20,000 annual radon-related lung cancer deaths. Because it is chemically inert, most inhaled radon is rapidly exhaled, but the inhaled progeny lodge in the lungs where they irradiate sensitive cells in the airways, enhancing the risk of cancer.[9] Radon concentrations are expressed in Pico-curies per liter (pCi/L). The average outdoor level is less than 0.5 pCi/L. The average U.S. indoor level is 1.3 pCi/L, but levels over 2,000 pCi/L have been measured. The EPA recommends remediation at levels above 4 pCi/L, although the risks of contracting lung cancer from radon at that level is about equal to your lifetime risk of drowning.

Smokers have a much higher risk of getting lung cancer (about 15 times greater than non-smokers) if there are elevated levels of radon in their home. The two factors are additive. If you inhale smoke, you also inhale more particulates of other things in the air. Infants, older adults, and people with compromised immune systems are at much higher risk with a combination of radon and tobacco smoke in the air.

Small amounts of radon can be released from building materials

---

8. https://blogs.duanemorris.com/esg/2023/09/24/new-ashrae-standard-241-for-indoor-air-quality-increasing-exterior-fresh-air-or-purifying-existing-indoor-air/
9. "EPA Assessment of Risks from Radon in Homes", June, 2003, https://www.epa.gov/sites/default/files/2015-05/documents/402-r-03-003.pdf
"Model Standards and Techniques for Control of Radon in New Residential Buildings" https://archive.epa.gov/epa/radon/model-standards-and-techniques-control-radon-new-residential-buildings.html

(including granite counter tops and concrete) and from the water. These levels are low enough and dissipate quickly enough so as not to be a concern. A whole dwelling ventilation system running continuously can remove those pollutants along with the rest of the chemical soup in the air.

As described previously, radon from the ground under the house should be treated as a separate ventilation issue from the rest of the air and pollutant sources in the house. As a part of new construction, many programs require the installation of radon mitigation systems under the slab with a pipe going all the way up through the roof of the house even before the house is tested. (EPA has national and state maps for estimates of radon levels by county. House by house measurement, however, is needed to determine if one particular house has radon-polluted air.)[10] If the system is installed for future use, it should still run all the way up through the roof and it should still be connected to the sub-slab system and the pipe must be labelled. It should not be terminated in the attic, and it should not be vented out through a wall. Both locations can cause problems with the pollutants flowing back into the house, and even if the piping is clearly marked, it can be confused with other piping and employed for other purposes. By venting out through the roof the pollutants are carried away from the house.

Ground moisture and other soil gases can enter the living space through diffusion, passing through the concrete walls into the living space. Air passing through the soil can pick up moisture and soil gases and move into the living space through small cracks and holes in the foundation. This is true if the basement is under negative pressure. That moisture can lead to mold and the growth of other organisms and the increased out-gassing of formaldehyde and other VOCs from building materials and furnishings. "Moisture entering the space from the ground is one of the most significant ways water vapor gets into houses. In fact, it often dwarfs the amount of moisture generated indoors by the occupants."[11] Keeping the water away from the foundation walls is a structural issue that results in an IEQ issue.

Pesticides and herbicides are poisons. They are formulated to kill creatures and plants. We apply them to our lawns and track them in on our shoes. The toxics are also drawn in through the air, moving through the soil. The herbicides spread on the lawn and even your neighbor's lawn can be drawn

---

10. EPA Map of Radon Zones, https://www.epa.gov/radon/epa-map-radon-zones
11. Bower, Understanding Ventilation, p 122

down through the soil and into your house. Chemicals such as chlordane that used to be injected into the ground around houses to prevent termites have been found in homes years after it was banned. Like the radon gas in the soil, chemicals spread on the lawn to make it beautiful and chemicals spread around the foundation walls to keep the termites, ants, and rodents away go into the soil around the house by design. Those gases are as likely as radon to get pulled into the house. Although not as common a health issue as radon, using and maintaining the radon mitigation system for other gases is a great strategy. If you suspect that pesticides and other chemicals are present in your basement, test kits are available for checking for a wide variety of pollutants including nitrogen dioxide, formaldehyde, and a variety of yeasts, bacteria, and fungus. Unfortunately, most of these tools are commercial grade and expensive.

Comfortable Air

The goal of any residential ventilation system is to surround the occupants with clean, unpolluted, comfortable air. Outside the house, people tolerate many conditions. We dress for the hot weather and the cold weather, the wind, and the rain. We don't expect the conditions to be constant.

Inside the house, however, we expect to live in a very narrow band of temperature and humidity. We expect our heating, cooling and ventilation systems to keep the air comfortable and safe. There are four factors that must be controlled to surround the occupants of the house with comfortable air: (1) temperature, (2) humidity, (3) air motion and distribution, and (4) the purity of the air or the minimization of the pollutant contents including odors, dust, toxic gases, and bacteria.

ASHRAE has defined "acceptable air quality" as, "air toward which a substantial majority of occupants express no dissatisfaction with respect to odor and sensory irritation and in which there are not likely to be contaminants at concentrations that are known to pose a health risk."[12]

ASHRAE Standard 55 defines thermal comfort as "that condition of mind that expresses satisfaction with the thermal environment". This standard is used around the world as the standard for designing, commissioning, and testing indoor spaces and systems.

---

12. ASHRAE Standard 62.2-2022

In the "Handbook of Fundamentals", Chapter 9, ASHRAE describes human comfort as emphasizing "that judgment of comfort is a cognitive process involving many inputs influenced by physical, physiological, psychological, and other processes." It also states that, "Surprisingly, although climates, living conditions, and cultures vary widely throughout the world, the temperature that people choose for comfort under similar conditions of clothing, activity, humidity, and air movement has been very similar."[13] Comfort conditions vary day to day, by age, by the adaption to the surroundings, by perceived outside conditions, by sex, and by seasonal and circadian rhythms. The heating or cooling system must allow occupants to effectively lose enough heat to permit the proper functioning the metabolic system and yet not lose heat so rapidly that their bodies become chilled. Our systems burn up the food we consume, warming our bodies so that they produce enough heat to keep our temperatures above that of our surroundings. As long as our bodies can effectively dissipate the heat produced at a rate equal to heat production, we remain comfortable.

The body dissipates heat to the ambient air moving past its surface by both conduction and convection, which is why both temperature and air motion are important comfort factors. The skin is also very effective at radiating heat to and absorbing radiant heat from surrounding objects. Our bodies are always giving up moisture to the surrounding air as long as the surrounding air is not saturated. Heating and evaporation of moisture into the air that enters the lungs also cools the core of the body. For these reasons, controlling the moisture content of the air is an important factor.

The mechanical equipment cannot automatically anticipate and adjust for all these issues and for all the occupants who will have their own momentary criteria, although controls are getting increasingly more "intelligent". Occupants like to have control over their environment. If they don't have any control and they don't understand why the system is doing what it is doing, they are likely to believe that it is defective and attempt to manually defeat it.

The heating and cooling equipment control thermal and humidity conditions and the majority of air movement through the house. The whole dwelling ventilation systems are there to remove pollutants (including humidity) and introduce fresh air into the home. Special purpose ventilation systems are there for cooling, radon, and soil gas removal, garage exhaust, attic ventila-

---

13. ASHRAE Handbook of Fundamentals, 2021, p9.1

tion, etc. And effective spot ventilation, like bathroom and range hood fans, removes moisture and pollutants at the source, improves air quality, and governs the fourth factor of indoor comfort.

Although some air motion in a room (in the 15 to 25 feet per minute range) contributes to a sense of the air being fresh, a "draft" or undesired local cooling of the human body is annoying. It causes people to want to raise the temperature or change clothing or location.

To minimize the possibility of drafts caused by the mechanical equipment, the vents (both the supplies and the returns) should be properly located and sized so that the air sweeps through the room effectively but most movement is out of the "occupied areas". This is true where bare skin will be cooled quickly, like the face or the hands or the entire torso in a bathroom.

Ventilation air supplied by HRV/ERVs or positive pressure ventilation systems is tempered but should still be delivered out of the occupied area because its temperature is commonly below skin temperature.

It is a particular challenge to supply large volumes of make-up air for clothes dryers and oversized range hoods (as described in Chapter 8). There is a serious energy cost of using electric coils to raise the temperature of the air in the room. Some make-up air can be supplied behind refrigerators where it will carry away some of the heat from the coils, but this may still cause unwanted drafts across the kitchen floor.

Another factor of air motion is the distribution of conditioned air through the house, designing the system so that there is adequate fresh air where occupants spend most of their time like bedrooms. Pockets of cold air under windows or on outside walls may allow the surface temperature to drop below the dew point, allowing mold to grow. Too much moving air can cause drafts, dry the air, and transport pollutants. Too little moving air can cause pockets where bacteria can grow and spaces that feel stale and uncomfortable.

People spend a very high percentage of their time indoors. It is critically important to their health, safety, and well-being that the systems conditioning the air surrounding them be effective and work as a system.

DALY - Disability Adjusted Life Year

Breathing "bad" or polluted air impacts living a long and healthy life. The World Health Organization *(WHO) has developed the DALY, a metric to quantify the burden of disease from mortality and morbidity.[14] One DALY equals approximately one lost year of "healthy" life. DALYs for a disease or health condition are calculated as the sum of the Years of Life Lost (YLL) due to premature mortality and Years of Life Lost due to Disability (YLD) for people living with the health condition or its consequences. There certainly is a difference between a day lived in full, normal health and a day burdened by disease or hunger or injury or asthmatic wheezing. Particulate matter ≤ 2.5 μm in aerodynamic diameter (PM2.5), acrolein, and formaldehyde accounts for the vast majority of DALY losses caused by indoor air particulates with impacts on par or greater than estimates for secondhand tobacco smoke and radon.[15] The improvement in air quality and reduction of these microscopic particulates due to improved mechanical ventilation is the new frontier and ultimate goal. When the question of the value of mechanical ventilation in a home arises, it is better to respond with an approximation of the reduction in the number of DALYs for the occupants.

---

14. https://www.who.int/data/gho/data/themes/mortality-and-global-health-estimates
15. Logue, M. et al A Method to Estimate the Chronic Health Impact of Air Pollutants in U.S. Residences, Environmental Health Perspectives, 2012 National Institute of Health/National Library of Medicine

Chapter 19

The Future of the Residential Ventilation Arts

This chapter is more about the advancement or state-of-the-art of residential ventilation than the future.

Residential ventilation has been around for a long time, and as building science and materials have changed, we have forgotten or chosen to ignore a lot of design features that were developed along the way. Some adventures in airflow are best left in the past (like double envelope houses), but some (like transoms which dynamically improved circulation) deserve another look. Clearly understanding the house and the occupants as an integrated and inter-reacting system leads to understanding the potentials of utilizing one system's waste as another system's treasure. Refrigerators, for example, expel waste heat. Could that waste heat be used to preheat incoming ventilation air? What would that mean to the operation of the refrigerator? How would it work when the incoming air was warm? Such questions inevitably lead to more questions. Unlike in the past, we now have tools to model innovative changes before we invest in them, before we build them, before we use our friends and neighbors as guinea pigs! We also have the tools to measure their performance once they have been built and installed.

If we can get the energy load down low enough, maybe we can figure out a way to effectively integrate all the comfort conditioning systems together, combining heating, cooling, and air conditioning in an energy efficient package. If the building needs less energy for conditioning, it may need less energy for conditioned air delivery and stale air removal. Smaller systems may allow for the use of smaller ducts and lower velocity airflows and more energy efficient delivery systems.[1]

The Passive House Institute [2] has been working on this for a long time. Passive House analysis is in the IECC codes as a path to compliance, but the level of rigor has not yet blended into mainstream building techniques.

Disaggregating the ventilation air may also lead to improved systems. Range hoods could provide their own make-up air. If people want to install those huge commercial hoods, they need to install huge, commercially sized, make-up air systems as well. Furnaces and water heaters should all provide their own combustion air. Most of these systems are moving to "sealed" combustion that doesn't need to draw air from the house at all. That eliminates all backdrafting issues and protects people from carbon monoxide poisoning. Central vacuums, fireplaces, wood, and pellet stoves could supply their own make-up air systems as well. Clothes dryers would work better if they drew in their own supply air. (It would be a challenge to create an effective heat exchanger that could return the waste heat from the dryer back into the living space while avoiding the lint build-up issues.) Heat pump electric dryers[3] are no longer exotic products and they don't need to vent to the outside or impact house pressure.

By compelling product manufacturers to think through their complete system process, fewer burdens are placed on the systems that condition and clean the air for the whole dwelling ventilation system.

There will undoubtedly be many, less obvious changes in ventilation design—new fan blades that are quieter and more efficient or perhaps fans without blades at all or better, more efficient motors, even fans that have neither blades nor motors! There will be better, more efficient closure systems and better controls, a myriad of tiny tweaks that all add up to more efficient systems. Even in a world as mundane as residential ventilation, things keep changing and hopefully improving.

---

1. Companies like Aldes are making multi-source ventilation systems which combines heat recovery ventilation with air purification: https://www.aldes-na.com/commercial-ventilation-product/e80-hf/
2. http://passivehouse.com/index.html
3. https://www.lg.com/my/lg-experience/helpful-hints/what-is-a-heat-pump-dryer/#:~:text=A%20heat%20pump%20dryer%20is%20a%20type%20of%20dryer%20that,a%20disadvantage%20for%20some%20users.

Airflow Rates

There is general agreement that mechanical ventilation matters in homes. There is a great deal of discussion on what the ventilation rate should be. How much air should be moved? Should it be constant or intermittent? Should the same levels apply to all homes or should there be regional rates? Certainly other parts of the world have different ventilation requirements, most higher than the U.S. rates.[4] (The EU health based recommended minimum air change rate is 0.5 ACH. That would be equivalent to a 133 cfm fan running continuously in a 2,000 square foot house.) As concerns for indoor pollutants increase, it is likely that ventilation rates will increase. Until there are better approaches for distributing the ventilation air throughout the house, higher rates may force more air to move throughout the building. As distribution and control systems improve and the cost of energy increases, rates may come down again.

We are getting a better appreciation for the amount of air that occupants need as we learn more about DALYs[5]. If houses were like personal space suits, the ventilation rate could be adjusted personally. But houses are not personal space suits. They contain multiple people, families, and friends. People perform different activities from exercising to sleeping to cooking. The required amount of fresh air goes up and down, but on average, it should meet the requirements of the occupants and the building. That average rate has been challenged by research worldwide, but the variation is small. Undoubtedly sophisticated controls and air movers can be created to flexibly adjust flow rates to meet the immediate and/or anticipated demand. But the fundamental question is why? If varying the rates improves the health of the occupants and the durability of the building, then it would be worth the cost.

---

4. McWilliams, Sherman, "Review of Literature Related to Residential Ventilation Requirements, INIVE EEIG, 2007
5. See Section 18.4

Fresh Air Sources

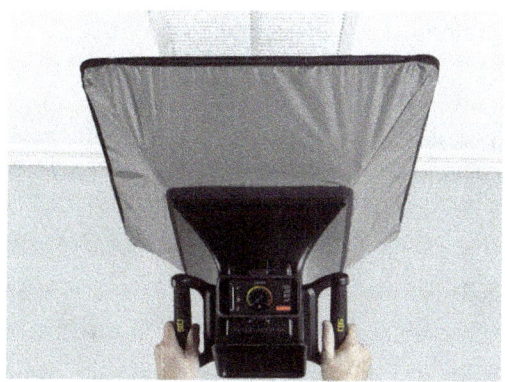

Figure 18.1 Flow Hood with Cell Phone

Traditional mechanical ventilation systems rely on the outside air being of better quality than air inside the house. Systems rely on the adage that "the solution to pollution is dilution distribution". But the air outside is not always better than the air inside. Air cleaning and purifying devices exist, and if those could be perfected, we wouldn't have to rely on the quality of the outside air at all. Our heating and cooling systems adjust the temperatures and the humidity of the air. Filters in these systems were originally designed to protect the equipment, not to clean the air moving through the house. There is a unique opportunity for the central air handling equipment to do it all: heat, cool, humidify, dehumidify, and filter. It could add a gentle odor of roses or cooking bacon. It could make the air soporific in the evening and invigorating in the morning. It could kill germs. And it could notify the occupants about what it is doing.

Much of this is already being done. Some companies are refining the earth air tempering idea that was pursued with "earth tubes". The Ground-Air heat exchangers[6] line the tubes with a proprietary silver particle-enabled antimicrobial inner layer that inhibits the growth of bacteria.[7]

Fresh air inlets—'smart holes'—that regulate the amount of incoming air have been around for a long time, but they are getting smarter. [8]The installa-

---

6. https://www.phstore.co.uk/PDF/Rehau/AWADUKT%20Thermo%20Domestic%20Installation%20Guide.pdf
7. https://www.rehau.com/gb-en/homeowners/ground-air-heat-exchanger-erth-tubes
8. https://www.aldes-na.com/ca_en/residential-ventilation-product/car3/

tion of these products requires an understanding of building pressures to be sure that they work as intended.

The air outside is not always pure, but in the future, maybe it will be[9].

Equipment & Installation

Termination fittings/hoods

There is certainly room for improvement of "termination fittings" like exterior hoods. Unconditioned air is not effectively stopped at the exterior of the building. Hoods are incredibly restrictive to airflow—they are made with too sharp a turn in order to minimize how visible they are on the outside of the house. Perhaps they should be made into an architectural element instead of trying to hide them. We used to stick television antennas on the top of our homes. A well-designed exhaust vent would be better than that. What about combining systems so that there would be fewer penetrations and hoods? In multi-family buildings, there are often three penetrations in the walls per apartment—bathroom exhaust, kitchen exhaust, and unit make-up air. If there are one hundred units in the project, that's three hundred hoods on the outside of the building. Maybe there is a way to improve ducting to make it smoother and less resistant to airflow. Or maybe there is a way to simplify installation so that the systems are installed perfectly every time. And let's step back to the design itself. How about perfect automatic system design?

HVI has a duct termination fittings certification. Certified products are listed in Section II of the Directory.[10] To achieve the desired and specified airflow, it is important to use termination fittings that have been proven to achieve the desired performance. Termination fittings can add exceptional resistance to the airflow, as you can see from the tables in Chapter 6.

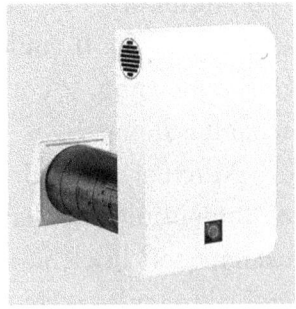

Figure 19.2 Zehnder Comfo-Air

Other Ventilation Related Equipment

---

9. Google is mapping air quality on a street by street basis. There are times when the solution to pollution in the home may not be dilution. https://www.blog.google/products/maps/lets-clear-air-mapping-our-environment-our-health/

10. https://www.hvi.org/hvi-certified-products-directory/section-ii-static-vents/

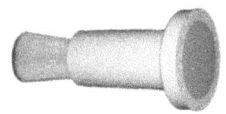

Figure 19.3 Daisy Ductless (Smart Ventilation)

Some companies are already combining ventilation with other devices. Aldes has developed the T.Flow thermodynamic water heater that recovers heat from extracted air through an air-to-air heat pump system that covers heating, cooling, and domestic hot water functions. Aldes also manufactures what they call a VentZone[11] that provides zone controlled exhaust ventilation from bathrooms that are in use that is particularly well suited for multifamily applications.

Panasonic has been pushing the window on residential ventilation products for a long time. They offer lots of options for lighting, heating, and control that make their products flexible and adaptable to a variety of situations.

HRV/ERV companies are developing sophisticated means from preheating the incoming air, moving beyond resistance coils to ground source and heat pump preheaters. These systems can be used to supply both fresh and conditioned air in very tight homes such as Phius designs.

The thing about future products is that they don't exist yet, and because of corporate competition, if companies told me about them, I would have to keep the information to myself. But the following table includes some interesting innovative products on the leading edge of the ventilation market. The more options you know about, the more informed choices you can make.

---

11. https://www.aldes-na.com/residential-ventilation-product/vz/

Product	Description
Broan-NuTone Evolve Premium Bath Fan	Advanced motor and TrueCFM™ technologies
Broan AI Series Fresh Air System	Uses AI to automatically adjust to changing indoor and outdoor conditions
Broan Fresh In supply fans	Algorithm that monitors outdoor conditions for optimal fresh air
Broan Bluetooth® Fans	Fans with stereo speakers and multi-color LEDs
Zehnder America ComfoAir 70 energy recovery unit	Single room through-the-wall ERV
Vents-US TwinFresh Comfo RA-50 ERV	Single room ERV up to 343 ft^2 that uses 5.61 watts
Vents-US Vents Micra 100 (Freshbox)	Single room ERV with a MERV 8 and MERV 14 filtration and Wi-Fi enables
Lunos e^2 ductless, through-the-wall HRV	In-Out low airflow units that are installed on either side of the room
Soler & Palau Total Recovery Low Profile ERV	A low ceiling ERV with MERV 8 filters designed for low ceiling residences and multifamily homes
Soler & Palau TRCeN/TRCe ERV	A resin core ERV for heat transfer
Soler & Palau TD-MIXVENT In-line mixed flow duct fan	Removable body

Table 19.1 Products

Controls

Electronics now allow us to control anything. Our cell phones can talk to our houses and our heating systems, our ventilation systems, and our refrigerators and dishwashers. We can automatically water the plants and feed the cat. It won't be long before we can communicate with the house and tell it to improve the air. We just have to figure out what that means, and since each of us is different, whose air are we improving?

Ventilation controls can be designed that recognized occupant levels in the house counting people coming in and going out or monitoring the level of CO_2 and increase the ventilation rate when a party is going on. (These have been available for a while but are generally priced out of the range of residential applications.) Integrated systems are available that cause bathroom fans to "talk" to each other, cycling from one to the next to make sure that there is some circulation in the house. Motion detectors and movement sensors delay off and cycling timers are all presently available for bathroom fans. Mixed gas sensors are available that measure a combination of gases to boost or activate HRVs and ERVs. "Smart" ventilation controls can take advantage of sophisticated electronics to do almost anything. A system that ran less when the outside air was colder could respond to the higher natural driving force from the greater temperature differential. Would the difference in run time be worth the extra cost? Just because it could be done doesn't mean it should be done!

What if there was a control that could evaluate the outside air conditions measuring the pollutant levels, the temperature, the humidity, particulates, and anything else that people should not be breathing? And if the outside air was "worse" than the inside air, the control activated an indoor air quality cruncher that reconditioned the existing air in the house? It might need to add some oxygen or something else to the air to purify it or make it smell better.

Do we really need to have a ventilation system that continuously delivers and removes the same amount of air all the time? A continuously operating system is simple and has less that can go wrong with it. It doesn't depend on operator knowledge to make adjustments. But from an energy efficiency standpoint, the ventilation system only needs to be working at a time and at a rate to get its job done.

A radon/soil gas mitigation system, for example, runs 24 hours a day, 7 days a week, sucking the soil gas out from under the house. But are the levels of soil gas and radon constant? Could the system be controlled so that the extraction rate varied in relation to the conditions? There are a lot of complexities to accomplish that, but it is something for the future to think about. What about garage ventilation? Does that flow rate need to be constant or could it be varied in relation to pollutant and pressure levels? Could the system "learn" when homeowners generally start and remove their cars, turn the system on in anticipation, anticipating when the occupants are coming home, and make sure that system runs long enough to get rid of all the gases? Should cars have CO sensors on them that would activate the ventilation system in the garage if the air surrounding them became polluted, or should they just shut themselves off so that the people in the house wouldn't die?

Airflow Measurement

The ability to measure performance will make the greatest changes in ventilation systems in the future. The problem in writing about the future is that each word ahead of this one was the future at some point. And now it's the past. Computer modeling is helping us to determine the effects of air distribution throughout homes based on assumed removal of contaminants. That, in turn, may lead to new approaches to fresh air delivery and pollutant removal systems.

Measurement tools can help us determine how well installed systems are working. Knowing what a ventilation system does in the test laboratory is very nice and a great place to start, but how is it actually working now that it has been installed? It is important to know how well the system is working when it has been installed and how well it continues to work. Building codes and green building programs describe what the installed system airflows need to be. Measuring the low flows of installed systems is difficult because of building and site pressures. Improvements in technology will help to bring down the cost of accurate and reliable testing equipment. Some manufacturers are building flow indicators into their equipment so that changes in performance can be monitored in real time. That means that homeowners have to have some understanding of what their ventilation system is for and how they should maintain it. That sort of "feedback" has proven to be an exceptionally good modifier of behavior.

The challenge is to measure really small airflows accurately. If the air is moving into or out of a fan in all directions simultaneously, in some cases flowing and in others just trickling, how can we capture all that movement, add it up, and come up with a consistent result? And how can we do all that instantaneously and inexpensively? If inspectors can't afford the measuring equipment, the results are not likely to be consistent and replicable.

Standards have to be written with reasonable levels of tolerance. A couple of cubic feet of airflow one-way or the other doesn't make much difference in a house.

Occupant Knowledge

Homeowner understanding and knowledge must change if there is going to be an impact on how we all use energy. Understanding smoke detectors and CO detectors and changing the furnace filters and setting thermostats and turning off lights in unused rooms are all occupant behavior issues that can have a major impact on how much energy we use. When the heating system was a massive fireplace in the middle of the house, everyone knew when it needed more wood. Central heating systems were relegated to the basement. Grilles and radiators were refined into artistic elements or hidden under boxes. Ventilation systems were made so quiet that it is impossible to know that they are running without some sort of indicator light. Home occupants just assume that the surrounding air will be magically warm or cool and clean and comfortable. Many don't know where their thermostat is, what it is for, or how to set it. Should we continue to make these things less obvious and more automatic, or should we force people to get more involved with the operation of their homes? Perhaps equipment manufacturers should do more to make their products more user friendly, less dependent on contractors to change filters, adjust settings, or replace batteries. Maybe we need nagging voices in machines that would say, "You haven't changed my filter in 12 months. It's not good for you to breathe this air. Wipe your feet when you come into the house and change my filter. Do it now before you forget!" (On the other hand, maybe voices in machines are not such a great idea. Remember the nagging seat belt voices in cars?)

* * *

AI version – Crystal Ball

Since this chapter is about the future of residential ventilation products, I thought it would be fitting to ask Artificial Intelligence about its opinion. The following is what AI came up with when I asked it in January 2025. The text is completely AI generated:

The Future of Residential Ventilation in the United States: Codes, Standards, and Technologies

The future of residential ventilation in the United States is set to be shaped by a combination of stringent building codes, evolving standards, and cutting-edge technologies aimed at improving indoor air quality (IAQ), energy efficiency, and occupant health. As environmental concerns and consumer awareness grow, residential ventilation systems are transitioning from basic, code-minimum solutions to smarter, more holistic systems that integrate seamlessly with modern building practices.

Code and Standard Evolution

The tightening of energy codes, such as those outlined by the

International Energy Conservation Code (IECC) and the American Society of Heating, Refrigerating, and Air-Conditioning Engineers (ASHRAE), will continue to drive advancements in residential ventilation systems. The following trends are anticipated:

1. **Stricter IAQ Requirements:** The next decade will see updates to ASHRAE Standard 62.2, which governs residential ventilation. Expect more stringent minimum airflow requirements and mandates for pollutant source control. This could include provisions for mitigating outdoor pollutants like wildfire smoke and localized air quality issues, driven by climate change concerns.
2. **Energy-Efficiency Integration:** Federal and state energy codes will increasingly require balanced ventilation systems, such as heat recovery ventilators (HRVs) and energy recovery ventilators (ERVs). These systems exchange heat or moisture between incoming and outgoing air, minimizing energy loss while ensuring fresh air supply.
3. **Resilience Standards:** Following natural disasters and public health crises, codes may mandate ventilation systems designed for resilience. Systems will likely need to provide consistent IAQ during power outages, extreme weather events, or airborne health emergencies.

Technological Advancements

The adoption of new technologies will transform residential ventilation, focusing on smart systems, health monitoring, and sustainability.

1. **Smart Ventilation Systems:** The integration of IoT (Internet of Things) technologies will enable advanced, demand-controlled ventilation (DCV). These systems will use real-time data from sensors to optimize airflow based on occupancy, CO_2 levels, humidity, and pollutant concentrations, reducing energy use and enhancing comfort.
2. **AI and Predictive Maintenance:** Artificial intelligence will play a critical role in monitoring and managing ventilation systems. Predictive algorithms will alert homeowners or building

managers to maintenance needs before system failures occur, ensuring consistent operation.

3. **Advanced Filtration and Air Purification:** With a heightened focus on health, ventilation systems will increasingly incorporate high-efficiency particulate air (HEPA) filters and UV-C light to eliminate pathogens and allergens. Advanced materials and technologies, like photocatalytic oxidation, will further enhance indoor air cleaning capabilities.

4. **Integration with Renewable Energy:** Ventilation systems will align with broader sustainability goals, integrating with solar or wind energy systems to operate efficiently off-grid. Battery-powered backup options will also gain popularity to ensure continuity during outages.

Market Trends and Adoption Drivers

Several factors will influence the pace of adoption for advanced residential ventilation systems:

1. **Consumer Awareness:** Homebuyers are becoming more educated about IAQ and energy efficiency. Builders and developers will respond by offering ventilation systems as key features in new construction.

2. **Affordability and Incentives:** The widespread adoption of advanced systems will be bolstered by decreasing costs of technologies and financial incentives. Federal and state programs may offer rebates or tax credits for installing energy-efficient ventilation systems.

3. **Focus on Retrofitting:** While new construction will lead the adoption curve, retrofitting existing homes with improved ventilation systems will gain momentum. This will be particularly relevant for aging housing stock in urban areas where IAQ challenges are pronounced.

Challenges and Opportunities

The transition to advanced residential ventilation will face challenges, including upfront costs, homeowner education, and the need for skilled labor to install and maintain complex systems. However, these obstacles present opportunities for innovation and workforce development.

Companies and professionals in the HVAC industry will play a crucial role in shaping this evolution, offering solutions that balance cost, efficiency, and performance. Collaborations with health and environmental experts will further refine standards and practices.

Conclusion

The future of residential ventilation in the United States is one of increasing sophistication, driven by evolving codes, advancing technologies, and heightened consumer awareness. By addressing the intersecting needs of health, energy efficiency, and environmental resilience, these systems will redefine the concept of "home," providing safer, cleaner, and smarter living environments for generations to come.

END OF AI INPUT.

* * *

That's not exactly Jules Verne or Star Trek, but as important as residential ventilation is, it will never be earth shattering, cutting edge technology. The industry will just get incrementally better and better at keeping the occupants of homes safe.

Appendix A - Acronyms and Abbreviations

Acronym Translations:

- ACCA: Air Conditioning Contractors of America
- ACH: air changes per hour
- ACH_{50}: air changes per hour at 50 Pascals of depressurization
- ACH_N: natural air changes per hour
- AFS: averaging flow station
- ASEF: apparent sensible effectiveness
- ASHRAE: American Society of Heating, Refrigerating, and Air-Conditioning Engineers

- Bhp brake horsepower
- BRE Building Research Establishment
- BTL building tightness limit
- Btu British thermal unit

- CATU Compact Air Treatment Unit
- CAZ combustion appliance zone
- ccf hundred cubic feet
- CDD cooling degree-days
- CEC California Energy Commission
- cfd computational fluid dynamics

- c.f. cubic foot
- cfm cubic feet per minute
- CFM_{50} cubic feet per minute at 50 Pascals of depressurization
- cps centipoise
- CO carbon monoxide
- CO_2 carbon dioxide
- CSA Canadian Standards Association

- DALY disability-adjusted life year
- dB decibel
- dBA decibels measured on the 'A' scale
- DCV demand-controlled ventilation
- ΔP pressure differential
- DTL depressurization tightness limit

- ECM Electronically commutated motor
- ELA effective leakage area (U.S.)
- EPA Environmental Protection Agency
- EqLA equivalent leakage area (Canadian)
- EER energy efficiency ratio (related to SEER)
- ERV enthalpy or energy-recovery ventilator
- ESL Energy Systems Laboratory
- ETL Electrical Testing Labs (Intertek)
- EQ Environmental Quality

- fpm feet per minute
- fms flow measuring station

- GAMA Gas Appliance Manufacturers' Association

- HDD heating degree-days
- HEPA High Efficiency Particulate Filter
- H_2CO formaldehyde
- H_2O water
- HRAI Heating, Refrigeration, and Air-Conditioning Institute of Canada
- HRV heat recovery ventilator

- HVAC heating, ventilating, and air-conditioning
- HVI Home Ventilating Institute

- IAQ Indoor Air Quality
- IAP Indoor Air Pollutants
- IEQ Indoor Environmental Quality
- IBC International Building Code
- ICC International Code Council
- IECC International Energy Conservation Code
- iwg (or i.wc.) inches of water on a pressure gauge or inches of water column
- IMC International Mechanical Code
- IPMC International Property Maintenance Code
- IRC International Residential Code for One and Two Family Dwellings

- KWh kilowatt-hour

- L/s liters per second
- L^3/h cubic liters per hour
- LEED Leadership in Energy and Environmental Design

- m^3/s cubic meters per second
- m.c. moisture content
- MCS Multiple Chemical Sensitivity
- MERV minimum efficiency rating value
- MET Lab Maryland Electrical Testing
- MPR Microparticle Performance Rating (3M Filtrete filters)
- MVC Minimum ventilation capacity

- NBC National Building Code of Canada
- nfa net free area
- NO_x Nitrogen oxide
- NL normalized leakage

- OTL overall tightness limit

- Pa Pascal
- PAV Powered Attic Ventilator
- pCi/L picocurie per liter
- ppm parts per million
- psi pounds per square inch
- psia pounds per square inch absolute
- psig pounds per square inch gauge
- PSV Passive Stack Ventilation
- PTAC Packaged Terminal Air Conditioner

- Q airflow

- RH relative humidity
- rpm revolutions per minute
- RSS reference sound source

- SEER Seasonal Energy Efficiency Ratio
- SLA Specific leakage area (ELA/floor area)
- SMACNA Sheet Metal and Air conditioning Contractors' National Association
- SWS Standard Work Specifications
- sp static pressure or system pressure
- sq. ft. square foot
- sq. in. square inch
- SRE sensible recovery efficiency

- TD or ΔT temperature differential
- TP Total pressure
- TRE total recovery efficiency

- UL Underwriter Laboratories
- USGBC United States Green Building Council

- VOC volatile organic compound
- VP Velocity pressure

- W watt

- w.g. water gauge
- WAP Weatherization Assistance Corporation
- Wh watt-hour
- WHO World Health Organization
- WRT with respect or reference to

- YLD Years Lost due to Disability
- YLL Years of Life Lost

Appendix B - Useful Formulas, Values, and Multipliers

Formulas:

Formula names are links to the location.

- Friction resistance of flex ducting Chapter 6
- Stack effect Chapter 7
- Jumper duct sizing Chapter 8
- Size of an under-door slot for pressure relief Chapter 8
- Straight through-the-wall grille covered pressure relief Chapter 8
- Airflow through a known size hole and pressure difference Chapter 9
- Airflow with known velocity and area Chapter 9
- Airflow measurement with a pitot tube Chapter 9
- Fan Law #1 Chapter 14
- Fan Law #2 Chapter 14
- Fan Law #3 Chapter 14
- Net Free Area Chapter 16
- HRV/ERV delivered air temperature Appendix H

Conversion values:

Multiply:	By:	To obtain:
BTU	0.29305	Watt-hours
Cubic Feet per minute (CFM)	0.471947	Liters/Second (L/s)
CFM	0.028317	Cubic Meters/min (m³/min)
CFM	1.699	m³/h
Fahrenheit (degree)	(T-32) x 0.555	Centigrade (degree)
Foot	0.3048	Meters
Foot	304.8	mm
Feet per minute (fpm)	0.00508	m/s
Gas		
Cubic Foot (natural gas)	1,028	BTUs
Therm	100,000	BTUs
Gallon of Propane	91,000	BTUs
Horsepower	42.42	BTUs/minute
Horsepower	0.7457	Kilowatts
Horsepower	746	Watts
Inch of water gauge (iwg)	248.64	Pascal
Inch of mercury (in. hg)	3,386	Pascal
Kilowatt-hours	3412	BTUs/hour
Oil Gallon	139,000	BTUs (100% efficiency)
Meters/second (m/s)	200	fpm (more accurately 196.9)
Watts	3.413	BTUs/hour
Watts	0.00134	Horsepower

Appendix C - Glossary

The following terms are defined relative to the content of this book. Some of them have other meanings. For example "defrost mechanisms" are used in refrigerators as well as in HRVs.

A

Absolute humidity: The weight of water in a given volume of air, commonly expressed in pounds of water per pound of dry air or grains of moisture per cubic foot. See also relative humidity.

Accidental pressure: A difference in air-pressure between the indoors and the outdoors induced by mechanical devices whose primary purpose is not ventilation.

Accidental ventilation: The unintentional movement of air into and out of a house caused by accidental pressures.

Air barrier: Material used to block the flow of air into a building.

Air change rate or **air changes per hour** (ACH): The number of times in one hour that the volume of air in a house is replaced with outdoor air, sometimes expressed at 50 Pa pressure difference (ACH_{50}) between the indoors and outdoors.

Airflow grid: A device that mounts inside a duct (often temporarily) that can be connected to an air-pressure gauge or manometer to sample a cross section of the airflow through a duct to determine the volume of flow.

Air handler: A cabinet for a conditioning system containing a blower that moves air through a system of heating/cooling ducts.

Air leakage: the uncontrolled exchange of air between the interior and exterior environments through unintentional openings in the thermal envelope of the building. See also infiltration and exfiltration.

Airtight construction: A building technique that reduces as many openings for unintentional airflow that results in a house with a small ELA. (Equivalent Leakage Area) A key component of a Zero Energy House (ZEH).

Air-to-air heat exchanger: A ventilation device designed to be balanced, capable of transferring heat (and sometimes moisture) between two air streams without merging the stream. See also heat recovery ventilator.

Ambient: Surrounding conditions.

Ambient temperature: The temperature that surrounds an object on all sides.

Anechoic chamber: A room designed to attenuate sound.

Adjusted Sensible Recovery Efficiency (ASRE): The net sensible energy recovered by the supply airstream as adjusted by case heat loss or heat gain, air leakage, airflow mass imbalance between the two airstreams and the energy used for defrost (when running the Very Low Temperature Test), as a percent of the potential sensible energy that could be recovered. This value should be used for energy modeling when wattage for air movement is separately accounted for in the energy model.

Adjusted Total Recovery Efficiency (ATRE): The net total energy (sensible plus latent, also called enthalpy) recovered by the supply airstream adjusted by case heat loss or heat gain, air leakage and airflow mass imbalance between the two airstreams, as a percent of the potential total energy that could be recovered. This value is used to predict and compare Cooling Season Performance for the HRV/ERV unit. This value should be used for energy modeling when wattage for air movement is separately accounted for in the energy model.

Aspect ratio: The ratio of the width to the depth particularly of a duct.

Atmospheric Pressure: The weight of air and its contained water vapor on the surface of the earth. At sea level this pressure is 14.7 pounds per square inch. (Based on NFPA 54)

Axial fan: A type of air moving device that has propeller-like blades, often used for window fans and moving air between spaces with little resistance.

B

Backdraft damper: A device that allows air to only flow in only one direction.

Backdrafting: Complete reversal of flow in the chimney of a fuel fired appliance, usually due to negative pressures indoors. Combustion products are forced back down the chimney into the living space.

Balanced ventilation: A ventilation strategy that results in the house experiencing a neutral pressure with an equal mechanical flow of air moving into and out of the space.

Balancing: The process of adjusting the flows of a ventilation system so that the house experiences a neutral pressure.

Balancing damper: A device that is mounted in the ducting that allows the ventilation system to be balanced. These generally include a "fixing" method that locks the damper in place once balance has been achieved.

Balometer: An airflow capture hood or flow hood used to measure air flow in an HVAC system.

Barometric damper (or draft regulator): A draft control device intended to stabilize the natural draft in an appliance by admitting room air into the venting system.

Biological pollutants: Air particulates and pollutants such as mold and pollen, that either are or once were alive or the by-products of metabolism.

Blower door: A large fan that mounts temporarily in a doorway used to pressurize or depressurize a house to evaluate its tightness.

Breathing zone: See headspace.

British thermal unit (BTU): The heat energy required to raise the temperature of 1 pound of water 1 °F, used in calculating building conditioning loads.

Building envelope: The exterior portion of a structure that keeps the weather out.

Building Tightness Limit (or Building Airflow Standard (BAS), Minimum Ventilation Level (MVL), Minimum Ventilation Rate (MVR): A term used for a house tightening limit used for ensuring adequate air quality for the occupants of the house.

Burner: A device for the introduction of fuel into the combustion zone for ignition.

Natural draft burner: A burner not equipped with a fan or blower.

Fan assisted burner: A burner with combustion air supplied by a mechanical device such as a blower at sufficient pressure to overcome the resistance of the burner only.

Forced draft burner: A burner with combustion air supplied by a mechanical device such as a blower at sufficient pressure to overcome the resistance of both the burner and the appliance.

Bypass: A pathway or hole through a building, usually hidden within the structure that bypasses the air boundary of the building envelope.

C

Capital cost: The installed or first cost of equipment (i.e. the equipment itself, incidentals expenses, and labor. (See also operating cost.)

Carbon dioxide (CO_2): A colorless, odorless gas released in exhaled breath, or by a combustion process.

Carbon dioxide sensor: A device that senses the carbon dioxide concentration in the air (usually in ppm or parts per million) and can be used to control a ventilation system based on human occupancy of a space.

Carbon monoxide (CO): A colorless, odorless, poisonous gas released during the incomplete combustion of carbon-containing fuels that in low concentrations causes headaches and nausea and flu-like symptoms and in high concentrations can cause coma and death.

Carbon monoxide detector: A device that senses carbon monoxide in the air and sounds an alarm when the concentration reaches a certain point.

Carcinogen: A substance that may cause cancer.

Centrifugal fan: A ventilating fan with blades that allow the spinning blades to throw off the air by centrifugal force.

Central exhaust ventilation: see Exhaust-Only Ventilation

Central supply ventilation: see Supply-Only Ventilation

Chase: A vertical space created to house pipes or ducts. A chase can be open all the way from the basement to the attic.

Chimney: A vertical structure or conduit that encases at least one flue and usually carries combustion by-products out of a house. See also ventilating chimney.

Chlordane: A persistent chlorinated hydrocarbon pesticide that is noticeable because of its odor used for the treatment of termites.e

Circulation fan: The blower in the air handler that draws the return air in from the house and pushes the conditioned air back to the rooms.

Coanda effect: The physical phenomena that describes how air or water in motion follows a curved surface.

Coaxial vent: A venting system consisting of an inner pipe to exhaust air within an outer pipe drawing in replacement air. Used for both combustion systems and heat exchangers.

Combustion air: Air that enters a house specifically to be used for satisfactory combustion of a fuel. See also ventilation air.

Combustion by-products: Gases and particulates released during the burning of a fuel. Includes inert gases that are part of the air but not excess air.

Comfort zone: The range of effective air quality conditions including temperature and humidity over which a majority (>50%) of adults feel comfortable.

Condensation: The change of a gas or vapor into a liquid, accompanied by the release of heat; the opposite of evaporation.

Conditioned space: The part of a house, within the building envelope, that is designed to be maintained at a comfortable temperature and humidity.

Conductance (thermal): The rate of heat flow through a unit area of a material per unit of temperature difference. Designated in a 'U' value. The lower the 'U' value the slower heat moves through the material, the better the insulation value.

Conduction (thermal): The process of heat transfer moving through a material from the warmer side to the cooler side.

Continuous duty: An electrical safety rating for motors, not the same as continuous use. Most motors are rated for continuous duty.

Continuous use: A rating that a fan is capable of running for an indefinite period of time, not the same as continuous duty. Not all motors are rated for continuous use.

Convection (thermal): The transfer of heat that takes place within moving gases and liquids. Moving warm air is continuously replaced by a flow of cooler air.

Cubic feet per minute (cfm): Free area in square feet times the face velocity in feet per minute (fpm).

Critical Exhaust Condition (CEC): The design condition used to determine the likely level of depressurization cause by the operation of the ventilation system plus the clothes dryer plus any exhaust appliance with an exhaust capacity larger then 160 cfm.

D

Disability-Adjusted Life Year (DALY): One DALY equals one lost year of "healthy" life.

Damper: A movable device, motorized or manually adjustable or reliant on gravity, used to vary or control the airflow in a duct. See also backdraft damper and modulating damper.

Decibel (dB): A logarithmic unit of measurement used to express sound intensity.

Defrost mechanism: A device used in HRVs and ERVs to melt ice that builds up in the core in cold climates.

Degree-day: A unit of measurement used to estimate fuel consumption and heating or cooling costs based on temperature and time. For heating this is generally set at 65 °F (18 °C). If the temperature drops below 65 °F (18 °C) by 1° for an hour, that would be 1 degree hour. Multiplying by 24 would be one degree day.

Dehumidistat: A control device that can be used to activate a ventilation or dehumidification system that makes contact as the relative humidity rises. Used to decrease the humidity in the space. See also Humidistat.

Delta Pressure (ΔP): The difference in pressure from one space to another. ΔP will also be expressed in relation to or with respect to (WRT) another space.

Delta Temperature (ΔT): The difference or change in temperature.

Demand-controlled ventilation (DCV): The process of automatically supplying air to, and removing air from, a space whenever needed by the occupants often associated with a CO_2 control.

Depressurization: When the air pressure inside a house is less than the atmospheric pressure outside the house. The rate at which air leaves the house exceeds the rate at which air enters the house.

Desiccant: A drying agent that absorbs moisture, used in some energy-recovery ventilators to enhance moisture transfer between airstreams.

Design temperature: The temperature used for sizing a heating or cooling system.

Dew point: The temperature at which air is saturated with moisture (100% relative humidity) and below which condensation will occur.

Diffuser: An outlet grille designed to spread out the airflow in a room for proper mixing.

Diffusion: The migration of molecules of a gas or a vapor (or a liquid) from an area of high concentration to an area of low concentration.

Dilution: The mixing of fresh air into polluted air to reduce the concentration of pollutants; also applies to liquids.

Dilution air: Air that is drawn together and mixes with combustion by-products prior to their being expelled from a house through a natural draft chimney.

Direct vent (sealed combustion): A type of fuel-fired appliance that takes its combustion air directly from the outdoors and ejects its combustion gases directly back to the outdoors through an independent sealed vent. The exhaust gas temperatures of these systems are usually low enough to allow the use of plastic vent piping.

Displacement ventilation: A method of moving air through a room, pushing the fresh, air in at the floor level and allowing to rise through the space, generally only used in specialized applications.

Distribution: Movement of air throughout the rooms of a house through ducting or through the rooms themselves.

Downdraft: An exhaust system that draws the air down and out of the building often applied to kitchen exhaust fans.

Draft: The pressure difference that causes a current of air or gases to flow through a flue, chimney, or space. Also an uncomfortable breeze or current of air in a room. See also natural draft.

Draft hood or draft cap: a draft control device having no moveable parts that may be built into a combustion appliance or vent connector that is designed to reduce the effect of stack action by drawing dilution air into the flue.

Dry bulb temperature: The temperature of the air indicated by an accurate thermometer. The common measurement of temperature, but referred to "dry bulb" to distinguish it from wet bulb temperature.

Drying potential: The ability of a substance to dry after it becomes wet.

Duct: A conduit for conducting air to intended spaces, made from a variety of materials and in a variety of shapes.

Duct, branch: A conduit for carrying air to or from only one grille or register.

Duct, trunk: A conduit for carrying air to or from multiple grilles or registers.

Ductboard: A fiberglass board material with an aluminum-foil facing on one side, used to construct ducts. Affectionately called "fuzzy-duct".

E

Earth tube: A pipe through the ground for moving air from the outdoors into the living space, used for tempering incoming air.

Effective leakage area (ELA): The size of a special, nozzle shaped opening that a house would have if all the small random holes between the indoors and the outdoors were combined into one hole. Used in the U.S. and based on a pressure of 4 Pa. It is the same concept as equivalent leakage area, but is calculated differently.

Effective length: The length of a duct or system path equal to the total of the actual duct length and the equivalent lengths of all the fittings. Used in system design.

Electrically (or Electronically) commutated motor (ECM): An ultra high efficiency, programmable brushless DC motor using a permanent magnet rotor and a built-in inverter. ECM motors are electrically efficient especially at low speeds. They usually include their own speed control.

Electrostatic air filter: An air filter made of plastic materials that capture particulate pollutants using static electricity.

Electrostatic precipitator: An air filter that uses a high voltage to cause particulates to become electrically charged and cling to metal plates having an opposite charge.

Energy-Recovery or Enthalpy Recovery Ventilator (ERV): An air-to-air exchanger that recovers both latent heat and sensible heat.

Enthalpy: The total amount of heat contained in air that is the sum of the sensible heat and the latent heat.

Entrain: To draw in used to describe the ability of airflow to carry particulates.

Equivalent length: The length of straight duct that would have the same resistance to airflow as a fitting. It is expressed in terms of feet of ducting of the same diameter of the fitting, which would have the same resistance to airflow.

Equivalent leakage area (ELA): The area of a single, square-edged hole that a house would have if all the individual random holes between the inside and the outside were combined into one hole. This number is primarily used in Canada and is based on a pressure of 10 Pa. It is the same concept as effective leakage area, but is calculated differently.

Evaporation: The changing of a liquid to a gas or vapor, by adding latent heat. See also condensation.

Exfiltration: Uncontrolled air leaving a house through random holes in the structure moved by building pressure differentials. See also infiltration.

Exhaust air: The air mechanically leaving a house through a ventilation system and not reused. See also supply air.

Exhaust grille: A grille through which "used" air leaves a room. See also supply grille.

Exhaust-Only or Central Exhaust Ventilation: A mechanical system that depressurizes a building in order to change the air, relying on gaps in the building shell to make up for the air removed.

Exchange rate: The speed at which indoor air is replaced with outdoor air

F

Fan: A device that moves air.

Filtration: The process of extracting pollutants from the air.

Flame rollout: Flames pushed outside a combustion chamber as a result of backdrafting.

Flat plate core: A device that is used in some HRVs or ERVs to transfer heat (and sometimes moisture) between two airstreams without mixing the two streams.

Flue: An enclosed conduit, pipe or passageway for conveying combustion gases out of a building; sometimes known as a stack.

Flue gases: A combination of combustion gases and excess air.

Forced draft: A mechanical system that uses a fan to inject air into the combustion chamber of a combustion appliance.

Formaldehyde: A gas found in indoor air, often used as a binder for building materials, consisting of 1 carbon atom, 2 hydrogen atoms, and 1 oxygen atom.

Free area: see Net free area (NFA)

Fresh air: Air that has not been polluted.

Fresh-air duct: A conduit used to guide unpolluted air into a building.

Furnace: A flue connected, space-heating appliance that uses warm air as the heating medium commonly including an air handler and the provision to attached return and supply ducting.

G

General ventilation: Distributed fresh air supply and return for the health and comfort of the building's occupants.

Grille: A duct covering on a wall or ceiling through which air moves to or from the conditioned space. Grilles are generally fixed and non-adjustable.

Grill: A grating that supports comestibles cooking over a fire.

H

Headspace: The breathing zone in a room. In a residence it usually extends from a few inches to about 6 feet off the floor.

Heat-recovery ventilator (HRV): A ventilation device capable of transferring heat between two airstreams without blending the streams. See also air-to-air heat exchanger and energy recovery ventilator (ERV).

HEPA filter: A very high-efficiency particulate air filter, often used in hospitals and laboratories. A HEPA filter is supposed to remove 99.97% of 0.3 micron particulates from the air flowing through it and 100% of the particulates larger than 1 micron.

Humidistat: A control device that activates and ventilation or humidification system that makes contact as the relative humidity falls. Used to increase the humidity in the space. See also dehumidistat.

Humidity: See absolute humidity and relative humidity.

Hydroxyl Radicals (OH): A powerful oxidant short lived highly toxic oxidant that not good to breath. It is the most reactive oxygen radical known.

It may be found in air "purifying" products with the marketing name of *nanoe*™.

Hygrometer: A device that measures relative humidity.

I

Inches of mercury (in. hg. or "hg.): A unit of atmospheric pressure measurement or a height of a column of mercury.

Inches of Water Column (IWC): A non-metric unit of pressure difference. One IWC is about 250 Pascals.

Inches of water gauge (iwg or "wg): A unit of atmospheric pressure measurement or a height of a column of water.

Induced draft: A system utilizing a fan or blower often located in the flue to exhaust air from the combustion chamber of a combustion appliance.

Infiltration: Uncontrolled air entering a house through random holes in the structure moved by building pressure differentials. See also exfiltration.

In-line fan: A ventilating fan made to attach a duct on both the inlet and the outlet sides.

Intentional ventilation: Purposeful air movement into and out of a building in a regular way, usually caused by a fan moving air through intentional openings.

Ionizer: A device that generates ions (usually negatively charged), ostensibly for cleaning the air to mimic natural ionization caused by lightning.

J

Jump duct: A short duct connection between two rooms through that "jumps" over the separating wall through which air can move when pressure imbalances occur. Also called a jump-over, jumper, or transfer duct.

K

Kilowatt hour (kWh): A unit for electrical energy measurement equal to 1,000 watts of power consumed over an hour.

L

Latent heat: The energy required in the change of state without a change in temperature or the amount of heat that must be removed from air to change the water vapor from a gas to a liquid or a liquid to a gas. See also enthalpy and sensible heat.

Local exhaust ventilation: A localized ventilation system near the source of air pollutants. See also general ventilation and spot ventilation.

M

Magnehelic gauge: An analog pressure-measuring device.

Make-up air: Outdoor air that enters a house to replace air that is exhausted from the house. It does not include air entering the house as combustion air or to replace air lost through exfiltration.

Manometer: A gauge for measuring air-pressure differences.

Media filter: A pleated filter that relies on a fibrous material, usually polyester or fiberglass, to physically strain particulates out of the air. See also electrostatic air filter and electrostatic precipitator.

MERV rating: A filter rating system developed by ASHRAE via Standard 52.2 (Minimum Efficiency Reporting Value). The higher the MERV rating the more effective the filter is at removing smaller particles.

Micron: A millionth of a meter.

Mildew: Fungus or mold that grows primarily on surfaces.

Minimum ventilation capacity (MVC): In the CSA F326 Standard this is a capacity set by room count (5 L/s per room except the Master Bedroom at 10 L/s, and 10 L/s for a basement area exceeding 2/3 of the total basement area. The same as Total Ventilation Capacity.

Mixed-gas sensor: A device that senses oxidizable gases in the air.

Modulating damper: A motorized closure system whose opening can be adjusted to regulate a volume of airflow.

Mold: A slimy or powdery growth caused by fungi. Molds require oxygen, moisture and a food source such as cellulose to grow.

Motion sensor: A device that senses movement that can be used to control a ventilation system by assuming room occupancy.

Multi-port ventilator: A ventilation device having a number of ports from running ducts to or from different rooms. See also single-port ventilator.

N

Natural draft: The negative pressure in a chimney caused by rising, warm combustion by-products often referred to simply as draft. This flow of gases relies on thermal buoyancy to vent the combustion products. The upward force must be greater than any resisting forces (including negative pressure) in the building envelope.

Natural pressure: The difference in air-pressure between the indoors and the outdoors induced by natural phenomena such as wind, stack effect, and diffusion

Natural ventilation: Random air movement into and out of a house caused by natural pressures through intentional openings like windows and unintentional cracks and holes.

Negative ions: Negatively charged atoms or groups of atoms that will cling to oppositely charge surfaces.

Negative pressure: See depressurization.

Net free area (nfa): "The amount of unobstructed open area of a grille, inlet, or outlet. HVI Certified products actually measure the flow through the opening rather than estimating the area blocked by the louvers. Sometimes known as the 'K' factor."

Neutral pressure: Air pressure that is neither positive nor negative with respect to another space.

Neutral pressure plane: The point of a house that experiences neutral pressure as a result of stack effect.

O

Olf: A unit of odor measurement equal to the amount of body odor produced by one person performing normal activities in one day.

Operating cost: The cost of operating equipment including electrical cost, conditioned air cost, and maintenance costs. See also capital cost.

Outgassing (off-gassing): The release of volatile gases from the surface of a solid material as a part of aging, decomposition, or curing.

Ozone (O3): An unstable form of oxygen (O2) consisting of three oxygen atoms, that can be produced in small amounts by electric motors, electrostatic precipitators, ionizers, etc.

Ozone generator: A device that creates ozone designed to react with air pollutants to neutralize them.

P

Partial-bypass filter: A filter that removes some contaminants from the air by extracting a portion of the return airflow, filtering it, and then returning it to the primary flow.

Particulate: A microscopic fragment of a solid or droplet of a liquid that is suspended in the air.

Parts per million (ppm): A unit of measurement commonly used to express the concentration of pollutants in the air.

Pascal (Pa): A metric unit of pressure measurement useful in diagnosing houses.

Passive ventilation: A non-mechanical general-ventilation strategy that utilizes natural or accidental pressures, that involves air movement through intentional inlets and outlets.

Permanent-split-capacitor motor: A type of electric motor that includes a primary winding and an auxiliary winding wired in series with a capacitor.

Pesticides: Chemical compounds formulated to exterminate living creatures.

Picocurie per liter (pC/l): A measurement unit of the concentration of radon.

Pitot tube: A device for measuring total pressure, static pressure, and velocity pressure within a duct.

Plenum: An element of the air-moving conduit where the air moving to or from the air-handling device is gathered.

Pounds per square inch (psi): A unit of pressure measurement. 1 psi equals 144 pounds per square foot.

Pressure drop: The static pressure loss caused by airflow through a duct, filter, or heat or energy exchanger core.

Pressurization: When the air pressure inside a house is greater than the atmospheric pressure outside the house. This occurs when the rate of air entering the house exceeds the rate at which air is leaving.

Primary ventilation system or whole dwelling ventilation system: The principal air moving system (usually mechanical) that circulates air through a building to control the overall air quality to ensure the health of the occupants and the building.

Psychometric chart: A chart that is used by engineers to graphically determine the moisture content of air at different temperatures.

R

Radon: A naturally occurring carcinogen often released as a radioactive gas from soil and rocks.

Radon daughters: The natural radioactive decay particulates of radon, some of which release harmful radiation and can lodge in the lungs.

Recirculate: To move air through a space without adding fresh air or removing polluted air.

Recirculating range hood: A range hood that has no duct and recirculates the air moving through it and is not connected to the outdoors.

Register: A duct termination fitting that can be adjusted to regulate the amount or direction of airflow.

Relative humidity (RH): The amount of moisture in the air, usually expressed as a percentage, compared to the maximum amount of moisture that air at that temperature can contain. See also absolute humidity.

Return air: Air moving from the living space that is drawn back to an air handler to be reconditioned.

Ridge vent: An opening at the ridge of the house usually covered by a cap that allows the attic air to flow out. The air flows in through vents located in the soffits. See also soffit vents.

Rotary core: A slowly rotating wheel that is used in some air-to-air heat exchangers to transfer heat and moisture between two airstreams.

S

Sealed combustion: A system used in some furnaces, boilers, fireplaces, and water heaters that are immune pressure imbalances in a house because it draws combustion air into a combustion chamber from the outdoors and expels combustion by-products to the outdoors within totally enclosed pipes and chambers.

Sensible heat: The amount of heat involved in raising or lowering the temperature of air not including the heat required to cause water vapor to change state (e.g. from a gas to a liquid): heat that can be "sensed". See also enthalpy and latent heat.

Sensible recovery efficiency (SRE): "A measurement of heat recovery that does not include latent that is useful in comparing the amount of energy passed between airstreams in a heat-recovery ventilator. It is corrected for the effect of motor heat gain, defrost energy, cross leakage gain and other effects like casing gain. It will usually be lower than apparent sensible effectiveness of the HRV.

Shaded pole motor: A type of motor whose starting torque is provided by a copper ring called a "shading coil" that delay the phase of magnetic flux.

Soffit vents: Intentional openings in the soffits that allow air to flow in and upward to the ridge vent and out of the attic, ostensibly to keep the roof surface cooler.

Sone: A linear unit of sound measurement used to express low level sound intensities. Two sones are twice as loud as one sone.

Sound attenuator: A sound muffler.

Source control: The principle of controlling the polluting materials in the living space.

Specific heat: The quantity of heat required to change the temperature of a substance by one degree.

Spillage: A situation where some combustion by-products spill into the living space rather than go up the chimney due to insufficient draft.

Spot ventilation: Ventilation for the direct removal of air pollutant near a source. See also local-exhaust ventilation.

Stack effect: The naturally phenomena of warm air exerting pressure on cooler air that results in warm air rising.

Static pressure: The amount of outward pressure exerted against the walls of a duct or airway, created by the friction and impact of air as it moves.

Supply air: The air entering a house through a ventilation system or HVAC system. See also exhaust air.

Supply grille: A grille through which air is delivered to a room. See also exhaust grille.

Supply-Only or Central Supply Ventilation: A positive pressure mechanical ventilation system that pressurizes the building relies on natural leakage to establish flow.

T

Temperature difference (TD or ΔT): The difference in temperature between two volumes of air.

Tempering: The conditioning of outdoor air so it will more closely match the temperature and humidity of the indoor air of the building it is entering.

Thermal boundary: The boundary that thermally separates the interior, conditioned space of a building from the exterior environment.

Through-the-wall vent: An intentional opening in an exterior wall through which a controlled quantity of air is allowed to move. See also trickle ventilator.

Total recovery efficiency (TRE): The energy recovered in an air-to-air heat exchanger that compensates for the fan energy and cross-leakage.

Total pressure: A non-existent pressure that expresses the sum of static and velocity pressures.

Total Ventilation Capacity Condition: The maximum amount of air that a ventilation system can supply to a space. (TVC is the ventilation rate which is required by the applicable code).

Transfer grille: A term used to describe the opening between rooms that allows for the equalization of pressure. See jump duct.

Trickle Ventilator: An intentional opening between the interior and the exterior of a building intended to equalize the pressure and provides for the transfer of polluted and fresh air.

Turbulent flow: The irregular swirling of air particles in an air-stream that offers more resistance than laminar flow.

V

Vapor diffusion retarder: A material used to block the flow of vapor through a structure.

Ventilating chimney: A vertical structure, pipe or conduit designed to passively carry ventilation air into or out of a house.

Ventilation: The process of intentionally supplying air to or removing air from or moving air around a house, most often with a fan, for the health and comfort of the occupants. See also controlled ventilation.

Ventilation air: Air that intentionally enters a house for the purpose of ventilating. See also combustion air.

Volatile organic compound (VOC): Molecular compounds

containing carbon that easily evaporate, often released from building materials and found as contaminants in indoor air. See also outgassing.

W

Wet bulb temperature: The temperature measured by the wet-bulb thermometer of a psychrometer.

Wetting potential: The ability of a substance to sequester moisture after it has dried out. See also drying potential.

Whole house fan or whole house comfort ventilator: A fan used to exhaust air from a space specifically for the purpose of enhancing the natural cooling effect of moving air through a house.

Appendix D - References

Adams, Nate, June, 2016, http://energysmartohio.com/uncategorized/which-indoor-air-quality-monitors-are-best-and-why/

Anderson, Bruce (with Michael Riordan). 1976. *The Solar Home Book*. Harrisville, NH: Cheshire Books.

ASHRAE Guideline 24-2008. 2008 *Ventilation and Indoor Air Quality in Low-Rise Residential Buildings*, Atlanta: American Society of Heating, Refrigerating and Air-Conditioning Engineers, Inc.

ASHRAE. 2008. *Handbook 2008, HVAC Systems and Equipment*. Atlanta: American Society of Heating, Refrigerating and Air-Conditioning Engineers, Inc.

ASHRAE. 2005. *Handbook 2005, Fundamentals*. Atlanta: American Society of Heating, Refrigerating and Air-Conditioning Engineers, Inc.

ASHRAE Standard 62.2-2022 *Ventilation and Acceptable Indoor Air Quality in Residential Buildings*. Atlanta: American Society of Heating, Refrigerating and Air-Conditioning Engineers, Inc.

Axley, J. 2001. Residential Passive Ventilation Systems: Evaluation and Design, AIVC Technical Note 54, 158 pp, Code TN 54.

Baldwin, Peter C. 2003, How Night Air Became Good Air, 1776 - 1930, Environmental History, Vol 8, No. 3 (July, 2003) pp. 412 - 429

Bean, R. 2009. Residential Indoor Air Quality Awareness. Mississauga: Heating, Refrigeration and Air Conditioning Institute of Canada.

Begley, Jr., E. 2008. *Living Like Ed*. New York: Clarkson Potter Publishers.

Billings, John S. M.D., LL. D., 1889, *The Principles of Ventilation and Heating and their Practical Application*, The Engineering & Building Record

Bleier, F. 1998. *Fan Handbook, Selection, Application and Design*. New York: McGraw-Hill.

Bower, J. 1995. *Understanding Ventilation*. Bloomington: The Healthy House Institute.

Brennan, T. and Turner, W. 1985. "Indoor Air Quality Problems & Solutions", Northeast Sun, June. 9-11.

Brennan, T. and Clarkin, M. 1985. *A Guide to Ventilating a House*. Albany: New York State Energy Research and Development Authority.

Brumbaugh, J. 2004. *HVAC Fundamentals*. Danvers: Wiley Publishing.

Buchan, William Paton, 1893. *Ventilation, A Text-book to the Practice and Art of Ventilating Buildings: with a Supplementary Chapter upon Air Testing*, J.S. Virtue and Co., Limited, London

California Department of Health Services, "Health Hazards of Ozone-generating Air Cleaning Devices, 1998", www.cal-iaq.org/03_fact.htm

Chen, Dr. B. and Wang, Dr. T and Maloney, Dr. J. and Ennenga, Prof. J. and Newman, M. 1984. *Measured Cooling performance of Earth Contact Cooling Tubes*. Progress in Solar Energy, American Solar Energy Society.

Corbett, Robert J. & Miller, Barbara. 1984. *Heat Recovery Ventilation For Housing: Air-to-Air Heat Exchangers*. The National Center for Appropriate Technology (DOE/CE/15095-9)

Cummings, J. and Withers, Jr., C. 2006. *Unbalanced Return Air in Residences: Causes, Consequences, and Solutions*. Florida Solar Energy Center, *ASHRAE Transactions*.

Dumont, R.S. and Makohon, J.T. 1997. Characterization of Volatile Organic Emissions from Building Materials for Indoor Environment Assessment. EEBA Journal, Winter/Spring. 12-16.

Edwards, R. 2005. Handbook of Domestic Ventilation. Amsterdam: Elsevier, Butterworth-Heinemann.

Emmerich, S. and Gorfain, J. and Huang, M. and Howard-Reed, C. 2003. Air and Pollutant Transport from Attached Garages to Residential Living Spaces. NIST, NISTIR 7072.

Emmerich, S. and Persily, A. 1996. Multizone Modeling of Three Residential Indoor Air Quality Control Options. Gaithersburg: NISTIR 5801.

Fugler, D, 2000, Is it Worth Putting in a Better Furnace Filter? Home Energy Magazine, May/June.

Fugler, D. 2004. The Impact of Vacuuming. IAQ Applications, ASHRAE, 5 (3): 1-3.

Greiner, T. and Schwab, C. 1998. Carbon Monoxide Exposure from a Vehicle in a Garage. Thermal Envelopes VII/Indoor Air Quality and Sustainability Practices. 209-216.

Greiner, T. 1998. The Silent Killer: Carbon Monoxide. Iowa State University, January.

Greiner, T, 2005. Wholistic approaches to CO. Affordable Comfort Conference, Indianapolis.

Grimsrud, D. 2004. Intermittent Ventilation and Standard 62.2. IAQ Applications, ASHRAE, Fall. 8 – 9.

Hayes, V. and Shapiro-Baruch, I. 1994. Evaluating Ventilation in Multifamily Buildings", Home Energy. July/August. 23-30.

Havrella, R. 1981. Heating, Ventilating, and Air Conditioning Fundamentals. New York: Gregg Division of McGraw-Hill Book Company.

Health Canada. 2007. Air Cleaners Designed to Intentionally Generate Ozone (Ozone Generators) – Questions and Answers https://www.canada.ca/en/health-canada/services/air-quality/indoor-air-contaminants/ozone.html

Hickory Consortium. 1999. Analysis of Current Practice and Advanced Ventilation Strategies for Residential Buildings. Building America Initiative, Deliverable 2.A.1, February.

Hood, I. 2004. *Garage Performance Testing*. The Sheltair Group for CMHC, January.

HRAI. 2004. Residential Mechanical Ventilation. Mississauga: Heating, Refrigeration and Air Conditioning Institute of Canada.

Indiana Community Action Association. 2007. Weatherization Assistance Program Indiana Field Guide, Chapter 5, Airflow".

Janssen, J. 1999. The History of Ventilation and Temperature Control. ASHRAE Journal, September. 47-52

Jennings, B. 1970. Environmental Engineering – Analysis and Practice. New York: International Textbook Company.

Kadulsky, R, 1988. Residential Ventilation: Achieving Indoor Air Quality. Solplan Review

Kadulsky, R, 2001. Attached Garages and Indoor Air Quality. Solplan Review, March.3-5.

Karg, R. 2001. Survey of Tightness Limits for Residential Buildings, July, 2001. For the Chicago Regional Diagnostics Working Group.

Kelley, M. 1995. *Ventilation System Performance in Energy Crafted Homes*, Building Science Engineering, November.

Krigger, J. and Dorsi, C. 2009. *Residential Energy*. Helena: Saturn Resource Management.

Lawrence, F.V. 1986. *Natural Energy Systems in Traditional Tibetan Buildings*. Sunstone Design.

Lstiburek, J. 2006. *Understanding Attic Ventilation*. Building Science Digest 102.

Manclark, B. 1999. *Oversized Kitchen Fans – An Exhausting Problem*. Home Energy Magazine, January/February.

May, J. 2001. *My House is Killing Me!* Baltimore: The Johns Hopkins Press.

McKone, T.E., and Sherman, M. 2003. *Residential Ventilation Standards Scoping Study*. LBNL Technical Assistance for PIER, LBNL-53800, October.

McWilliams, J. 2002. *Review of Airflow Measurement Techniques*. Energy Performance Buildings Group, LBNL-49747.

McWilliams, J, and Sherman, M. 2007. *Review of Literature Related to Residential*

Ventilation Requirements. Lawrence Berkeley National Laboratory. INIVE EEIG.

Offerman, F. et al 2008. *Window usage, ventilation, and formaldehyde concentrations in new California homes*, Indoor Air 2008 Conference, August.

Palmiter, L. and Brown, I. 1989. *The Northwest Infiltration Survey*. ECOTOPE; Washington State Energy Office

Parker, D, and Sherwin, J. 2000. *Performance Assessment of Photovoltaic Attic Ventilator Fans*. Florida Solar Energy Center (FSEC), FSEC-GP-171-00. http://www.fsec.ucf.edu/en/publications/html/FSEC-GP-171-00/

Pekkinen, J. 1993. *Thermal Comfort and Ventilation Effectiveness in Commercial Kitchens*. ASHRAE Journal, July. 35 – 38.

Raymer, P. 2005. *Make Room For The Caddy*. Home Energy Magazine, March/April. 21-23.

Rizzi, E. 1980. *Design and Estimating for Heating, Ventilating and Air Conditioning*. New York: Van Nostrand Reinhold Company.

Rizzuto, J, 1989. An Investigation of Infiltration and Indoor Air Quality. NYSERDA 90-11.

Rizzuto, J. et al. 1985. Indoor Air Quality, Infiltration and Ventilation in Residential Buildings. NYSERDA 85-10.

Rose, W. and TenWolde, A. 2002. Venting of Attics & Cathedral Ceilings. ASHRAE Journal, October: 26 – 33.

Rudd, A. 2006. Ventilation Guide. Westford: Building Science Press.

Rudd, A. and Bergey, Daniel. 2014. Ventilation Effectiveness and Tested Indoor Air Quality Impacts. DOE, Buildings Technologies Office, February, 2014

Seppänen, O. and Fisk, W. and Mendell, M. 2002. Ventilation Rates and Health. ASHRAE Journal, August. 56 – 58.

Sherman, M. and Walker, I. Can Duct-Tape Take The Heat? Energy Performance of Buildings Group, Lawrence Berkeley National Laboratory, University of California, LBNL- 41434.

Sherman, M. and Walker, I. 2007. *Energy Impact of Residential Ventilation Standards in California*. Environmental Technologies Division, LBNL- 61282.

Sherman, M. 2008. *On the Valuation of Infiltration towards Meeting Residential Ventilation Needs*. Environmental Energy Technologies Division, Lawrence Berkeley National Laboratory, University of California, LBNL- 1031E.

Shurcliff, W. A. 1981 *Air-to-Air Heat Exchangers for Houses*. Published by the author

Sonne, J and Parker, D. 1998. *Measured Ceiling Fan Performance and Usage Patterns: Implications for Efficiency and Comfort Improvement*. ACEEE Summer Study on Energy Efficiency in Buildings, Vol. 1.

Steven Winter Associates. 2006. *Evaluation of Three Ventilation Systems in Chicago Homes, Final Report for Field Evaluation of PATH Technologies*. March, 2006

Tohn, Ellen, 2016, *Occupant Health Benefits of Residential Energy Efficiency*, E4TheFuture

Tooley, J. 1995. *Duct Diagnostics*. Affordable Comfort Conference, March, 1995.

Vent-Axia, *Fan Selector*. https://www.vent-axia.com/tools-services/fan-selector.

Walker, I. 2003. *Garbage Bags and Laundry Baskets – Homemade air flow diagnostic tools get professionally tested*. Home Energy Magazine, November/December. 20-23

Walker, I. 2014. *Houses are Dumb without Smart Ventilation*, Lawrence Berkeley National Laboratory, May, 2014
http://escholarship.org/uc/item/22m9243j#page-1

World Health Organization (WHO). 2007. *Development of WHO guidelines for indoor air quality: dampness and mould, Working group meeting*. 2007.

Yberg, I. 2004. *Indoor Air – The Silent Killer*. Växjö: Svensk Ventilation.

Yberg, I. 2005. *Shortness of Breath – A hand book about the air in our homes*. Växjö: Svensk Ventilation.

Appendix E - Organizations & Resources

This section includes trade associations, places to learn, and organizations that are working with energy efficient, tight housing that require mechanical ventilation. Please note that because the world changes so fast, addresses, phone numbers, web sites and even names may have changed.

* * *

Conferences:

Better Buildings: Better Business - Wisconsin Conference
   The heart of the conference revolves around networking with a thousand or so building professionals dedicated to constructing high quality, energy efficient homes.
   https://b4conference.org/

BuildingEnergy NYC
   Conference and trade show sponsored by the Northeast Sustainable Energy Association (NESEA)
   https://www.nesea.org/buildingenergy-conferences-trade-shows
   50 Miles Street
   Greenfield, MA 01301
   Phone: 413-774-6051

Energy and Environmental Building Association (EEBA)

Annual Conference - EEBA provides education and resources to transform residential design, development and construction industries to deliver energy efficient and environmentally responsible buildings and communities.

www.eeba.org
6520 Edenvale Boulevard, Suite 112
Eden Prairie, MN 55346
Phone: 952-881-1098

Energy OutWest

A biennial building science conference and training session held in one of the western states.

http://www.energyoutwest.org/
360.890.4440

Greenbuild

Annual conference focusing on international green building technologies sponsored by the USGBC.

https://greenbuildexpo.com/

Home Performance Coalition (Formerly Affordable Comfort, Inc.)

HPC presents some of the most informative building science conferences around the country.

http://www.homeperformance.org/
1187 Thorn Run Ext. Suite 340
Moon Township, PA 15108
Phone: 412-424-0039

JLC Live New England

Conference and trade show for residential construction professionals in Providence, RI.

https://ne.jlclive.com/

* * *

Organizations:

Air Infiltration and Ventilation Center (AIVC)

The AIVC offers industry and research organizations technical support aimed at optimizing ventilation technology. AIVC offers a range of services and facilities, including comprehensive database on literature standards, guides, technical notes and ventilation data. www.aivc.org

INIVE eeig
Lozenberg 7
B-1932 Sint-Stevens-Woluwe
Belgium
Phone: +32 2 655 77 11

BuildingGreen, LLC

An organization committed to improving the environmental performance and reducing the adverse impact of buildings. (Publisher of Environmental Building News and GreenSpec)

www.buildinggreen.com
122 Birge Street Suite 30
Brattleboro, VT 05301
Phone: 802-257-7300

Building Performance Institute (BPI)

BPI offers nationally-recognized training, certification, accreditation and quality assurance programs.

www.bpi.org
107 Hermes Road, Suite 110
Malta, NY 12020
Phone: 877-274-1274

Canadian Mortgage and Housing Corporation (CMHC)

CMHC is Canada's national housing agency whose mission is to enhance the quality, affordability and choice of housing in Canada. CMHC has an excellent resource

library that include a great deal of data and articles on residential ventilation and IAQ issues for both Canada and the U.S.

www.cmhc-schl.gc.ca

700 Montreal Road
Ottawa, Ontario, Canada K1A 0P7
Phone: 613-748-2000

Delmar Cengage Learning
On-line learning for the Building Trades and Construction and numerous other fields.
www.informationdestination.cengage.com

Earth Share
Helping individuals and organizations care for our environment for more than 20 years
http://www.earthshare.org/
7735 Old Georgetown Road, Suite 900, Bethesda, MD 20814
Phone: 800-875-3863 / 240-333-0300
Fax: 240-333-0301
Email: info @ earthshare.org

The Engineering Toolbox
A wide array of engineering information, tools, charts and conversion factors.
www.engineeringtoolbox.com

Enterprise Green Communities
The first national green building program developed for affordable housing.
www.greencommunitiesonline.org
10227 Wincopin Circle, Suite 500
Columbia, MD 21044
Phone: 410-715-7433

Interstate Renewable Energy Council (IREC)
An independent not-for-profit organization that makes clean, efficient, sustainable energy possible for more Americans through forward-thinking regulatory reform, quality workforce development and consumer education.
http://www.irecusa.org/
PO Box 1156

Latham, NY 12110-1156
Phone: 518-621-7379
info@irecusa.org

National Center for Healthy Housing
NCHH is a nonprofit based in Columbia, MD dedicated to creating safe and healthy homes for children.
www.nchh.org
10320 Little Patuxent Parkway, Suite 500
Columbia, MD 21044
Phone: 410-992-0712

National Comfort Institute
www.nationalcomfortinstitute.com
PO Box 2090
Sheffield Lake, OH 44054
Phone: 800-633-7058

National Renewable Energy Lab (NREL) - Standard Work Specifications
Basic details on installing just about everything in a house
https://sws.nrel.gov/

Northeast Sustainable Energy Association (NESEA)
www.nesea.org
50 Miles Street
Greenfield, MA 01301
413-774-6051

North American Technician Excellence (NATE)
www.natex.org
2111 Wilson Blvd., Suite 510
Arlington, VA 22201
Phone 877-420-NATE

Residential Energy Dynamics
Tools and explanations particularly for mechanical ventilation
http://www.residentialenergydynamics.com/

Residential Energy Services Network (RESNET)

RESNET supports the HERS (Home Energy Rating System) index of home efficiency that is recognized by financial institutions, for federal tax incentives and the EPA's Energy Star™ Program.

    www.natresnet.org
    PO Box 4561
    Oceanside, CA 92052-4561
    Phone: 760-806-3448

United States Department of Energy

The programs at the DOE are extensive and in flux. This is a great place to start searching for government info.

    https://energy.gov/energysaver/ventilation

United States Environmental Protection Agency (EPA)

Instigator, manager, and purveyor of the Energy Star programs including Energy Star for Homes Indoor Air Plus. Includes a listing of all the ventilating fans that are classified as ENERGY STAR at: https://www.energystar.gov/

    1200 Pennsylvania Ave. NW
    Washington, DC 20460
    Phone: 888-782-7937
    www.energystar.gov

U.S. Green Building Council (USGBC)

Instigator, manager, and purveyor of the LEED programs.
    www.usgbc.org
    Washington, DC
    Phone: 800-795-1747

Yestermorrow Design/Build School

Yestermorrow inspires people to create a better, more sustainable world by providing hands-on education that integrates design and craft as a creative, interactive process.

    www.yestermorrow.org
    189 VT Route 100
    Warren, VT 05674
    Phone: 802-496-5545

Appendix E - Organizations & Resources 405

* * *

Trade Associations:

Air-Conditioning, Heating and Refrigeration Institute (AHRI)

A national trade association of manufacturers of central air conditioning, warm-air heating, and commercial and industrial refrigeration equipment.

https://www.ahrinet.org/
2111 Wilson Blvd, Suite 500
Arlington, Virginia 22201
Phone: 703-524-8800

Air Conditioning Contractors of America (ACCA)

A national trade association of heating, air conditioning, and refrigeration systems contractors. Publishers of Manual J and Manual D.

www.acca.org
2800 Shirlington Road Suite 300
Arlington, VA 22206
Phone: 703-575-4477

Air Diffusion Council (ADC)

An organization that was formed to promote the interests of the manufacturers of flexible air ducts and related air distribution equipment. Detailed flexible ducting installation materials.

www.flexibleduct.org
1000 E. Woodfield Road Suite 102
Schaumburg, IL 60173
Phone: 847-706-6750

Air Movement and Control Association International, Inc. (AMCA)

AMCA is a not-for-profit association of the world's manufacturers of fan, louvers, dampers, air curtains, airflow measurement devices, ducts, acoustic attenuators and other air system components. It is primarily a commercial product organization.

www.amca.org
30 West University Drive
Arlington Heights, Illinois 60004

847-394-0150

American Gas Association (AGA)
The AGA develops residential gas operating and performance standards and maintains system performance and statistical records.
www.aga.org
151400 North Capitol Street, N.W.
Washington, DC 20001
Phone: 202-824-7000

American Society of Mechanical Engineers (ASME)
A non-profit technical and educational association offering educational and training services and conducting technology seminars and on-site training programs
https://www.asme.org/
Three Park Ave
New York, NY 10016
Phone: 800-843-2763

Heating, Refrigeration and Air Conditioning Institute of Canada (HRAI)
Skill-Tech Academy – Ventilation training and IAQ resources (not just for Canada!)
www.hrai.ca
2800 Skymark Avenue, Building 1, Suite 201
Mississauga, Ontario, Canada L4W 5A6
Contact HRAI for further information at 1-800-267-2231 or 905-602-4700 ext. 246

Home Ventilating Institute (HVI)
HVI is a nonprofit trade association representing residential ventilation products sold in North America. HVI certifies the performance of residential ventilation products through a very carefully controlled testing process.
www.hvi.org
1000 N Rand Rd.
Suite 214
Wauconda, IL 60084
Phone: 847-526-2010

Indoor Air Quality Association, Inc.

A nonprofit, multi-disciplined organization, dedicated to promoting the exchange of indoor environmental information, through education and research for the safety and well being of the general public.

www.iaqa.org
12339 Carroll Ave.
Rockville, MD 20852
Phone: 301-231-8388

International Building Performance Simulation Association

IBPSA advances and promotes building and environmental performance simulation to improve the design, construction, operation, and maintenance of the built environment worldwide.

https://ibpsa.org/
PO Box 939
Britton, SD 57430

Heating, Air-conditioning & Refrigeration Distributors International (HARDI)

HARDI is a national trade association of wholesalers and distributors of air conditioning and refrigeration equipment.

www.hardinet.org
3455 Mill Run Drive Suite 820
Columbus, OH 43026
Phone: 614-345-4328
Toll Free: 888-253-2128

National Association of Home Builders (NAHB)

NAHB is a trade association that helps promote the policies that make housing a national priority.

www.nahb.org
1201 15th Street, NW
Washington, DC 20005
Phone: 202-266-8200

National Association of the Remodeling Industry (NARI)

NARI's core purpose is to advance and promote the remodeling industry's

professionalism, product & vital public purpose.
>   www.nari.org
>   780 Lee Street Suite 200
>   Des Plaines, Illinois 60016
>   Phone: 800-611-NARI (6274)

Sheet Metal and Air Conditioning Contractors National Association (SMACNA)

An international trade association of union contractors who install ventilating, warm-air heating, air-conditioning, and air handling equipment.
>   www.smacna.org
>   4201 Lafayette Center Dr.
>   Chantilly, VA 20151
>   Phone: 703-803-2980

* * *

Test, Certification, Professional, and Standards Organizations:

American Society of Heating, Refrigerating, and Air-Conditioning Engineers (ASHRAE)

ASHRAE is an international professional organization concerned with the advancement of the science and technology of heating, ventilation, air conditioning, and refrigeration. ASHRAE maintains Standard 62.2 for residential ventilation.
>   www.ashrae.org
>   1791 Tullie Circle NE
>   Atlanta, GA 30329
>   Phone: 800-527-8400

Canadian Standards Association (CSA)

CSA is the Canadian equivalent of UL. The test products to both Canadian and U.S. standards, issue the CSA mark and require product maintenance inspections.
>   http://www.csagroup.org/
>   178 Rexdale Boulevard

Toronto, ON Canada M9W 1R3
Phone: 866-797-4272

International Code Council (ICC)
A membership association dedicated to building safety and fire protection and the developer of codes used to construct residential and commercial buildings, including homes and schools.
www.iccsafe.org
500 New Jersey Avenue, NW
Washington, DC 20001-2070
Phone: 888-422-7233

Intertek Testing Laboratories (ETL)
The ETL mark is a compliance mark for North American safety standards.
http://www.intertek.com/contact/
480 Neponset Street, Suite 9C
Canton, MA 02021
781-821-2355

MET Laboratories (Eurofins)
Product safety approvals and regulatory certification of electrical products.
http://www.metlabs.com/
33439 Western Ave.
Union City, CA 94587

Texas A&M Energy Systems Laboratory (ESL)
The test and research facility for the heating ventilation and air conditioning industry. Used by HVI for the Certification of ventilation products.
https://esl.tamu.edu/
Texas Engineering Experiment Station
Riverside Campus – Building 6502
3100 S.H. 47 Bryan, TX 77807
Phone: 979-845-6334

Underwriter Laboratories, Inc. (UL)

UL is an independent, nonprofit product safety testing and certification organization.

www.ul.com
333 Pfingsten Road
Northbrook, IL 60062
Phone: 8467-272-8800

Appendix F - Equipment Sources

Fans and Ventilation Equipment:

Note that many of these companies are members of the Home Ventilating Institute and have certified products. Contact information for all the HVI related companies can be found at: https://www.hvi.org/hvi-member-listing/

Active Ventilation Products, Inc.
    Manufacturer of a variety of attic and roof ventilation products.
    www.roofvents.com
    P.O. Box 1521
    Newburgh, NY 12551-1521
    Phone: 800-247-3463

Aero Pure
    Manufacturer of a variety of ventilation products.
    www.aeropurefans.com
    1006 Bankton Circle
    Suite B
    Hanahan, SC 29410
    Tel: 843.377.8642
    Fax: 843.377.8643

Airia Brands, Inc.
Manufacturers of the Lifebreath HRVs and ERVs.
www.lifebreath.com
511 McCormick Boulevard
London, ON N5W 4C8
Phone: 519-457-1904

Air-King
Manufacturer of a wide range of residential ventilation products.
www.airkinglimited.com
820 Lincoln Ave.
West Chester, Pa 19380
Phone: 610-436-1454

American Aldes
Manufacturer of a wide range of unique ventilation products.
https://www.aldes-na.com/residential-ventilation/
4521 19th Street Court East Suite 104
Bradenton, FL 34203
Phone: 800-255-7749

Brink Flair
Manufacturer of high performance HRV/ERV products.
www.475.supply/
334 Douglass St.
Brooklyn, NY 11217
Phone: 800-995-6329

Broan-NuTone
Manufacturer of a variety of consumer products including numerous ventilation fans.
www.broan-nutone.com
926 West State Street
Hartford, WI 53027-1098
Phone 262-673-4340

Build Equinox

Appendix F - Equipment Sources 413

The manufacturer of the CERV, fully integrated HVAC system.
http://www.buildequinox.com/
1103 N. High Cross Road
Urbana, IL 61802
Phone: 773-492-1893

Deltabreez

The manufacturer of quiet bathroom fans.
https://www.deltabreez.com/
46101 Fremont Boulevard
Fremont, CA 94538
Phone: 877-685-4384

DewStop

The manufacturer of ventilation control systems.
https://www.dewstop.com/
GTR Technologies, Inc.
1420 Lumsden Road
Port Orchard, WA 98367
Phone: 360-876-2974

Enervex

The manufacturer of the premier chimney top fan systems.
https://enervex.com/
1685 Bluegrass Lakes Parkway
Alpharetta, GA 30004 USA
Phone: 800-255-2923

Fantech

Manufacturer of in-line fans and air-to-air heat exchangers
www.fantech.net
Systemair
Lenexa, KS
Phone: 800-747-1762

Flaktwoods

Manufacturer of iris dampers and associated ventilation products

http://www.flaktwoods.com/products/
Herne Headquarters
Südstraße 48
44625 Herne
Germany
+49 2325 468 00
info@flaktgroup.com

Heyoka Solutions, LLC

Products for ventilation and building analysis, product development, education, and the home of the author of this book.
www.HeyokaSolutions.com
157 Palmer Ave.
Falmouth, MA 02540
Phone: 866-389-8578

Greenheck

Mostly commercial fans & dampers. Some innovative residential products.
http://www.greenheck.com/
PO Box 410
Schofield, WI 54476
Phone: 715-359-6171

Hunter

The manufacturer of bathroom fans and other ventilation products.
www.hunterhomecomfort.com
2260 Northwest Parkway, Unit I
Marietta, GA 30067
Phone: 888-880-FANS

Imperial Air Technologies, Inc.

Manufacturer of the Greentek and Imperial lines of ventilation products.
www.imperialgroup.ca
480 Ferdinand Boulevard
Dieppe, NB E1A 6B9
Phone: 888-724-5211

Lipidex (AirCycler)
   Manufacturer of ventilation control systems.
   www.aircycler.com
   411 Plain Street
   Marshfield, MA 02050
   Phone: 781-834-1600

Lunos
   Through-the-wall HRV system.
   www.475.supply/
   334 Douglass St.
   Brooklyn, NY 11217
   Phone: 800-995-6329
   718-622-1600

Minotair Ventilation, Inc.
   Manufacturer of multi-function air exchangers
   https://www.minotair.com/home_us/
   282D Industrial Road
   Gatineau, QC J8R 3N9
   Canada
   819-777-2454
   855-888-2292

Nu-Air Ventilation Systems, Inc.
   Manufacturer of a variety of air-to-air heat exchangers and controls
   www.nu-airventilation.com
   16 Nelson Street
   Windsor, NS B0N 2T0
   Phone: 902-798-2261

Panasonic Ventilation Systems
   A source of extremely quiet, efficient and well made fans and ventilation related products.
   https://na.panasonic.com/
   One Panasonic Way 1H-3
   Secaucus, NJ 07094

Phone: 866-292-7292

Quality Aluminum Products
Manufacturer of aluminum siding, soffits, fascia, trim coil and rain carrying products.
www.qualityaluminum.com
Flat Rock
Michigan, U.S.
Phone: 734-783-0990

Renewaire, LLC
Manufacturer of air-to-air heat and energy exchangers and bath fans.
www.renewaire.com
4510 Helgesen Drive
Madison, WI 53718
Phone: 800-627-4499

Reversomatic
The manufacturer of a variety of residential & commercial ventilation products.
www.reversomatic.com
790 Rowntree Dairy Road
Woodbridge, ON L4L 5V3
Phone: 800-810-3473

SmartVentilation, Inc.
Manufacturer of innovative fan products
http://smartventilation.com/

Soler & Palau U.S.A.
Manufacturer of in-line fan products.
www.solerpalau-usa.com
6393 Powers Ave.
Jacksonville, FL 32256
Phone: 800-961-7370

Spruce Environmental Technologies

The manufacturer of in-line and radon mitigation fans & products.
www.spruce.com
3 Saber Way
Ward Hill, MA 01835
Phone: 800-355-0901

Therma-Stor

Manufacturer of excellent dehumidification equipment.
http://www.thermastor.com/
Therma-Stor LLC
4201 Lien Rd.
Madison, WI 53704
Phone: 800-533-7533

Universal Metal Industries

Manufacturer of a wide range of residential ventilation products including bath fans and range hoods.
https://universalmetalproducts.com/
800 W. Grant
Phoenix, AZ 85007-2409
Phone: 800-875-3654

Venmar Ventilation

Venmar makes heat exchangers, range hoods and other residential ventilation products.
https://www.nortekair.com/about/our-brands/venmar/
550 Lemire Blvd
Drummondville, (Quebec) Canada J2C 7W9
Phone: 800-567-3855

Ventamatic Ltd

Manufacturer of the NuVent residential ventilation products and numerous other fans.
www.bvc.com
100 Washington Street
Mineral Wells, TX 76068
Phone: 800-433-2626

Vent Axia

A British ventilation manufacturer that includes exceptional system design information on their web-site

www.vent-axia.com
Fleming Way
Crawley, West Sussex RH10 9YX
United Kingdom
U.S. Phone: 800-735-7026

Ventilation Systems USA

The manufacturer of a range of ventilation & make-up air products
www.vents-us.com
11013 Kenwood Road
Cincinnati, OH 95242
Phone: 513-348-3853

Zehnder America

The manufacturer of HRV/ERVs
www.zehnderamerica.com
540 Portsmouth Ave.
Greenland, NH 94502 Phone: 603-422-6700

* * *

Fresh Air Make-up Systems

Electro Industries, Inc.

Tempered fresh air make-up systems and make-up air heaters.
https://electromn.com/make-up-air-2/
2150 West River Street
Monticello, MN 55362
Phone: 800-922-4138

EP Sales

Make-up air systems particularly EPS systems.
http://www.epsalesinc.com/products.php
7878 12th Ave. South

Bloomington, MN 55425
Phone: 952-854-4400

Fantech
Manufacturer of make-up air systems.
www.fantech.net
Systemair
Lenexa, KS
Phone: 800-747-1762

Hoyme Manufacturing, Inc.
Motorized damper make-up air systems
www.hoyme.com/
4512 39 St
Camrose, AB T4V 2N5, Canada
Phone: 780-672-6553

Rehau - United Polymer Solutions
Piping for Ground-Air Heat Exchangers
https://www.rehau.com/uk-en/product-listing
Hill Court, Walford
Ross-on-Wye
Herefordshire HR9 5QN

Renson
Manufacturer of trickle vents and other unique ventilation products.
https://www.renson.eu/en-us/renson-usa-1.html
400 Continental Blvd
El Segundo, CA 90245, USA
Contact: Mr. Julien Brugmans
Cell: +1 (310) 746-6069

Titon Inc.
British manufacturer of "trickle vents".
www.titon.co.uk
PO Box 241
Granger, IN 46530

Phone: 574-271-9699

* * *

Test Equipment and Indoor Air Quality Products and Supplies:

Aerobiotix
   Whole home multi-pollutant HVAC component.
   350 Fame Road
   West Carrollton, Ohio 45449 USA
   https://aerobiotix.com/
   +1 888 978 7087

Air Chek, Inc.
   Source of radon equipment and facts.
   www.radon.com
   1936 Butler Bridge Road
   Mills River, NC 28759-3892
   Phone: 800-247-2435

AirAdvice, Inc.
   Air quality analysis systems that can be used for indoor air diagnostics for homes and businesses.
   www.airadvice.com
   707 SW Washington Street, Suite 800
   Portland, OR 97205
   Phone: 888-959-4686

Aircuity, Inc.
   Manufacturer of integrated sensing and control solutions for buildings, particularly schools and commercial spaces.
   www.aircuity.com
   39 Chapel Street
   Newton, MA 02458
   Phone: 617-641-8800

CERV - BuildEquinox
"Smart" Ventilation equipment
www.buildequinox.com
1103 N. High Cross Road
Urbana, IL 61802
1-773-492-1893

Energy Conservatory
Tools for measure pressures in and through houses and ducts.
www.energyconservatory.com
2801 21st Ave. South Suite 160
Minneapolis, MN 55407
Phone: 612-827-1117

HomeAirCheck
IAQ test kits for chemical identification and analysis of contaminants in the air.
https://www.homeaircheck.com/indoor-air-quality-testing/?gad_source=1
Prism Analytical Technologies, Inc.
2625 Denison Drive
Mt. Pleasant, MI 48858
Phone: 877-243-5247

Infiltec
A great source of information and material for radon mitigation and blower door equipment.
www.infiltec.com
108 South Delphine Ave.
Waynesboro, VA 22980
Phone: 888-349-7236

Onset Computer Corporation
Full line of data loggers and data logging software for short and long term building performance analysis.
www.onsetcomp.com
470 MacArthur Bldvd.

Bourne, MA 02532
Phone: 800-564-4377

Retrotec

Blower doors, duct testers and tools for measuring pressures through houses.

https://www.retrotec.com/
1060 East Pole Road
Everson, WA 98247
Phone: 360-738-7683

TruTech Tools

A wide variety of building and system diagnostic tools.
www.trutechtools.com
PO Box 19013
Akron, OH 443319
Phone: 888-224-3437

Appendix G - Digital Tools & Applications

There are a number of on-line tools that aid in the design and installation of ventilation systems. Some of these are product/brand connected.

* * *

RedCalc from the Pacific Northwest National Laboratory (LBNL) and hosted on the Building America Solution Center website (https://basc.pnnl.gov/redcalc) is a gold mine of building science tools. The residential ventilation calculators quickly and simply solve the ventilation rate puzzles from the ASHRAE 62.2 Standard for both new and existing buildings. But there are also exceptionally useful tools for airflow measurement, insulation, domestic hot water, moisture, electrical use, and weather data. The tools include in depth explanations of how to use them. These are free tools.

* * *

KWIK Model 3D is an application for quickly and easily creating a 3D computer model of duct designs with no CAD software. It features HVAC design features and ACCA approved Manual J load calculations via "Energy-Gauge Loads" a product of the Florida solar Energy Center. This is reasonably priced tool.

* * *

AirCycler Annual Ventilation Cost Calculator This handy app provides an estimate of ventilation cost of ventilating with or without an AirCycler control. It can be used to compare the cost of operating an exhaust-only or heat recovery system either as a stand-alone or air handler connected product. This is a free tool.

* * *

<u>ASHRAE Duct Fitting Database Lite</u> is a free app from the App store (ASHRAE DFDB Lite) that allows for pressure loss calculations for 14 select supply, common, and return/exhaust ASHRAE duct fittings in both I-P and SI units. This mobile app can be used in the field for quick duct pressure loss calculations. The inputs can be adjusted by touch, and installation is automatic.

The full duct fitting database is a cloud based program accessed by annual subscription. It includes loss coefficient tables for more than 200 round, rectangular, and flat oval duct fittings. "Featuring pictorial outlines of each fitting, this database is useful to design engineers dealing with a variety of duct fittings. For any given fitting, enter the flow rate and fitting information and obtain loss coefficient data and associated pressure loss." This is not a free tool.

* * *

Broan/NuTone

Broan/NuTone has developed a couple of handy applications for Duct Length and HRV/ERV performance. These were added to their site in October, 2024

Duct Length Calculator This tool can be used for Broan range hoods or bathroom fans to determine the maximum allowable duct length for a specific airflow. "This tool may be used to comply with the requirements of 2015 IRC Section M1506.2 and 2018 IRC Section M1504.2.

Performance Calculator This tool allows the input of design criteria to select the right Broan HRV/ERV product, obtain efficiency metrics, and verify ASHRAE 90.1 compliance. The tool pulls in the information about the climate from the ASHRAE information. These are free tools.

SeeStack - The Energy Conservatory

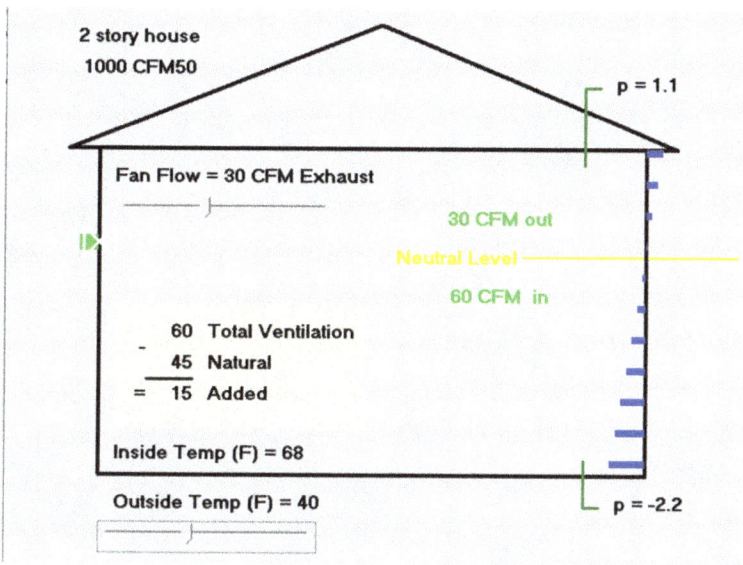

SeeStack is a stack effect simulator available for free for Windows computers from The Energy Conservatory. Pressure on the wall of the house is simulated by vectors - the longer the blue vector the greater the pressure. The temperatures and the airflows can be adjusted and the yellow neutral pressure plane moves up and down between the vectors. The type of ventilation as well as the rate and direction of flow can be changed along with the tightness of the house and the number of stories.

In the snap shot pictured here, the inside temperature is 68, the outside temperature is 40F, and a 30 cfm exhaust fan is running. Because there is still natural leakage, only 15 cfm of additional airflow needs to be accounted for in energy calculations.

Appendix H - Manual BV

Why use balanced ventilation?

Since a house can be ventilated with a simple exhaust fan and still meet code and ASHRAE 62.2 ventilation requirements, why go to the effort and expense of installing balanced ventilation—a heat (HRV) or energy (ERV) recovery ventilator or some other form of balanced ventilation? Although there can be savings in the conditioned air cost between an exhaust fan and an HRV/ERV, the difference is small—typically less than $100/year[1]. And since the first cost is much higher, cost cannot be the determining issue. The advantage of using an HRV/ERV is neither the cost of conditioned air saving nor the energy savings.

Many programs require HRV/ERV systems now and there has to be a good reason for it. That reason is building pressure. Exhaust- and supply-only ventilation systems intentionally put the dwelling under negative or positive pressure, increasing infiltration or exfiltration. Those pressures can drive moisture into the structure. Exhaust-only systems compete for replacement air with furnaces, water heaters, range hoods, clothes dryers, any mechanical equipment that relies on the flow of air through the system to function.

---

1. AirCycler has a nice tool for estimating the operating cost of various residential ventilation systems. https://www.aircycler.com/pages/calculator

There are two principal reasons for using a properly designed, installed, and commissioned HRV/ERV system:

1. They are <u>balanced</u>. There is little to no driving force on either side of the dwelling's pressure boundary.
2. They distribute new air throughout the dwelling and remove old air from high polluting spaces such as bathrooms and kitchens.

The design, installation, and commissioning of the HRV/ERV system MUST achieve those two fundamental benefits — balance and distribution - and that is the reason behind this Manual BV.

The Heating, Refrigeration, and Air Conditioning Institute of Canada (HRAI) in their Skilltech Academy has a comprehensive course and supporting design manual for Residential Mechanical Ventilation detailing the application of HRV/ERV systems[2]. This Appendix just highlights the fundamentals.

This Appendix draws information from the work that William Shurcliff documented in 1981 in the early days of heat exchangers in his book *Air-to-Air Heat Exchangers for Houses*. And in 1984, the Department of Energy funded the creation of a document called *Heat Recovery Ventilation for Housing—Air-to-Air Heat Exchangers*.

In 1990, the Home Ventilating Institute developed their Standard 929 to support a course in the application of heat recovery ventilators. Its structure is like the HRAI manual.

Many of the background steps included in the ACCA, HRAI, and HVI design manuals have been covered elsewhere in this book and will not be duplicated here.

Many elements of heat recovery and energy recovery ventilators are the same and there have been a variety of attempts to combine them in descriptions, such as AAX and HERV. Rather than return to the label William Shurcliff used in his book of AAX, I have used the popular HRV/ERV term to simplify referring to both types simultaneously.

It is important to note that when those 1980s documents were written, the motors in HRV/ERV systems were permanent split capacitor (PSC), single speed types. Most new HRV/ERV systems use electronically commutated

---

2. https://www.hrai.ca/technical-manuals

motors, many of which have virtually infinite speed adjustment capabilities, allowing the systems to adapt to various issues in the installation. However, it can make them even more challenging to balance and verify the installed system airflows.

Once again, the purposes of a balanced ventilation system are **balance** and **distribution.** Everything else is just like putting socks on a pig.

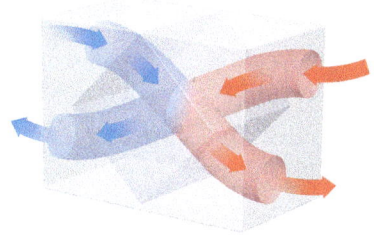

Figure H.1 Exchanger Airflow Path (Broan-NuTone)

* * *

HRV or ERV?

There are few hard and fast rules whether to select a heat recovery ventilator (HRV) or an enthalpy recovery ventilator (ERV). Most manufacturers produce both types of products. The quality of the product cores has reached a point where, from the core design, the two versions are interchangeable. Selection commonly depends on personal preference. Climate and the quality of construction also play a role. It is important to understand the difference between the two devices and make an educated choice.

- In a climate dominated by cooling with hot, humid weather, an ERV will remove moisture from the incoming airstream and lower the air conditioning latent heat load.
- A very tight structure in a heating dominated climate might want an HRV to remove as much of the moisture trapped inside the house as possible.
- An HRV requires a condensate drain, requiring external plumbing.

- Referring to the airflow at the sensible recovery efficiency at 32°F will provide a good airflow performance reference for either type of product.

Quick Start

Important: Read and understand the product installation manual thoroughly prior to installation.[3]

1. Determine the airflow and required efficiency and select a system.
2. Select an installation design—stand-alone or air handler connection.
3. Select controls.
4. Locate the HRV/ERV in a serviceable location.
    a. Close to outside to limit in/out duct runs.
    b. HRV proximity to condensate drain.
5. Mount the HRV/ERV to limit vibration transfer and noise.
6. Locate the supply (fresh air) grilles in the bedrooms and living room, etc.
7. Locate the exhaust (old air) grilles in the bathrooms and kitchen (not over range).
8. Insulated supply air duct <u>from</u> outside (no damper).
9. Exhaust air <u>to</u> outside.
10. If HRV: condensate to drain.
11. Program the controls.
12. Run the system.
    a. Verify balanced pressure and flows.
    b. Verify delivered new air performance.
13. Document the design, installation, and operation details.

* * *

---

3. BetterBuiltNW Infographic of HRV best practices: https://betterbuiltnw.com/assets/uploads/resources/HRV-Systems-Best-Practices-poster.pdf

Developing a Ventilation Plan

Good Practice

In designing an effective HRV/ERV system, several fundamental elements need to be considered. These are covered elsewhere in this book.

Fundamental Design Details:

- Application/installation complexities - Chapter 6
- Average air change vs Effective air change - Chapter 4
- Building Pressures - Chapter 7
- Contaminant sources - Chapter 18
- Filtration - Chapter 17
- Knowledge and skill of the designers, installers, occupants - Chapter 2
- Maintenance and commissioning - Chapter 9
- Pressure balance issues - Chapter 7
- Relative humidity - Chapter 17

Fundamental Design Considerations

For an HRV/ERV to function properly and deliver the best air quality to the dwelling, it should NOT be ducted through the heating and cooling (HAC) air handler. The HRV/ERV and the HAC systems are different products with different purposes. Combining them is like trying to use the dishwasher to make dinner—they're both kitchen appliances and both have heating elements, but they serve different purposes. It is strongly discouraged to draw exhaust air from the HAC ducting and supply the fresh air directly back into the HAC duct system.

Joining the ducting of the two systems can cause a severe imbalance of supply and exhaust ventilation airflows, as the HRV/ERV operates at low to high speeds, as well as the variable speed operation of the furnace and air conditioner. It is challenging to assure the design airflows remain in balance when the two systems are operated at varying blower speeds, resulting in a large variation of static pressure in the HAC ducting system. The imbalance in the dwelling may cause unpredictable levels of infiltration and exfiltration.

If the HRV/ERV is set up to operate only when the HAC system is running, then mechanical ventilation is not provided when most needed—in milder weather but when the windows remain closed. Ventilation is likely to be excessive in severe weather, when the air handler operates more frequently.

Determining the flow rate to meet the ASHRAE 62.2 Standard is based on continuous operation. To establish an equivalent intermittent flow rate, requires that the operational schedule of the HAC air handler be known which would be impossible if the air handler is controlled by a thermostat unless a control is used to force the HAC air handler to operate in harmony with both the thermal and ventilation requirements of the dwelling. The equivalent ventilation rate when the two systems are combined will be significantly higher.

The ASHRAE 62.2 standard was written for single, dedicated ventilation systems — moving the air from the inside to the outside of the dwelling. It does not have a provision for combined devices.

Operating the HAC air handler to run continuously is strongly discouraged in climates with warm summers and high humidity whether the fresh air is introduced into the system. If the blower continues to run for extended times after the cooling thermostat is satisfied, the water remaining on the air-conditioning coil and in the drain pan re-evaporates. During this time, the air continues to be cooled by the cold AC coil and by the evaporation of water, so the space temperature continues to decrease while the relative humidity increases. In the next cooling cycle, this humidity has to be condensed again, so any efficiency gain in evaporating this water is offset by the next cycle and by the loss of comfort at higher relative humidity.

If the two systems are connected, during the summer months, the outdoor humidity supplied through the HRV/ERV may cause condensation on the interior surfaces of the HAC equipment and the supply plenum and ducting. These surfaces will be around 60F and outdoor air dew points in the summer in much of the US are well above this temperature. These are the very conditions that promote mold growth.

* * *

HRV/ERV Fundamentals

The purpose of an air-to-air heat exchanger (HRV/ERV) is to provide fresh air while exhausting stale air from the dwelling. By combining those two functions, some of the energy from the exhaust air stream can be transferred to the incoming air stream, tempering the condition of the incoming fresh air. Air-to-air heat exchangers do not *produce* heat; they only *exchange* heat from one airstream to the other. Equally important, by working with both air streams and balancing the flows, the system does not put the dwelling under unbalanced pressure, reducing infiltration and exfiltration.

The HRV/ERV commonly has two blowers or two blower wheels spun by one motor. They also include filters and the exchanger core housed in an insulated box. It usually has four duct fittings and controls. Many designs include balancing dampers that can be adjusted and locked along with pressure taps to assist in measuring the balance of the system after installation. A heat recovery ventilator (HRV) also includes a condensate drain attachment.

Heat exchanger core

The heart of the HRV/ERV is the exchanger core. Residential equipment falls into one of four categories: plate, rotary (heat or desiccant wheel), ceramic tube, and heat pipe.

Plate type

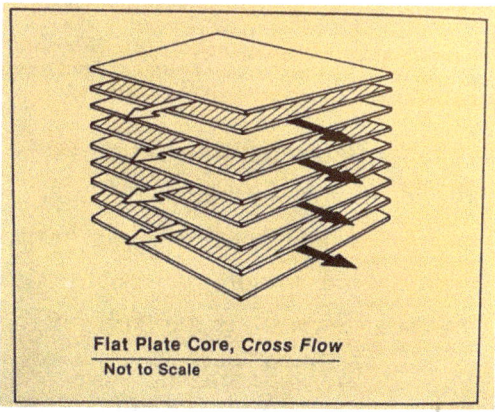

Figure H.2 Plate Heat Recovery Ventilation for Housing National Center for Appropriate Technology Archive 1984

The plate type of heat recovery core is constructed of thin sheets or plates of metal, paper, or plastic forming channels. The plates keep the supply and exhaust air from mixing. If the air channels are arranged so that the exhaust air flows in the opposite direction to the supply flow, it is referred to as a counter-flow heat exchanger core. If the core is arranged so that the exhaust air flows at a right angle to the supply flow, the core is referred to as a cross-flow heat exchanger core. Although it does not transfer heat quite as efficiently as the counter-flow arrangement, it is simpler to fabricate. Some units combine the characteristics of both counter and cross-flow patterns.

Counter Flow heat exchangers can have a longer path inside the exchanger core to increase the exchanger efficiency.

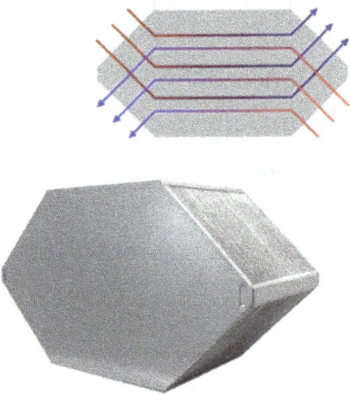

Figure H.2a Counter Flow Heat Exchanger Core (Holtop)

Rotary

The rotary HRV/ERV (often referred to as a heat or desiccant wheel) is designed around a cylinder or core formed with small air passages from one end to the other. This "heat wheel' rotates slowly between the exhaust and supply air streams. In the heating season, the exhaust air warms the core as it passes through the tiny passageways. As the core rotates into the supply air stream, the flow of air in the small passageways is reversed and the heat stored in the core is absorbed by the colder supply air. Carefully fitted seals along the edges and face of the wheel prevent the leakage of exhaust air into the supply air section of the HRV/ERV.

Ceramic tubes

Ceramic tube heat exchangers combine a series of ceramic tubes that take advantage of the fast heating and cooling characteristics of the ceramic material. Compared to traditional metal heating elements, ceramic cores can more effectively transfer heat energy to the air. These cores are commonly used in single room ERVs using a bi-directional fan to move the air in and out of the room in short periods of time, absorbing and releasing heat with each pass.

Heat Pipes

A heat pipe is a permanently sealed tube partially filled with a liquid refrigerant. When one end of the tube is surrounded by warm air, heat from the air is transferred to the tube, causing the liquid to evaporate. The vapor that is formed will move to the other end of the tube, and if that end is surrounded by cold air, heat is removed from the vapor, and it returns to liquid form. A wick along the inside of the tube then draws the liquid back to the warm end of the heat pipe and the cycle is repeated. A heat pipe core has a series of heat pipes passing through a plate which separates the exhaust air from the supply air.

Fans

Although heat exchangers with no accompanying fans are available, most HRV/ERV units include two fans or blowers, or a single motor with two blower wheels. Axial or propeller fans may be used in single room products, where the static pressure of the system is low. Ducted units with higher system static pressures commonly use centrifugal blowers. Some of these fans are driven by electronically commutated (ECM) motors that vary their speed and resulting flow rate based on the pressure drop they are experiencing.

Filters

HRV/ERV components are commonly mounted in an insulated casing or cabinet which accommodates mounting brackets and vibration isolators that will reduce the transmission of sound to the floor, ceiling, or wall. Some casings are designed for "quick" access to the exchanger core or filter to allow cleaning or replacement. Because of the limited space in the casing, filters are often thin and have a low MERV rating, although some units include MERV 8 or MERV 11 filters and offer optional HEPA filtration.

Casing or Housing

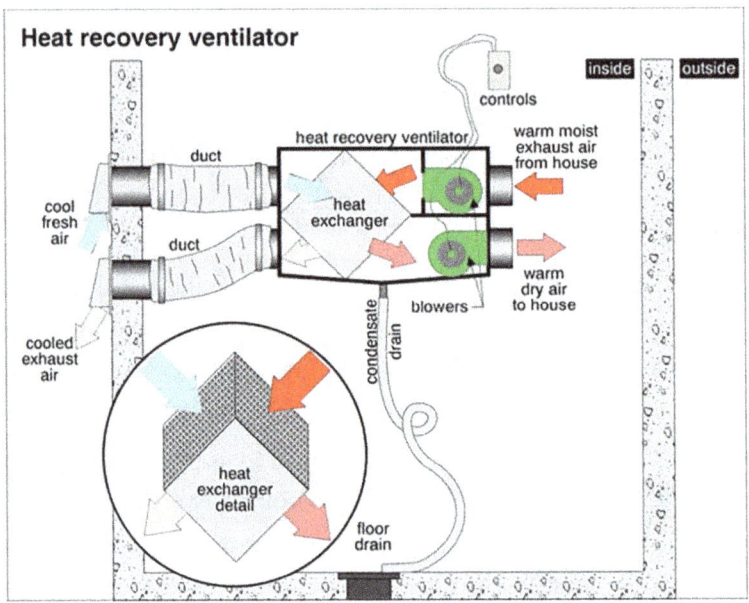

Figure H.3 Condensate[4]

Stand-alone HRV/ERV components are contained in a well-insulated box that provides air passages for the two streams along with the exchanger core and filters. The core can be extracted for cleaning and service. Casings include mounting brackets and vibration isolators that will reduce the transmission of sound to the mounting surface. HRV units include a drain-pan on the exhaust section that collects the condensate and is connected to the external drain. A drain hose must include a "U" trap or loop to prevent air from being sucked into or out of the HRV through the drain pipe. Some HRVs include a second drain on the bottom of the supply section to remove moisture that may accumulate because of high outdoor humidity during summer operation or because of the entry of snow during winter operation.

Through-wall single room systems are like a section of pipe passing directly from the inside to the outside of the building. Many of these housings include a power cord that can be plugged in to a receptacle simplifying installation and maintenance.

Balancing Dampers

Built-in balancing dampers permit the supply and exhaust airflows to be balanced by the installer. They are usually on the warm side of the unit.

---

4. Home Inspection Consultants Inc. https://www.homeinspect.ca/

Dampers may be integrated into the design so that they block passive flow when the system is not running.

Some products now use built-in automatic balancing systems, measuring the flow with either pressure sensors or vane anemometers that control the speed of the ECM motors and strive to keep the system constantly in balance.

Controls[5]

Controls range from simple ON/OFF and HIGH/LOW operation to sensors that respond to ambient conditions, including moisture and carbon dioxide, to timers. Most manufacturers offer a range of controls for their systems. To select the best system for a particular application depends on how the occupants want the system to work.

The simplest approach is to hard wire the system so that it runs all the time with an emergency override to shut it off. If the system is designed with independent ducting and installed correctly, having a continuous flow of tempered fresh air flowing through the house is a good thing. The cost is minor.[6] And it is simpler than constantly adjusting the operation.

However, control for changing conditions, such as increased building occupancy, heavy moisture conditions, forest fire smoke, or other changing IAQ conditions, could be a good thing.

There is a growing number of HRV/ERV controls as sensors, electronics, and scientific understanding of IAQ grows. Some controls work with just the HRV/ERV while others control all aspects of the indoor air quality in the house. The following is a limited cross section of devices.

AirCycler

To assure thorough mixing of fresh air throughout the home, a cycle timer such as the Aircycler product periodically turns on the HVAC blower to complete the ventilation cycle. This device wires in parallel with the thermostat, to periodically operate the furnace blower. It avoids redundant fan operation by starting a timed off cycle at the end of blower operation for a heating, cooling, or previous ventilation cycle. Then it turns the blower on again to meet the prescribed ventilation program. This approach reduces the electrical

---

5. Control technology is advancing rapidly. The information here is a snap shot of devices which are presently available
6. https://www.aircycler.com/pages/calculator

cost of constant furnace fan operation and drafts during the winter, while assuring good mixing of fresh air throughout the home.

Broan AI Controls

These controls offer bidirectional communication between the unit and the wall control to get detailed maintenance information and they can be paired with auxiliary control(s). They operate according to outdoor temperature and indoor temperature and humidity. The dehumidistat will deactivate if the outdoor temperature exceeds 75F (24C). They can operate the system at three different speeds. The control has scheduling capability so that it can provide different operating modes throughout the week, but it is advisable, as previously discussed, to set it and forget it. The control also includes an indicator for when filter maintenance is required and includes a system error log to simplify maintenance. Broan also manufactures auxiliary controls to allow system adjustment from bathrooms, laundry rooms, or workshops.

Fantech HRV/ERV Controls

The ECO-Touch IAQ control recognizes cleaning solvents, cooking odors and particulates, or elevated levels of CO_2 and increases the HRV/ERV's airflow rate based on the total VOC levels. It is only compatible with Fantech products.

Zehnder Controls

Zehnder offers a range of control products, including CO_2 sensors which can be in each living space. Their ComfoSense C control provides for four ventilation flow rates, scheduler, summer bypass, frost protection indicator, and service and maintenance alert.

* * *

Freeze Control

If the incoming supply air is very cold, the moisture condensing out of the exhaust air may freeze to the heat exchange core. Depending on the type of HRV/ERV, this could begin when outdoor temperatures fall below 23F (-5°C). If the ice accumulates, the air passageways in the heat exchange core will eventually become plugged.

Some HRVs have an electric preheat coil in the incoming air stream of the unit. This preheat coil raises the outside air temperature above the temperature at which freezing is likely to occur. Other HRVs automatically shut off the flow of cold supply air through the core whenever ice builds up on the exhaust section of the HRV. In most, the supply fan is stopped, while the exhaust fan continues to run, blowing warm air over the iced surface. In some units, the exhaust air is blown directly outside, while in others the exhaust air is directed back into the house through the supply air side of the core.

Supply air by-pass is another technique that is used by some manufacturers, while others include a system of imbalanced flow conditions with greater exhaust flow than supply flow. Melting the accumulated ice in the HRV generates the liquid that needs to leave the unit via the drain pan and condensate hose.

ERV exchangers may use recirculation, exhaust only, preheat, or bypass for defrost functions.

Pre-conditioners

Products are available with built-in electric pre-heating elements that will kick in if the incoming air temperature would be too cold to be delivered to the space. And there are geothermal preconditioning units that use a ground loop similar to a geothermal heat-pump. Because of the ground connection, these conditioners can also do an effective job of dehumidifying the air reducing the need to air conditioning in many situations. (Note that in some cases utility incentives for HRV/ERV may not apply if the unit includes a pre-conditioner.)

Verify the delivered air temperature from the HRV/ERV with the formula:

$$Temp_{Delivered} = Temp_{Outdoor} + ((Temp_{Exhaust} - Temp_{Outdoor}) \times SRE)$$

SRE is Sensible Recovery Efficiency of the HRV/ERV. An HRV/ERV with an SRE of 75% would deliver 53 °F air to the room if the outdoor air was 32 °F and the exhaust air from the HRV/ERV was 60 °F so a pre-conditioner might be needed.

Ventilation Efficiency

It must always be kept in mind that an HRV/ERV is, first and foremost, a ventilator. Ventilation efficiency is the ability of an HRV/ERV to efficiently remove stale or old air from all areas of the house while replacing the stale air with new, outside air based on the assumption that, on average, the outside air is less contaminated than the indoor air. Ventilation efficiency is related to:

1. The capability of the HRV/ERV to move sufficient exhaust and supply air at the design airflow rate against the pressure drop of the ductwork. Obstructions to airflow are created by the ductwork, the number of elbows and other fittings, the filters, screens, and grilles.
2. The capability of the HRV/ERV to effectively separate the exhaust and supply air streams, to prevent "cross leakage". If the supply air leaving the HRV/ERV for distribution within the house is a mixture of old air and new air, the real ventilation rate will be reduced accordingly.
3. The capability to distribute the new air supply throughout the living areas of the house.

Ventilation efficiency is a measure of how well the HRV/ERV system exhausts the pollutants before they spread throughout the house and how well the HRV/ERV distributes new air within the house. The solution to pollution is dilution distribution. It is critical to ensure that the new air distribution system has been effectively planned and installed.

The three requirements that must be met by an efficient ventilation system are:

1. Providing the desired amount of new air to each room in the dwelling;
2. Providing good diffusion (mixing) of the air once it is supplied to the room;
3. Exhausting air from the rooms with the highest concentrations of moisture and contaminants.

The first and third items relate to the air handling capability of the HRV/ERV and the design of the ductwork, while the second relates to the location and type of supply grilles and their effect on the mixing of new air with the room air (air diffusion).

Heat Recovery Efficiency

Heating and air conditioning address the concept of "heat" and "cold". However, only "heat" can be transferred from one place to another. Heating or cooling is adding or removing heat from the air in the dwelling.

HRV/ERV devices take advantage of the natural second law of thermodynamics, which says that heat moves to cold and wet moves to dry—things that are warmer will cool and things that are wetter will dry. This can be defined in terms of Sensible Heat, Latent Heat, and Total Heat.

Sensible heat is the energy that is added to air that causes the temperature of the air to increase. (It is the type of heat that we perceive when we walk inside the house on a cold winter day.)

The transfer of water to air is referred to as humidification. The energy required to evaporate the water needed to humidify the air is termed **Latent Heat**. For example, swimmers feel the loss of latent heat when they come out of the swimming pool and are cooled quickly by evaporation, even though the surrounding air is warm.

The **Total Heat** in the air is the sum of the sensible heat and the latent heat in moist air—a process referred to as Enthalpy.

The exchanger core of the HRV/ERV transfers heat (either sensible heat only or sensible and latent heat) from one airstream to the other. It makes sense that the quantity of heat extracted from the exhaust air should be equal to the quantity of heat added to the supply air. This temperature change may be indicated by an equal reduction in the temperature of one airstream with the increase in the temperature of the other airstream.

However, this is not always the case, because of air leakage of heat added by the fan motors. Therefore, since it is the increase in supply air temperature that reduces the home heating bill, it is this temperature rise that one should measure when evaluating the sensible heat recovery of an HRV/ERV.

The efficiency of sensible heat recovery for a particular HRV/ERV is described as the amount of heat transferred to the supply air expressed as a fraction of the amount of heat available in the exhaust air. For example, if the temperature difference between the inside and outside air was 60°F, and the HRV/ERV increased the incoming supply air temperature by 45°F, the efficiency would be 45 divided by 60 = 0.75 or 75%.

The Home Ventilating Institute maintains a product directory of HRV/ERV products, listed in Section 3 of the Directory. Definitions for terms related to HRV/ERV performance are carefully defined in the Cover Pages of that section.

Max Rated Sensible Recovery Efficiency at 0 degrees C (SRE):

The Sensible Recovery Efficiency is the "net sensible energy recovered by the supply airstream as adjusted by electric consumption, case heat loss or heat gain, air leakage, airflow mass imbalance between the two airstreams and the energy used for defrost (when running the Very Low Temperature Test), as a percent of the potential sensible energy that could be recovered plus the exhaust fan energy. This value is used to predict and compare Heating Season Performance of the HRV/ERV unit."

Adjusted Sensible Recovery Efficiency (ASRE)

This value removes equipment elements and should be "used for energy modeling when wattage for air movement is separately accounted for in the energy model."

Total Recovery Efficiency

"This value is used to predict and compare cooling season performance for the HRV/ERV unit."

Adjusted Total Recovery Efficiency (ATRE)

"This value should be used for energy modeling when wattage for air movement is separately accounted for in the energy model."

Efficacy @ Max Rated SRE cfm/W

This reflects how energy efficient the product's motor is at moving the air at its maximum rated SRE. This value is sometimes mandated by codes and energy efficiency programs.

Warnings Regarding Pressure Impact

Combustion Appliances and spillage susceptibility

Residential ventilation systems work by exchanging the air inside the dwelling with outside air. In doing so, they impact the indoor pressure. Other devices such as atmospherically vented boilers, furnaces, water heaters, clothes dryers, range hoods also impact the indoor pressure.

On their own, a perfectly balanced HRV/ERV should have little to no impact on indoor pressure by design. However, in the process of system design, building pressures must be considered. There are two pressurization limits defined by HRAI: the TVCC and the CEC.

The TVCC is the Total Ventilation Capacity Condition, which includes all fans which are part of the mechanical ventilation system.

The CEC is the Critical Exhaust Condition, which includes the TVCC, the dryer, and all other exhaust fans which have an airflow of 160 cfm or greater.

In the process of ventilation system design, the potential for causing the backdrafting or spillage of atmospherically vented appliances must be considered. If the HRV/ERV is not balanced, small negative pressures on the building can cause atmospherically vented combustion appliances to spill deadly combustion gases into the house. The RedCalc Depressurization Analysis tool available on the Building America Solution Center site has a tool to quickly calculate the depressurization caused by ventilation.

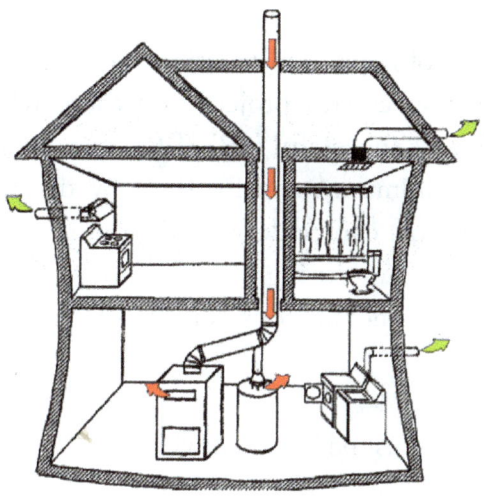

Figure H.4 Potential Backdraft Routes (EPA)

Plugging in the blower door measurement for the house and the potential exhaust flow cfm results in a depressurization value which can then be compared to the following BPI chart. Alternatively, if the depressurization of the building is known (in Pascals), the tool can indicate the volume of exhaust airflow.

The Building Performance Institute (BPI) defines the Combustion Appliance Zone (CAZ) depressurization limit for:

Appliance Type	Max Depress.
Atmospheric water heater only (Category I, natural draft), open-combustion appliances	−2 pa
Atmospheric water heater (Category I, natural draft) and atmospheric furnace (Category I, natural draft), common-vented, open-combustion appliances	−3 pa
Gas furnace or boiler, Category I or Category I fan-assisted, open-combustion appliances	−5 pa
Oil or gas unit with power burner, low- or high-static pressure burner, open combustion appliances	−5 pa
Wood-burning appliances	−7 pa
Open-combustion furnaces or boilers with fan-powered horizontal venting	−15 pa
Pellet stove with draft fan and sealed vent	−15 pa
Direct-vent, sealed combustion appliances with forced draft.	−25 pa

Table H.1 CAZ Depressurization

System Design

As with other elements of house construction and the installation of mechanical systems, the most successful projects are those which have been well thought out in advance. A successful HRV/ERV installation must begin at the design stage, leaving minimum room for error by the system installer. The clearer the information that can be developed prior to starting the project, the less likely problems will occur during the installation process.

There are a few fundamental considerations for the ducting and locating the HRV/ERV:

- The HRV/ERV must be installed where it is maintained above freezing temperatures.
- It must be installed where it is easily accessible for maintenance and filter changes.
- It should be relatively close to an exterior wall to minimize the length of insulated duct to the exterior vent hoods or termination fittings.
- The outdoor duct connections need to be insulated and covered with a complete vapor barrier to prevent indoor moisture from condensing on the inner duct, saturating the insulation layer. The duct connections to the HRV/ERV and the exterior termination fittings must be designed to maintain this vapor barrier over the insulation.

- The external fresh air intake must be about 6 feet or more from any exhaust device, including the discharge from the HRV/ERV. It should not be installed where noxious gases from outdoor sources are likely to be present, such as the exhaust of an automobile in a driveway.
- If attaching to an air handler;
    - Connect the supply to the forced air return.
    - Use an injection port design to ensure the air flows in the right direction.[7]
    - Pull exhaust air from the bathrooms.
    - The air handler must have an EC motor.

Design steps:

1. Determine the minimum and peak ventilation capacity required by the HRV/ERV system installation.
2. Select an HRV/ERV capable of meeting the mechanical ventilation requirements and ASHRAE 62.2 requirements for performance.
3. Decide on the system configuration—stand-alone or connected to the HAC ducting.
4. Locate the HRV/ERV and size the supply air registers and the exhaust air grilles on the house plans.
    a. Supply air should be delivered on the opposite side of the room from the entry door or exhaust air.
    b. Install exhausts in bathrooms, supplies in bedrooms, and both in the main living areas.
    c. HRV/ERV supply and exhaust air vents should be > 10 feet apart.
5. Locate the HRV/ERV and lay out the supply and exhaust air duct runs on the plans.
6. Size ductwork and select fittings.
7. Specify manual and automatic HRV/ERV controls.

---

7. The large blower in the air handler is much more powerful that the small blowers in the HRV/ERV. By using a 90 elbow inside the supply trunk pointed in the direction of the flow, the HRV/ERV air is surrounded by household conditioned air supporting the flow rather than fighting it.

8. Verify that the HRV/ERV system, when operating at the same time as other systems and appliances, will not negatively impact any other system and keep it from drafting properly.
9. Confirm that the HRV/ERV will not be supplying makeup or combustion air to any appliance.

* * *

Design Procedure

Step 1: Determining the ventilation requirements.

These design steps are based on the HRV/ERV serving a solitary purpose: whole dwelling ventilation. This system runs continuously to exchange the old air with new air throughout the house via dedicated ductwork. In that configuration, it is like other basic appliances in the house. Dishwashers or ovens are dedicated to the one task they were designed and manufactured to accomplish.

Dedicated HRV/ERV systems can be designed, installed, balanced, commissioned, and maintained to provide balanced and continuous ventilation and not tasked with jobs they were not designed to do.

ASHRAE 62.2 requires local exhaust ventilation from bathrooms and kitchens. Bathroom exhaust can be integrated with the HRV/ERV, although the flow rate from the bathroom is likely to be lower than a dedicated bathroom exhaust fan, meaning that mirrors won't clear off as quickly.

An HRV/ERV can remove air from a kitchen area, but **NOT from over the range**. A kitchen exhaust grille should include a MERV 3 cleanable filter to protect the HRV/ERV from grease particulates in the kitchen air.

Ventilation Capacity

ASHRAE 62.2 specifies the amount of air (Q_{tot}) required for the whole dwelling ventilation system described in Chapter 3 of this book. The process for determining the minimum whole dwelling ventilation rate for an HRV/ERV is the same as for other whole dwelling ventilation systems. Sizing the system to the ASHRAE 62.2 standard can be accomplished by using the tables or formulas in the standard or by using the RedCalc tool available from PNNL https://basc.pnnl.gov/redcalc .

$$Q_{tot} = 0.03 A_{floor} + 7.5(N_{br} + 1)$$

where

Q_{tot} = fan flow rate in cfm (cubic feet per minute)
A_{floor} = floor area in square feet
N_{br} = number of bedrooms (not less than one)

This can be adjusted with the infiltration credit based on blower door testing (or estimation), location, and building height. Other rate change factors are included in the latest version of the Standard (2025 as of this writing).

Canadian Ventilation Capacity

Although it is not recognized by US codes, an alternative to this is to use an approach described in the Canadian F326 Standard, which is based on room use ventilation—a Total Ventilation Capacity or TVC approach. This can be further modified through the use of a pollutant or harm based approach.

The TVC is determined using a room count method where each room in the house is assigned a supply airflow in cfm:

- 20 cfm for a primary bedroom on the assumption that it will be occupied by two adults;
- 20 cfm for a family room or large basement room that is finished or unfinished;
- 10 cfm for all other habitable rooms, not including entrances, hallways, landings, storage room, closets, etc.
- 10 cfm for each room use for room such as kitchen/dining rooms.

The system must be capable of providing these airflows continuously so that the HRV/ERV minimum average airflow for any 24-hour period will meet the TVC.

Harm-based ventilation rate design – pollutants – Calculating the Room Contents Factor

ASHRAE 62.2 is working on a "harm based" approach to sizing the ventilation system known as IAQP, sizing the airflow based on three Contaminants of Concern: very small particles—PM2.5, formaldehyde, and nitrogen dioxide. This selection was primarily based on looking at harm intensities and typical indoor concentrations after a paper by Morantes et al[8]. This approach would size the ventilation rate based on the contaminant level for a particular dwelling, rather than a national average. The process would require understanding the dwelling and its contents during the design process and plugging the information into a sizing formula. As of this writing, it is designated as Appendix D to ASHRAE 62.2-2022.

Step 2 Specifying an HRV/ERV

There are an enormous number of choices for HRV/ERV products. The system must meet the following fundamental criteria:

1. UL, ETL, CSA or other approved laboratory certification for safety;
2. HVI Certification of Performance;
3. Compliance with all applicable local codes;
4. Type of HRV/ERV – Heat Recovery Ventilator or Energy Recovery Ventilator

Pertinent information is included on the product data sheets and websites. Comparative operating information can be found in the HVI's Certified Product directory.[9]

Prod Cat	Brand	Model	Net supply at 100 PA (L/s)	Net supply at 0.4 iwg (cfm)	Max Rated Sensible Recovery Efficiency at 0 deg C	Net Airflow @ Max Rated SRE (L/s)	Net Airflow @ Max Rated SRE (cfm)	Power Con. @ Mx Rated SRE (watts)	Efficacy @Max Rated SRE (L/s/w)	Efficacy @ Max Rated SRE (cfm/w)
ERV	Brand1	Model1	56	119	67	31	66	30	1.03	2.2
HRV	Brand2	Model2	47	100	68	30	64	26	1.15	2.4
ERV	Brand3	Model3	86	182	74	85	180	146	0.58	1.2
HRV	Brand4	Model4	119	252	75	30	64	18	1.66	3.5

Table H.2 Fundamental Design Elements - Sample from Section III of the HVI Product Directory

Product Category ERV, HRV, CATU (Compact Air Treatment Unit)
Brand Manufacturer of the product
Model Specific model name

---

8. https://papers.ssrn.com/sol3/papers.cfm?abstract_id=4409736
9. https://www.hvi.org/hvi-certified-products-directory/section-iii-hrv-erv-directory-listing/

Net supply at 100 PA Airflow at 100 Pascals of pressure in liters/second
Net supply at 0.4 iwg Airflow at 0.4 iwg in CFM
Max Rated Sensible Recovery efficiency
Efficiency (SRE) at 0 degrees C
Net Airflow @ Max Rated SRE Airflow in L/s at the rated SRE
Net Airflow @ Max Rated SRE Airflow in cfm at the rated SRE
Power Consumed at SRE Power consumed in watts
Efficacy @ at SRE (L/s/w) Efficacy in L/s/w
Efficacy @ at SRE (cfm/w) Efficacy in cfm/watt

Looking at the first two example products on Table H.3, they are quite similar in performance, although one is an ERV and one is an HRV. Looking at the "Net supply at 0.4 iwg (cfm), the ERV moves 119 cfm while the HRV moves 100 cfm. However, when looking at the recovery efficiencies, the ERV has an SRE of 67 and the HRV has an SRE of 68 and at that efficiency, the Net Airflow for the ERV is 66 cfm using 30 watts and the HRV is 64 cfm using 26 watts.

It is important to note the airflow at the Max Rated SRE, rather than the range of airflows that the manufacturer may list on the product literature. For example, this ERV manufacturer promotes "131 cfm 67% SRE" performance in the product title, but listing "67% (66 CFM)" in the specifications—about half the airflow. It is the combination of efficiency and airflow that is important to how the product will function when it has been installed.

Step 3 system configuration—stand-alone or connected to the HAC ducting

Optimum performance will be achieved if the HRV/ERV is installed with its own dedicated ductwork.

- The system will provide the best distribution of new air throughout the living space along with the optimum removal of old polluted air from polluting locations such as bathrooms and kitchens.
- The system can be designed by *harm based* criteria.
- It can be run continuously to satisfy the varying conditions.
- The typical power consumption of an HRV/ERV (around 30

watts) is a fraction of the power consumption of a companion 500 watt air handler, which a connected design requires.
- System balancing and airflow performance verification are much simpler with a stand-alone system.
- Airflows for connected systems have to be considerably higher and controls more sophisticated, expensive, and complex to set-up and maintain.

Connecting the system to the HAC air handler is a compromise.

Step 4 Locate the HRV/ERV and size the supply air registers and the exhaust air grilles

Interior Grilles and Registers

For an independent HRV/ERV system, the preferred method of supplying outside air is through a high sidewall or ceiling outlets which discharge the air horizontally. When the supply air is discharged in this manner, it clings to the warmer ceiling because of the Coanda effect and warms before descending into the occupied areas of the room. High sidewall registers should be within 6 to 12 inches from the ceiling and should incorporate louvers that project or throw the air slightly upwards and across the ceiling. A long and narrow grille will allow for a better spread across the ceiling.

Rooms should have either both a supply outlet and exhaust inlet or a supply outlet and a means of pressure relief, such as a transfer grille or jumper duct. (See Chapter 8) Door undercuts and most in-door transfer grilles have considerable resistance to the high airflow of conditioned air systems. Because ventilation airflows are lower, however, they may work satisfactorily for stand-alone HRV/ERV systems.

The system must be designed and installed so that the temperature of the supply air and its manner of introduction into each room avoids discomfort in the occupied zone by the occupants. The air temperature entering the room should be a minimum of 60F (16°C).

Supply diffusers should be located as far as practical from the exit point of the room to facilitate circulation and encourage replacement of the 'old' air with 'new' air.

Grilles and diffusers commonly are the stamped metal HVAC type or molded round adjustable plastic style. The steel grilles have a lower equivalent length—a lower resistance to airflow—and won't throw the low-flow ventilation air as far out into the room.

Termination fitting or exterior hoods

Exterior termination fittings or hoods on the outside of the house, whether intake or exhaust must be:

- Protected from precipitation
- Corrosion resistant
- Accessible for cleaning and service
- Protected from animal entry (Insect protection must be provided inside the HRV/ERV with a filter. Insect screening on the termination fitting will greatly affect the airflow.)
- If the termination fitting includes a backdraft damper, it should only be used on the exhaust side of the system.

The intake termination fitting - because it will introduce the 'new' or fresh air in the house - must be located to avoid contamination from sources such as:

- Exhaust air openings such as dryer or range hood vents
- Driveways or other automotive exhaust sources
- Trash locations
- Gas meters or oil fill pipes
- Attics and crawl spaces
- Under decks or other places that might contain odiferous air.

Termination fittings must be above the expected depth of snow accumulation—minimum distance of eighteen inches above grade, and they must be labeled so that the consumer is aware that the fitting is supplying fresh air to the house. Intake air termination fittings should be located forty inches from a corner of a building to avoid pressure pockets created wind circulation around the house and they should have fixed louvers with no backdraft damper.

Exhaust termination fittings must not discharge into:

- Enclosed, unheated spaces
- Attics
- Garages

- Crawl spaces
- Porches or sheds

They must not exhaust into adjacent buildings or onto walkways where condensation can freeze and cause a safety hazard.

Step 5 Locating the HRV/ERV

The HRV/ERV must be installed where it is maintained above freezing temperatures. Vented attics are challenging locations both because of the temperature swings, which will impact the heat transfer efficiency and the serviceability. The HRV/ERV must be installed where it is easily accessible for maintenance and filter changes. It should be relatively close to an exterior wall to minimize the length of the insulated ducting to the termination fittings. An HRV must be near a drain. Room should be provided for servicing and considering sounds and vibrations that might be generated by the unit, it is advisable to avoid locating the HRV/ERV under a bedroom.

* * *

Duct Design for Independently Ducted HRV/ERV Systems[10]

---

10. Kwik Model 3D is a duct design tool for HVAC systems but can also be applied to the duct design for HRV/ERV duct systems. https://kwikmodel.com/

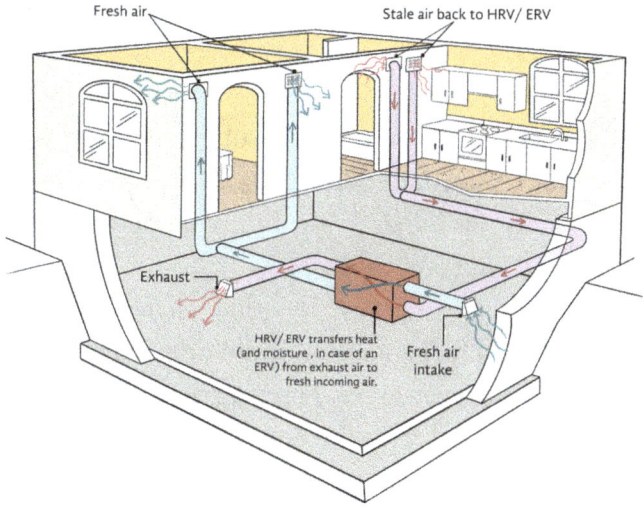

Figure H.5 Fully Independently Ducted HRV/ERV

As described in Chapter 6, there are three elements that impact the static pressure or resistance to airflow in the duct design:

- Actual length
- Equivalent length
- Effective length

The actual length is the measured distance between point A and point B, like the distance measured by a tape measure between the HRV/ERV and the exhaust termination fitting.

The equivalent length is the straight duct equivalent of each fitting. The shape of the duct fitting provides resistance to the airflow as it has to change direction.

The effective length is the sum of the actual length and the equivalent length.

- **Step 1:** Start the duct design process by sketching out the duct runs to and from the HRV/ERV and to and from each supply and exhaust point. Identify all the fittings and determine the equivalent length of each duct run, starting at the grille and working through to the HRV/ERV. As air is forced through a duct system, the External Static Pressure (ESP) capability of the

HRV/ERV is used up in overcoming the resistances imposed by the ducts and fittings. This resistance to airflow causes a loss of air pressure (pressure drop) from one end of the system to the other.
- **Step 2:** Determine the actual length of each duct run from the grille to the outside termination fitting. The length of the duct runs can be scaled off the drawing, but remember to include the vertical duct runs in your total.
- **Step 3:** Calculate the effective length of each run from the outside termination fitting to the supply or exhaust grille or register in the living space remembering that the effective length equals the actual length plus the equivalent lengths.
- **Step 4:** Apply Steps 1, 2, and 3 to each duct run in the system, even though several runs may share the same trunk duct. Tabulate the results.

Duct insulation

All ducts carrying cold air through warm spaces and warm air through cold spaces must be insulated and have a sealed vapor barrier on the warm side of the insulation. The temperature of the air in ventilation ducting is as crucial as the temperature of the air in conditioned air ducting and should be treated with the same consideration and care. Supply and exhaust ducts in unconditioned spaces need to be insulated to a minimum of R-8 if they are at least 3 inches in diameter. Ducts smaller than three inches in attics need a minimum of R-6 insulation. Supply and exhaust ducts in any other unconditioned space, such as a basement or crawlspace outside the building pressure boundary and/or thermal envelope or garage, need a minimum of R-6 insulation if they are at least three inches in diameter, and R-4.2 if they are smaller than that. Be wary of thin duct insulation products like foil-faced bubble wrap that claim to meet these R-values through the use of radiant barriers and air spaces.

The vapor barrier on the ductwork must be carefully sealed. Use the right tape. Use a pressure-sensitive vapor retarder tape designed for ductwork. Seal all the seams, both lengthwise and between pieces with tape. Overlap the insulation by two to three inches. Don't compress the insulation. In hot humid climates, the insulation and vapor barriers are critical not only to reduce chances of water damage from condensation but also to reduce the chance of mold, mildew, and bacteria growth on or in damp ducts.

The ducts connecting the HRV/ERV to and from the outside termination fittings are particularly important to insulate and seal, since those ducts will carry unconditioned outside air.

* * *

Duct Design for HRV/ERV Systems Attached to Air Handlers[11]

Using the conditioned air ductwork for ventilation saves money and saves space—but there are performance and operating cost compromises. There are several issues to bear in mind in choosing this installation approach:

- Conditioned air duct systems move much more air than HRV/ERV devices and therefore require much larger ducts. Larger ducts results in lower airflow velocity if the HRV/ERV is running on its own without the help of the big air handler blower.
- The static pressure (flow resistance) is much higher through the air handler system (filter, heat exchanger, air conditioning coil, etc.) than it is through a duct connected to a return grille. The HRV/ERV airflow connected to the return side of the air handler is more likely to flow back up the return duct to the closest and largest grille in the system if the air handler blower isn't running.
- The exhaust fan in the HRV/ERV is working against the negative pressure in the return plenum. If the return plenum pressure is sufficiently low with the HVAC blower running, it can reduce or even stall the exhaust airflow.
- At the same time, if the HRV/ERV supplies air to the return plenum, the supply blower has the help of the HVAC blower to supply excessive fresh air whenever the HVAC system is operating, dragging air in through the open HRV/ERV intake. This situation also makes it difficult to assure the HRV/ERV will remain balanced.

---

11. https://www.greenbuildingadvisor.com/article/integrating-hrvs-with-air-handlers

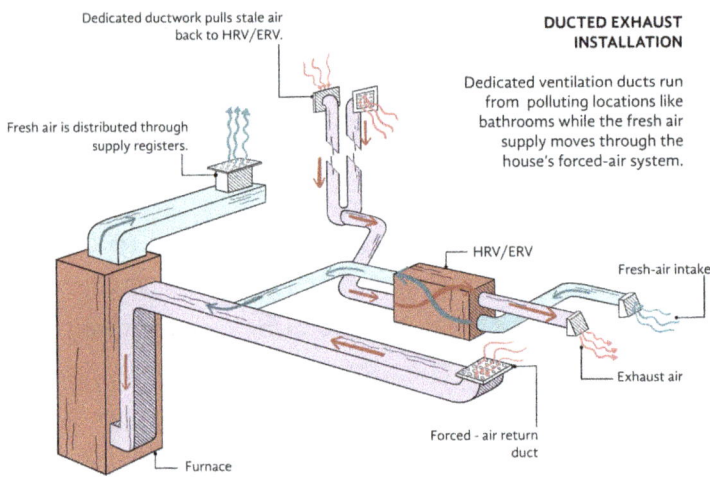

Figure H.6 HRV/ERV Connected to Air Handler with Independently Ducted Exhausts

If the choice is to connect the HRV/ERV to the air handler, the best configuration is to draw the stale air out of the high polluting areas like the bathrooms and the kitchen area and inject the fresh air (new air) into the return side of the air handler. The minimum mixed air temperature entering the furnace casing must be at least 60°F (16°C).

NOTE: The ASHRAE 62.2 Standard allows for intermittent operation of the whole dwelling ventilation system if the airflow rate is increased so that the average volume of flow is equivalent to the continuous rate. For example, if the system is operated half the time, the flow rate has to be doubled. Consequently, if the ducting for the HRV/ERV is connected to the conditioned air ducting (HVAC) and interlocked with the operation of that system, the flow rate through the HRV/ERV must be increased to match the operating time of the HVAC system.

If a typical air handler runs for 20 minutes per cycle, the air flow from HRV/ERV would need to be triple the ASHRAE 62.2 ventilation rate.[12]

---

12. https://completecomfortgo.com/how-long-air-conditioner-run/

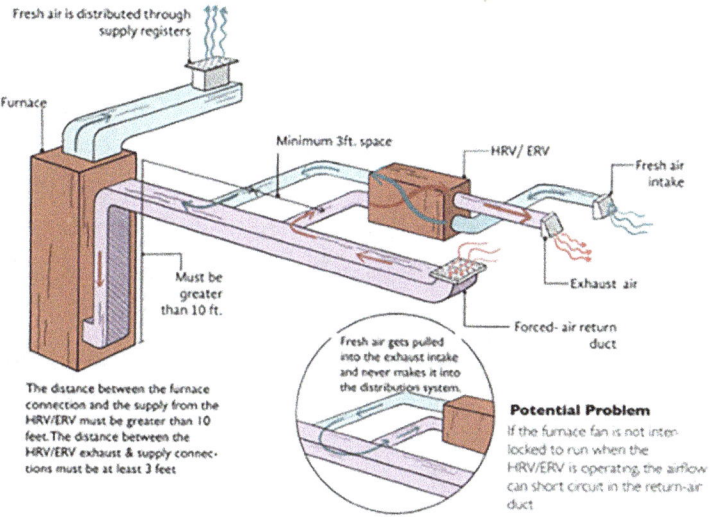

Figure H.6 Connected to Air Handler

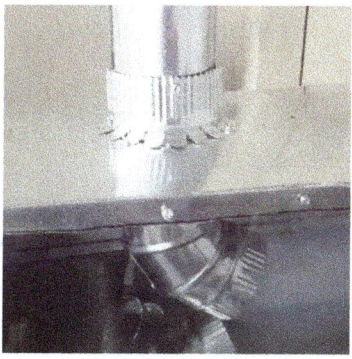

Figure H.7 Airflow Injection Port (Manclark)

Connecting both the supply and return from the HRV/ERV to the air handler is a compromise. The air from the HRV/ERV entering the trunk should be guided into the flow of the airstream by using an injection port or turning vane to ensure the proper direction of flow and reduce the chance of short circuiting the airflow path.

* * *

HRV/ERV System Commissioning

Testing airflows

HRV and ERV manufacturers realize the importance of having their products work in a balanced manner and some of them provide flow taps on their systems or offer flow stations (a short length of duct and an air-velocity sensing grid). Along with the flow station, an analog (like a magnehelic gauge) or a digital manometer is needed to measure the pressure. The following procedures describe balancing a fully installed system and assume that the house is complete, the HRV or ERV is fully installed, and any other appliances that move air into or out of the house (like a clothes dryer or range hood) are fully installed and operational.

These systems will have multiple supply and exhaust points. Note that flow-measuring products such as flow hoods like balometers are not effective at measuring low supply airflows.

The "Garbage Bag Test" mentioned earlier can get a good indication of the system balance.

1. Use a large garbage bag that is 48 inches long (1.2 m) and tape the opening to a wire coat hanger to keep it open.
2. Crush the bag and then hold it over the exhaust hood. The exhaust air will inflate the bag in approximately 8 seconds. (If it takes less than that, set the control on the HRV/ERV to a lower flow setting and do the test again.)
3. Swing the bag through the air to inflate it, and then hold it over the intake hood. The bag should deflate as quickly as it inflated for the exhaust side.

If you find the bag inflates much more quickly than it deflates, try to determine the cause. Make sure all the duct connections are tight and that the filters are clean. It's amazing what you can find inside an HRV/ERV housing when the system has been running for a while. If those observations don't turn up any obvious problems, the system may need to be rebalanced using more sophisticated equipment.

Heat Recovery Ventilation for Housing National Center for Appropriate Technology

An alternative to the garbage bag test is the Hanging String. This must be done on a day when the winds are calm and outdoor and indoor temperatures are similar. All the windows and doors are securely closed, and one window is opened slightly. The HRV/ERV is turned on at high speed, and one person checks the airflow at the open window while the other person adjusts the balancing dampers until the flow is balanced.

House setup for commissioning

Testing the flow through a stand-alone HRV or ERV (not connected to either side of an HVAC system):

1. Open all interior doors in the house;
2. Doors and windows to the exterior must be closed;
3. Fireplace dampers must be closed;
4. The air handlers and all exhaust fans, including the clothes dryer and central vacuum (any device that will impact the pressure inside the house with respect to the outside) must be turned off;
5. Filters and the core of the ventilator must be clean;
6. Supply and exhaust termination fittings on the outside of the house must be clear and open;
7. HRV clear of ice and drain pan not full of water;
8. Install flow measuring stations[13] in the supply and exhaust connections from and to the outside (or use the flow taps on the ventilator unit provided by the manufacturer);
9. Turn the HRV/ERV on high speed;
10. Measure the velocity pressure with a single channel of the

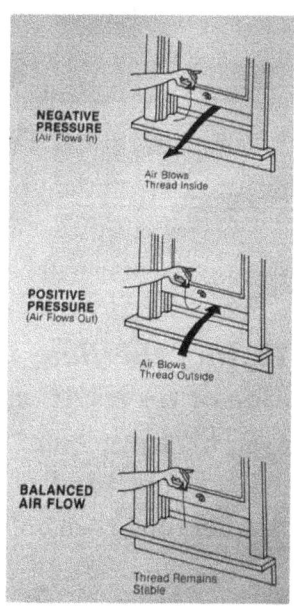

Figure H.8 Heat Recovery Ventilation for Housing
National Center for Appropriate Technology 1984

---

13. Air turbulence can have a significant effect on the measurements, so the flow measuring station should be located far enough away from turbulence producing elements (like elbows, dampers, or the fans themselves to get accurate readings. As a rule of thumb, the flow measuring station should be located a minimum of 12 inches (300 mm) away from dampers and 30 inches away from axial (propeller) fans or the outlets of blowers.

manometer connected to the two ports on the flow station[14]. (Zero the gauge if required. A magnehelic gauge must be vertical, not lying on its back. A slight tap on the gauge may be required before zeroing.);

11. Wait for the gauge to stabilize;
12. Convert the reading to cfm using the calibration label attached to the flow station or by using the conversion formula $V = 1096.2 \times (V_p/0.075)0.5$ where V equals the velocity in feet per minute and V_p is the velocity pressure in inches of water gauge;
13. Multiply the V_p by the area of the ducting;
14. Repeat the process for the other air stream. The two flows should be within 10% of each other. The average flow of the two air streams will be the ventilation rate through the system.

Testing the flow through an HRV or ERV connected to either side of an HVAC system.

This will require two tests: one with the air handler turned off and one with the air handler turned on. If the ventilator only runs when the air handler runs, then only Test 1 needs to be performed:

Test 1 Air Handler turned on:

1. HRV or ERV must be fully installed and connected;
2. Open all interior doors in the house;
3. Doors and windows to the exterior must be closed;
4. The air handlers and all exhaust fans, including the clothes dryer and central vacuum (any device that will impact the pressure inside the house with respect to the outside) must be turned off;
5. Filters and the core of the ventilator must be clean;
6. Filter in the air handler must be clean;
7. Supply and exhaust termination fittings on the outside of the house must be clear and open;
8. HRV clear of ice and drain pan not full of water;

---

14. Connecting both taps on a single channel of the manometer will provide the difference between the input and the reference taps i.e. the difference between the Total Pressure and the Static Pressure which is the Velocity Pressure.

9. Install flow measuring stations in the supply and exhaust connections from and to the outside (or use the flow taps on the ventilator unit provided by the manufacturer);
10. Turn the HRV/ERV on high speed;
11. Turn the air handler fan on;
12. Measure the velocity pressure with a single channel of the manometer connected to the two ports on the flow station;
13. Convert the reading to cfm using the calibration label attached to the flow station or by using the conversion formula $V = 1096.2 \times (V_p/0.075)0.5$ where V equals the velocity in feet per minute and V_p is the velocity pressure in inches of water gauge;
14. Multiply the V_p by the area of the ducting;
15. Repeat the process for the other air stream. The two flows should be within 10% of each other. Note the average flow of the two air streams. This is the whole dwelling ventilation rate if the ventilator only runs when the air handler is running.
16. If the ventilator is operated on an independent control, continue with Test 2.

Test 2 Air Handler turned off:

1. Air handler fan must be turned off
2. Repeat steps 2–10 above;
3. Turn the HRV/ERV on high speed;
4. Measure the velocity pressure with a single channel of the manometer connected to the two ports on the flow station;
5. Convert the reading to cfm using the calibration label attached to the flow station or by using the conversion formula $V = 1096.2 \times (V_p/0.075)0.5$ where V equals the velocity in feet per minute and V_p is the velocity pressure in inches of water gauge;
6. Multiply the V_p by the area of the ducting;
7. Repeat the process for the other air stream. The two flows should be within 10% of each other. Note the average flow of the two air steams;
8. The average of the two tests (with the air handler on and the air handler off) is the whole dwelling ventilation rate.

Balancing steps using flow stations.

Install the flow measuring stations (Note that it is advisable to use two stations, one in each flow stream because as the system is balanced, several readings will need to be made in both streams): Air turbulence can have a significant effect on the measurements so the flow measuring station should be located far enough away from turbulence producing elements (like elbows, dampers, or the fans themselves) to get accurate readings. As a rule of thumb, the flow measuring station should be located a minimum of 12" (300 mm) away from dampers and 30" (750mm) away from axial (propeller) fans or the outlets of blowers ("squirrel cage").

The flow measuring stations should be installed in the ducting, referring to the arrows on the station for airflow direction. (Note that not all flow-measuring stations are direction sensitive.) The joints between the station and the ducting should be sealed.

Take the flow measurements:

1. Turn the HRV/ERV on high speed.
2. Measure the flow with the manometer. (Zero the gauge if required. A magnehelic gauge must be vertical, not lying on its back. A slight tap on the gauge may be required before zeroing.)
3. Wait for the gauge to stabilize.
4. Convert the reading to airflow volume using the calibration label attached to the flow station.
5. When the reading has been made, if it is with an analog gauge, remove the gauge, disconnecting the hoses and check that it returns to zero. If not, re-zero the gauge and retake the reading.
6. Repeat the procedure for the other air stream.

Balance the system:

If the airflows are out of balance by ten percent or more, a balancing damper in the air stream with the greater flow can reduce the flow to bring it into balance. (If a balancing damper is used, the position of the damper should be locked in place once balance has been achieved.) If the higher flow rate is on the supply side, adjustable room grilles can throttle down the volume. Note that the delivered airflow must still meet the design requirements once the flow has been reduced.

Some products now have internal automatic balancing capabilities, sensing the pressures and adjusting the fan speeds. Some systems will indicate unbalanced system conditions and whether the supply or return side is the limiting element so that the installer can adjust the installation to improve airflows.

Balancing steps using a Pitot tube:

When it is difficult to remove sections of duct to install flow stations, measurements can be made using a pitot tube which only requires drilling a small (about 3/16") hole in the ducting. This procedure can be used effectively when the HRV/ERV is connected to the HVAC system or air handler that should also be running at high speed during the testing. This will provide the maximum pressure that the HRV/ERV will have to overcome.

1. Drill the measurement hole away from sources of turbulence (as with the flow measuring stations described previously);
2. Point the pitot tube into the airflow;
3. Connect the gauge. The connection at the top of the pitot tube (measuring the velocity pressure), should be connected to the high pressure side of the gauge (Input). The connection at the side of the Pitot tube (measuring the static pressure) should be connected to the low pressure or reference side of the gauge. The gauge should be capable of reading from 0 to 0.25 iwg (0 to 62.5 Pa).
4. Read the pressure on the supply side and then repeat the procedure on the exhaust side.
5. Determine which flow is the greatest.
6. Install and adjust a balancing damper in that stream to balance the flows. (Adjustable room grilles can sometimes substitute for a balancing damper.) Note that in heating climates, if an imbalance must be allowed, slightly higher exhaust than supply will increase the supply air temperature.

Testing controls

Part of the commissioning process must be a system operational check. Depending on the sophistication of the controls, some of that test may be part of the first boot of the system, but it is still good practice to verify to the extent feasible that the system is performing as designed.

System Maintenance

HRV/ERV's have more components and require more attention. They drag out the bad air, push in the fresh air, and run all that through the exchanger element. The outside air will contain dust, pollen, and other particulates depending on the location and the local environment. If the system is not cleaned and maintained, it won't continue to work as it was designed to work.[15]

> The Canadian Mortgage and Housing Corporation (CMHC) has a clear, simple description of basic HRV/ERV maintenance, including a maintenance checklist that you can copy and paste on the front of the unit to keep track and remind you of service issues.[16]

Refer to the product manual, shut off the power, and open up the housing for HRV/ERV air handler. That will provide you with access to the exchanger core and the filters. Clean out any detritus or dead bugs that might have collected in the housing. Clean and/or replace the filters. The grille in the kitchen should include a filter that should be maintained (cleaned or replaced) when the system filter is maintained. Additional filter boxes can be added to the lines to allow for the insertion of more effective filters.[17]

Pull out the core and carefully clean it. If it is not very dirty, you can shake it, brush it, or vacuum it off. If it is very dirty, you may need to rinse it off but be sure to check the product instructions before getting the core wet. Be sure it is completely dry before putting it back in the unit.

Check the fans to make sure both the supply and exhaust fans are still working.

---

15. Fantech system maintenance video or https://broan-nutone.com/en-us/broan-ai-series-fresh-air-systems
16. https://www.cmhc-schl.gc.ca/professionals/industry-innovation-and-leadership/industry-expertise/indigenous-housing/develop-manage-indigenous-housing/maintenance-solutions/how-to-maintain-heat-recovery-ventilator
17. Chapter 17 includes a section on furnace filters and MERV filter ratings. Those same ratings can be applied to ventilation systems.

Check on the condensate drain and pans. Make sure they are not blocked and that the pans are clean. (Whatever is in those pans may eventually evaporate and be part of the airstream.) Make sure that there is a proper trap in the drain. If the HRV/ERV is connected to the air handler of the heating and cooling system, make sure that those connections are still solid. If they have been taped, consider resealing those joints with mastic. Some HRV/ERV's are designed to be coupled to the home's air handler without a "closed connection" (known as an "indirect connection") between the two but deliver the outside air near an inlet vent on the return side of the air handler's ducting. Often all of the incoming air is not "captured" by the opening in the return particularly if the two systems are not control interlocked so that they both operate at the same time so that the air handler fan is pulling in the air from the HRV/ERV at the same time as HRV/ERV's blowers are running. This will cause over ventilating the basement and under ventilating the house. And if the air handler is in an unconditioned basement, garage, or attic, it will depressurize that space sucking in and distributing any other nearby pollutants. This sort of connection should be discouraged and repaired.

Check on the exterior hoods or termination fittings and make sure that they are not blocked or have plants or leaves or snow piling up in front of them. Make sure animals are not living in them and that their protective screens are still in place. Check the backdraft damper on the exhaust fitting. (There should not be one on the supply fitting!) Make sure that there are no contamination sources like trashcans or rotting leaves under a deck near the intake. Homeowners will occasionally add insect screens to the intake vent out of a concern for insects being drawn into the system. These screens are very restrictive to airflow and will clog quickly. They are likely to be unnecessary because air and insects drawn into the system have to pass through the ducting, the system filter, the system core, through the blower and out into the house. Hopefully, the particulate filters in the system will be effective enough before something the size of an insect will make it all the way into the house.

Check the ducting:

- Poorly taped connections—poor tape, tape falling off, open connections;
- Poor sealing of the vapor diffusion retarder at the HRV/ERV and at the outside wall;

- Compressed ducting and insulation by hanging straps and unsupported runs;
- Missing insulation;
- Crushed flex where it has been squeezed into wall cavities;
- Poorly sized ducting and meandering duct runs.

Check the frost prevention system. The combination of cold outside air hitting warm humid air from the house will often result in frost build-up on the exchanger core. The defrost cycle in most systems activates when the temperature in the incoming air drops below 25°F (-5°C). Some systems have an internal motorized damper that temporarily blocks incoming fresh air, allowing only house air to circulate through and defrost the core. Other systems have an automatically timed supply fan shutdown. These systems are difficult to test unless the incoming air temperature is quite cold, but you can make sure that if there is an internal damper that it looks clear of dirt and debris. Do not move it manually, as you are likely to strip the motor gears.

One final reminder: More than any other component in the house, ventilation systems in homes are there to keep the occupants and the building healthy. They must be maintained to accomplish that.

Symptom	Cause	Solution
Poor Air Flows	<ul><li>¼" (6mm) mesh on the outside hoods is plugged</li><li>Filters plugged</li><li>Core obstructed</li><li>House grilles closed or blocked</li><li>Dampers are closed (if installed)</li><li>Poor power at the site</li><li>Ductwork is restricting HRV/ERV</li><li>Improper speed control setting</li><li>HRV/ERV airflow unbalanced</li></ul>	<ul><li>Clean exterior hoods or vents</li><li>Remove and clean filter</li><li>Remove and clean core</li><li>Check and open grilles</li><li>Open and adjust dampers</li><li>Have electrician check supply voltage at the house</li><li>Check duct installation</li><li>Increase the speed of the HRV/ERV</li><li>Have contractor balance HRV/ERV</li></ul>
Supply air feels cold	<ul><li>Poor location of supply grilles, the airflows may be drafting on the occupants</li><li>Outdoor temperature extremely cold</li></ul>	<ul><li>Locate the grilles on the walls or under the baseboards</li><li>Install ceiling mounted diffusers or grilles that do not spill the supply air directly on the occupants</li><li>Turn down the HRV/ERV supply speed</li><li>Add a small duct heater (1kw) to temper the supply air</li><li>Rearrange the furniture or open closed doors that are restricting the circulation of air in the home</li><li>If the supply air is ducted into the furnace return, the furnace blower may need to run continuously to distribute ventilation air comfortably</li></ul>
Dehumidistat is not operating	<ul><li>Improper low voltage connection</li><li>External low voltage is shorted out by a staple or nail</li><li>Dehumidistat misadjusted or turned off (Ideal RH 35% - 55%)</li></ul>	<ul><li>Check that the correct terminals have been used</li><li>Check external wiring for a short</li><li>Adjust dehumidistat to the desired setting</li></ul>

Humidity levels are too high and condensation is appearing on the windows	• Dehumidistat is set too high • HRV/ERV is undersized to handle intermittent operation, a hot tub, an indoor pool, etc. • Lifestyle of the occupants • Moisture coming into the home from an unvented or unheated crawl space • Moisture is remaining in the bathroom and kitchen areas • Condensation seems to form in the spring and fall • HRV/ERV is set at too low a speed	• Set dehumidistat lower • Cover pools, hot tubs when they are not in use • Avoid hanging clothes to dry, storing wood or venting clothes dryer inside. (Wood for heating may have to be moved outside.) • Vent crawl space and place a vapor diffusion retarder on the floor or seal up the crawl space and condition it • Ducts from the bathrooms should be sized to remove moist air effectively. Use bath fans after showers • On humid days in the changing seasons, some condensation may appear • Increase the speed of the HRV/ERV
Humidity levels are too low	• Dehumidistat set too low • Blower speed of HRV/ERV is too high • Lifestyle of the occupants • HRV/ERV airflows may be out of balance	• Set dehumidistat higher • Decrease the HRV/ERV blower speed • House may have too many air leaks. This should be considered and addressed before adding any additional humidity to the space. • Have a contractor balance airflows.
HRV/ERV and/or ducts are frosting up	• HRV/ERV airflows are out of balance • Malfunction of the defrost system	• Note: minimal frost build-up is expected on cores before unit initiates the defrost cycle functions • Have HVAC contractor balance the airflows • If the unit has a self-test feature for the defrost cycle

Condensation or ice build-up in insulated duct to the outside	• Incomplete vapor diffusion retarder around insulated duct • A hole or tear in the vapor diffusion retarder covering	• Tape and seal all joints • Tape any holes or tears in the vapor diffusion retarder covering • Ensure that the vapor diffusion retarder is completely sealed
Water in the bottom of the HRV/ERV	• Drain pans plugged • Improper connection of the drain lines • HRV/ERV is not level • Drain lines are obstructed • HRV/ERV core is not properly installed	• Clean out the drain pans • Check the connections • Check for kinks in the lines • Make sure water drains properly from the pans

Table H.3 HRV/ERV Trouble Shooting (American Aldes)

Consumer/Owner Information

How to live with an HRV/ERV

A properly installed and efficiently operating HRV/ERV can be a lifesaver distributing fresh air throughout the house while simultaneously removing the stale, used air. It is the homeowner's responsibility to regularly maintain it, clean the filters, inspect the exchanger core, be sure that the intake and exhaust ports are clear and the backdraft damper on the exhaust port works properly. The condensate drain from the HRV must also be clear and functional, and the condensate pan inside the housing is free of dust, dirt, and dead insects.

If the system is not functioning properly or not running at all, the HRV/ERV is just a box of fans.

Acknowledgments

As I went through the process of updating of this book (the second edition was published eight years ago), my appreciation for the importance of residential ventilation only grew. I also recognized the enormous body of knowledge that has accumulated over the intervening years spurred on by the devastation of the Covid-19 pandemic that trapped people in their homes and changed our lives forever in ways that we can only begin to imagine. I have been privileged to get to know, and be guided by, some of the best minds.

There is the huge crowd of wonderful people living and dead I cited in the first and second versions of this book and others that I didn't have a chance to: Rana Belshe, John Bower, Terry Brennan, Chris Clay, Anthony Cox, John Davies, Bob Davis, Dennis Dietz, Steve Emmerich, Vic Flynn, Don Fugler, Paul Francisco, Tom Greiner, Dave Grimsrud, John Harrell, John Holton, Nick Hurst, Phil Kaluza, Rick Karg, Mark Kelley, Steve Klossner, John Krigger, Tim Lenahan, Dennis Livingston, Joe Lstiburek, Mike Lubliner, Bruce Manclark, Jeff May, Paddy Morrissey, Neil Moyer, Joe Nagan, Ken Nelson, Rick Olmstead, Collin Olson, Danny Parker, Duncan Prahl, David Price, Travis Rasch, Judy Roberson, Armin Rudd, Max Sherman, Bill Spohn, Doug Steege, Don Stevens, John Tooley, Bruce Torrey, George Tsongas, Iain Walker, Eric Werling, and Dave Wolbrink.

Many thanks to you all.

All of these folks and more have taught me more than I could ever relay. If you get a chance to sit in on any of their sessions at a conference, seize the opportunity.

Paul H. Raymer
Falmouth, MA
April, 2025

Paul H. Raymer

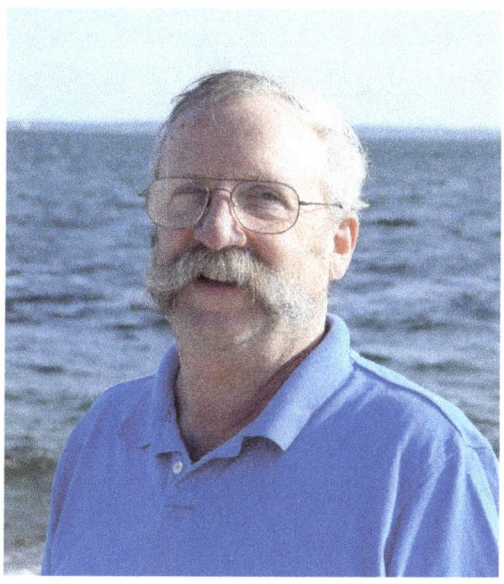

Paul H. Raymer has been working with building science for more than forty-five years. Because he likes solving complex problems with reasonable solutions, he developed and brought to market more than twenty products, most of them related to mechanical ventilation in homes. He has taught building science courses to diverse audiences from home owners, home inspectors, and weatherization specialists to architects and engineers. He has been a member of the ASHRAE 62.2 SSPC residential ventilation committee for more than 20 years. He has the honor and pleasure to call many of the best and brightest minds in the building science industry "friend".

Salty Air Publishing Newsletter & Website

Salty Air Publishing, bi-weekly newsletter
Subscribe here

Salty Air Publishing Website
https://www.paulhraymer.com/

www.ingramcontent.com/pod-product-compliance
Lightning Source LLC
Chambersburg PA
CBHW080516030426
42337CB00023B/4541